THE POTENTIAL FOR NUTRITIONAL MODULATION OF AGING PROCESSES

F N P

PUBLICATIONS IN FOOD SCIENCE AND NUTRITION

The American Health Foundation Series

THE ROLE OF FOOD PRODUCT DEVELOPMENT IN IMPLEMENTING DIETARY GUIDELINES, G.E. Livingston, R.J. Moshy and C.M. Chang

ENVIRONMENTAL ASPECTS OF CANCER: ROLE OF MACRO AND MICRO COMPONENTS OF FOODS, E.L. Wynder, G.A. Leveille, J.H. Weisburger and G.E. Livingston

NUTRITIONAL STATUS ASSESSMENT OF THE INDIVIDUAL, G.E. Livingston

THE POTENTIAL FOR NUTRITIONAL MODULATION OF THE AGING PROCESSES, D.K. Ingram, G.T. Baker, III, and N.W. Shock

Other Food and Nutrition Books

NITRITE-CURED MEAT, R.G. Cassens
CONTROLLED/MODIFIED ATMOSPHERE/VACUUM PACKAGING OF FOODS, A.L. Brody
QUALITY ASSURANCE OF FOODS, J.E. Stauffer
THE SCIENCE OF MEAT AND MEAT PRODUCTS, 3RD ED., J.F. Price and B.S. Schweigert
HANDBOOK OF FOOD COLORANT PATENTS, F.J. Francis
ROLE OF CHEMISTRY IN THE QUALITY OF PROCESSED FOODS, O.R. Fennema, W.H. Chang and C.Y. Lii
NEW DIRECTIONS FOR PRODUCT TESTING AND SENSORY ANALYSIS OF FOODS, H.R. Moskowitz
PRODUCT TESTING AND SENSORY EVALUATION OF FOODS, H.R. Moskowitz
SHELF-LIFE DATING OF FOODS, T.P. Labuza
RECENT ADVANCES IN OBESITY RESEARCH, VOL. V, E. Berry, S.H. Blondheim, H.E. Eliahou and E. Shafrir
RECENT ADVANCES IN OBESITY RESEARCH, VOL. IV, J. Hirsch *et al.*
RECENT ADVANCES IN OBESITY RESEARCH, VOL. III, P. Bjorntorp *et al.*
RECENT ADVANCES IN OBESITY RESEARCH, VOL. II, G.A. Bray
RECENT ADVANCES IN OBESITY RESEARCH, VOL. I, A.N. Howard
ANTINUTRIENTS AND NATURAL TOXICANTS IN FOOD, R.L. Ory
UTILIZATION OF PROTEIN RESOURCES, D.W. Stanley *et al.*
FOOD INDUSTRY ENERGY ALTERNATIVES, R.P. Ouellette *et al.*
VITAMIN B_6: METABOLISM AND ROLE IN GROWTH, G.P. Tryfiates
HUMAN NUTRITION, 3RD ED., F.R. Mottram
FOOD POISONING AND FOOD HYGIENE, 4TH ED., B.C. Hobbs *et al.*
POSTHARVEST BIOLOGY AND BIOTECHNOLOGY, H.O. Hultin and M. Milner

THE POTENTIAL FOR NUTRITIONAL MODULATION OF AGING PROCESSES

Proceedings of an International Conference
Sponsored by the
AMERICAN HEALTH FOUNDATION
Co-Sponsored by
NATIONAL INSTITUTES ON AGING
FOOD AND DRUG ADMINISTRATION
THE GERONTOLOGICAL SOCIETY OF AMERICA
September 13–15, 1988
New York, New York

Edited by

Donald K. Ingram, Ph.D.
NATHAN W. SHOCK LABORATORIES
GERONTOLOGY RESEARCH CENTER
NATIONAL INSTITUTE ON AGING
BALTIMORE, MARYLAND

George T. Baker, III, Ph.D.
BAKER AND ASSOCIATES
AND
NATHAN W. & MARGARET T. SHOCK AGING RESEARCH FOUNDATION
SILVER SPRING, MARYLAND

*Nathan W. Shock, Ph.D.**
GERONTOLOGY RESEARCH CENTER
NATIONAL INSTITUTE ON AGING
BALTIMORE, MARYLAND

*DECEASED

FOOD & NUTRITION PRESS, INC.
TRUMBULL, CONNECTICUT 06611 USA

FOOD & NUTRITION PRESS, INC.
Trumbull, Connecticut 06611 USA

Library of Congress Catalog Card Number: 90-071070
ISBN: 0-917678-26-5

Printed in the United States of America

CONTRIBUTORS

ALI, RIDA, Ph.D., Bristol Meyers International, New York, NY 10154

AMES, BRUCE N., Ph.D., Division of Biochemistry and Microbiology, University of California, Berkeley, CA 94720

ARCHER, JONATHAN, The Jackson Laboratory, Bar Harbor, ME 04609

BAKER, III, GEORGE T., Ph.D., Baker and Associates and Nathan W. & Margaret T. Shock Aging Research Foundation, Silver Spring, MD 20904

BLATT, L., Ph.D., Department of Psychology, Boston University School of Medicine, Boston, MA 02215

BRESNAHAN, ELAINE, Ph.D., Gerontology Research Center, National Institute on Aging, Francis Scott Key Medical Center, Baltimore, MD 21224

CADWALLADER, L., Bowman Gray School of Medicine, Winston-Salem, NC 27103

CAMPBELL, L., Bowman Gray School of Medicine, Winston-Salem, NC 27103

CARBONELL, R. J., Ph.D., Del Monte USA, Coral Gables, FL 33134

CUTLER, RICHARD, G., Ph.D., Gerontology Research Center, National Institute on Aging, Francis Scott Key Medical Center, Baltimore, MD 21224

DAVIS, BARBARA, J., Ph.D., Departments of Neurology and Neurobiology, University of Rochester School of Medicine, Rochester, NY 14627

DRAPER, H. H., Ph.D., Department of Nutritional Sciences, College of Biological Science, University of Guelph, Guelph, Ontario, Canada

EDEN, STAFFAN, M.D., Ph.D., Department of Geriatric Medicine, University of Gothenburg, Gothenburg, Sweden

ETIENNE, P., M.D., CIBA-GEIGY US, Summit, NJ 07901

FABRIS, NICOLA, M.D., Ph.D., Immunology Center, Department of Gerontology and Geriatric Research, INRCA, Ancona, Italy

FERNANDES, GABRIEL, Ph.D., Departments of Medicine, Microbiology, and Physiology, The University of Texas Health Science Center at San Antonio, San Antonio, TX 78284

FLEENOR, D., Bowman Gray School of Medicine, Winston-Salem, NC 27103

GOLD, PAUL E., Ph.D., Department of Psychology and Neuroscience Program, University of Virginia, Charlottesville, VA 22903

HALLFRISCH, JUDITH, Ph.D., Gerontology Research Center, National Institute on Aging, Baltimore, MD 21224

HAMILL, ROBERT W., M.D., Department of Neurology and Neurobiology, University of Rochester, Rochester, NY 14627

HARRISON, DAVID E., Ph.D., The Jackson Laboratory, Bar Harbor, ME 04609

HATANO, SUICHI, M.D., Faculty of Social Welfare, Shukutoku University, Chiba, and Department of Epidemiology, The Institute of Public Health, Tokyo, Japan

HOLEHAN, ANNE, M., Ph.D., The Institute for Human Ageing, University of Liverpool, Liverpool, England

HUNTER, J. EDWARD, Procter and Gamble Co., Winton Hill Technical Center, Cincinnati, OH 45239

INGRAM, DONALD K., Ph.D., Gerontology Research Center, National Institute on Aging, Francis Scott Key Medical Center, Baltimore, MD 21224

KANNEL, WILLIAM B., M.D., Section of Preventive Medicine and Epidemiology, Boston University School of Medicine, Evans Research Foundation, Boston, MA 02118

KERR, S., Bowman Gray School of Medicine, Winston-Salem, NC 27103

LANDFIELD, P., Bowman Gray School of Medicine, Winston-Salem, NC 27103

LIPSCHITZ, DAVID A., M.D., Ph.D., Geriatric Research, Education and Clinical Center, John L. McClellan Memorial Veterans Hospital, and Division on Aging, University of Arkansas for Medical Sciences, Little Rock, AR 72205

LIVINGSTON, G. E., Ph.D., Food Science Associates, Dobbs Ferry, NY 10522

MASORO, EDWARD J., Ph.D., Department of Physiology, The University of Texas Health Science Center at San Antonio, San Antonio, TX 78284

McCARTER, ROGER, Ph.D., Department of Physiology, The University of Texas Health Science Center at San Antonio, San Antonio, TX 78284

McNEILL, THOMAS H., Ph.D., Ethyl Percy Andrus Gerontology Center, University of Southern California, University Park, Los Angeles, CA 90089

MELLSTROM, DAN, M.D., Ph.D., Department of Geriatric Medicine, University of Gothenburg, Gothenburg, Sweden

MERRY, B. J., Ph.D., The Institute for Human Ageing, University of Liverpool, Liverpool, England

MOCCHEGIANI, EUGENIO, Ph.D., Immunology Center, Department of Gerontology and Geriatric Research, INRCA, Ancona, Italy

MUZZIOLI, MARIO, Ph.D., Immunology Center, Department of Gerontology and Geriatric Research, INRCA, Ancona, Italy

NANDY, K., M.D., Ph.D., Department of Anatomy, Boston University School of Medicine, Boston, MA 02215

NANDY, L., Department of Psychology, Boston University School of Medicine, Boston, MA 02215

NANDY, S., Department of Psychology, Boston University School of Medicine, Boston, MA 02215

PROVINCIALLI, MAURO, Ph.D., Immunology Center, Department of Gerontology and Geriatric Research, INRCA, Ancona, Italy

RICHARDSON, ARLAN, Ph.D., Department of Chemistry, Illinois State University, Normal, IL 61761

RICHIE, JR., JOHN P., Ph.D., American Health Foundation, Valhalla, NY 10595

ROTH, GEORGE S., Ph.D., Gerontology Research Center, National Institute on Aging, Francis Scott Key Medical Center, Baltimore, MD 21224

SAMUELSON, AMY, Ph.D., Nabisco Brands, East Hanover, NJ 07936

SHOCK, NATHAN W., Ph.D., Gerontology Research Center, National Institute on Aging, Francis Scott Key Medical Center, Baltimore, MD 21224

SVANBORG, ALVAR, M.D., Ph.D., Department of Geriatric Medicine, College of Medicine, University of Illinois at Chicago, Chicago, IL 60612, and Department of Geriatric Medicine, University of Gothenburg, Gothenburg, Sweden

VINSANT, S., Bowman Gray School of Medicine, Winston-Salem, NC 27103

WEINDRUCH, RICHARD, Ph.D., Biomedical Research and Clinical Medicine Program, National Institute on Aging, Bethesda, MD 20892.

WILLIAMS, GARY M., M.D., American Health Foundation, Valhalla, NY 10595

WILLIAMS, T. FRANKLIN, M.D., National Institute on Aging, National Institutes of Health, Bethesda, MD 20892

YAMAOKA, KAZUE, Ph.D., Faculty of Jurisprudence, Teikyo University, Tokyo, and Department of Epidemiology, The Institute of Public Health, Tokyo, Japan

ZS.-NAGY, IMRE, M.D., VILEG, Hungarian Section, University Medical School, Debrecen, Hungary, and VILEG, Italian Section, Department of Gerontological Research, INRCA, Ancona, Italy

ACKNOWLEDGMENTS

The organizing committee extends its appreciation to the members of the advisory committee for this international conference for their helpful suggestions in program development and for their active participation in the conference. The members of this committee were:

Richard C. Adelman, Ph.D.	University of Michigan, USA
Rida Ali, Ph.D.	Bristol-Meyers International, USA
Vincent J. Cristofalo, Ph.D.	University of Pennsylvania, USA
Marco Ermini, Ph.D.	Mundipharma, Switzerland
Stanley Gershoff, Ph.D.	Tufts University, USA
Yves Guigoz, Ph.D.	Nestle, Switzerland
Carel Hollander, M.D., Ph.D.	Merck Sharp & Dohme, France
Anita Owens, M.A., R.D.	RJR Nabisco Inc., USA
David P. Rose, M.D., Ph.D.	American Health Foundation
Donald M. Watkin, M.D., M.P.H.	U.S. Department of Transportation

In addition, we should like to acknowledge the following organizations without whose generous financial support this International Conference on Longevity and Aging would not have been possible.

Best Foods Company
Bristol-Meyers International
RJR Nabisco Brands, Inc.
The Procter & Gamble Company

Finally, we wish to express our thanks to the offices and staff of Mr. Richard Klarberg for necessary and timely administrative assistance in preparation and implementation of this conference.

Organizers
George T. Baker, III, Ph.D.
Donald K. Ingram, Ph.D.
Guy E. Livingston, Ph.D.
Nathan W. Shock, Ph.D.

PREFACE

This book is dedicated to our co-editor, colleague and friend, Dr. Nathan W. Shock. Dr. Shock died of cancer on November 12, 1989, at the age of 83. The book represents one of the last of the many contributions he made throughout his most illustrious career, a career which spanned over half of this century and included approximately 350 publications. Most significantly, it was through his pioneering vision, perseverance, integrity and the quality of his science that the field of gerontology is recognized today as a legitimate area of scientific inquiry.

This volume reports the proceedings of a conference held between September 13–15, 1988, at the Ford Foundation Building in New York City. The conference was sponsored by the Food and Nutrition Council of the American Health Foundation, the National Institute on Aging/National Institutes of Health, the Food and Drug Administration and the Gerontological Society of America, as well as by major industry: Best Foods, Bristol-Meyers International, RJR Nabisco Brands, Inc., and Proctor & Gamble Company.

The conference emerged from the combined efforts of several individuals. The need for such a conference was recognized by Drs. Guy E. Livingston and Rida Ali, Chairman and Vice Chairman of the Food and Nutrition Council of the American Health Foundation, respectively. In the fall of 1986, Dr. Livingston approached Dr. Shock, then Scientific Director Emeritus at the Gerontology Research Center, for his opinions on the potential need and organization of such a conference. Dr. Shock, in turn, solicited our thoughts on the matter. After a meeting in January 1987, with Drs. Livingston, Ali, Wynder (President of the American Health Foundation) and others from the American Health Foundation and subsequent consultation with a number of colleagues, many of whom are represented on the Advisory Committee for the conference, there was a general consensus to organize a conference on nutrition and aging. The focus of the conference, however, was not to be on nutrition or diet among the elderly but, at the insistence of Dr. Shock, rather on the more fundamental effects of nutritional variables on aging processes. Such a focus followed Dr. Shock's long-held view that the primary goal of gerontology is to understand the basic mechanisms underlying the biological phenomenon of aging. Moreover, research had unquestionably demonstrated that nutritional variables could have either positive or negative effects on the processes of aging.

In adherence to Dr. Shock's concept that research in gerontology should be developed along interdisciplinary lines, we organized the conference to cover research ranging from population demography and epidemiology to biochemistry and molecular genetics. Such an organizational format recognized the value of each approach. At the population level, the involvement of nutritional variables in the etiology of specific diseases, such as cancer and heart disease, are well illustrated in different populations in Section II. The next step was to consider whether and how aging processes could be affected by nutrition. Animal models of the effects of caloric restriction on a number of age-related phenomena ranging from genetic expression to learning and memory are well documented in Sections III and, in part, Section V. In addition, the involvement of specific nutrients, such as trace minerals and specific lipids, on age-related processes are presented and discussed in Sections IV and V. Many of these effects were being tested in light of specific hypotheses, including glycolysation, oxygen radicals and other variants of metabolic theories of aging. Section V also presents some of the identifiable nutritional variables that have been shown to exert effects on the central nervous system with advancing age.

Finally, consistent with the mission of the American Health Foundation as a public advocate for good nutrition and health in general, several representatives from the food industry were invited to discuss issues raised during the conference. The commitment of industry to improving the quality of food products to enhance the health of our society was renewed in these discussions. However, it was also recognized that the role of nutrition in the aging processes was only beginning to be realized by industry.

Thus, we feel that the product of these combined efforts to explore the potential for nutritional modulation of aging processes is a fitting tribute to Dr. Nathan W. Shock's relentless pursuit of excellence in the science of gerontology. The contributors represent outstanding scientists from around the world who have conducted research on the phenomena of aging and nutrition at various levels of biological organization. The research reported in this volume establishes that nutrition is a highly potent environmental variable that can modulate a number of aging processes, including longevity and physiologic performance. Furthermore, the conference facilitated the identification of commonalities of findings and pointed toward new directions in research. Although the application of many of the findings to specific clinical strategies or general human nutrition presented in this volume might take several decades to emerge, the volume itself will hopefully serve as a benchmark in the realization of the potential for nutritional modulation of aging processes. As such, it will be another in a long list of major contributions by Dr. Nathan W. Shock to biomedical science, in general, and the field of geronology, in particular.

DONALD K. INGRAM, Ph.D.
Baltimore, Maryland

GEORGE T. BAKER, III, Ph.D.
Silver Spring, Maryland

CONTENTS

INTRODUCTION

T. FRANKLIN WILLIAMS, M.D.
National Institutes of Health
National Institute on Aging
Bethesda, Maryland

POTENTIAL IMPORTANCE OF NUTRITION IN AGING

How does nutrition impact on the processes of aging? To begin with the obvious, food is basic to life; appropriate nutrition is fundamental to the entire life span, including aging. But there are two important general questions in relation to aging. First, what constitutes good nutrition throughout the life span, possibly with special features at different stages in life, in order to help assure good health in functioning and to minimize diseases in the later and very late years? Second, in addition to maintaining good health, can nutritional modifications modify aging itself, that is, modify the aging processes including the possibility of extending the life span?

It is often difficult to keep these two questions separate. Certainly, severe malnutrition, or deficiencies in certain key dietary components, will produce disease, disability, and early death. Dietary modifications in humans, such as less fat intake (especially saturated fat) and weight control, will lead to improvement in the risk factors for the diseases that are the major causes of death, that is, heart disease and cancer. The role of nutrition is illustrated by marked differences in nutritional patterns and related mortality in different world populations.

Thus, in the sense of minimizing disease and early death, nutritional choices are important and make a difference. We clearly need to learn more about just what details are most important in later years. To address such issues longitudinal studies in different human populations, as well as careful metabolic studies, are necessary. We already have promising examples, several of which will be reported in this conference.

With regard to modifying aging itself, specifically, extending the life span, the evidence in rodents is unequivocal that dietary restriction has a major effect. How does this happen? What features of aging—what biomarkers of aging—are involved? To help answer these questions the National Institute on Aging is supporting a series of careful studies, in a number of academic centers, utilizing special colonies of dietary restricted rodents. Among other questions, we need to learn how dietary restriction markedly reduces certain disease conditions in these aging animals, such as cancers and renal disease.

In addition, does this phenomenon apply in other species, and in particular in humans and other primates? This is a particularly difficult question to address, both because of the difficulty in maintaining comparable groups in an experimental design and because of the time periods that would be involved; our grandchildren might begin to learn the answers. It appears to me that we need to look for proxies, for other, more limited and specific, features of aging and disease in which we can measure changes in shorter time intervals. Again, longitudinal studies are necessary.

Our Institute puts a high priority on support for further research on nutrition and aging, in addition to the biomarkers studies. We have commissioned a series of conferences and special program announcements, dealing with such aspects as the role of nonenzymatic glycosylation in aging, an NIH-wide conference on the Maillard reaction on aging, and other relevant initiatives.

This conference, with its distinguished participants, provides up-to-date information on these and related questions, as well as helps point the way to future research. In closing, I want to thank the Organizing Committee and the Advisory Committee for this well-planned and significant conference.

SECTION I

Concepts in Aging Research

CHAPTER 1

THEORETICAL CONCEPTS GOVERNING GERONTOLOGICAL RESEARCH

GEORGE T. BAKER, III, Ph.D.
Baker and Associates
and
Nathan W. & Margaret T. Shock Aging Research Foundation
Silver Spring, Maryland

and

NATHAN W. SHOCK, Ph.D.[1]
Gerontology Research Center
National Institute on Aging/National Institutes of Health
Francis Scott Key Medical Center
Baltimore, Maryland

INTRODUCTION

This article is written as a general overview of principles governing research in aging. We believe there are basic tenets unique to gerontological research that need elucidation as an introduction to current concepts in the field.

TIME AS A DEFINING PROPERTY OF AGING

The goal of gerontological research is to identify the basic mechanisms of aging so that interventions can be designed that will alter the rate and expression of aging in individuals. Conceptually, aging represents the irreversible changes in a structure, performance or function that take place with the passage of time in all members of a given species. Thus, time is a primary variable in the study of aging.

[1]Deceased Nov. 12, 1989.

Effective research on aging requires a definition of aging as the net result of multiple biological, biochemical, physiological and behavioral processes that occur with advancing time. Thus, aging must be regarded as an on-going process that is common to all members of a species. The study of aging requires discrete sets of measurements made throughout the life span of an organism. The power of any study of aging increases with the number of points in time at which observations are made. When measurements are confined to the early periods of the life, the results of these time-dependent changes are related primarily to growth and development which are components of the phenomenon of aging. The study of gerontology, however, requires a number of observations after this period of biological maturity. These measurements which characterize aging must be made under strictly defined environmental conditions in animal experimentation and with an understanding of age-independent effects such as that of cohort and period, particularly in human experimentation. The most confounding variable in any study of aging, whether animal or human, is the increasing prevalence of disease with advancing age which must be separated from the processes of aging.

AGE DIFFERENCES VERSUS AGE CHANGES

The method most commonly used to measure aging is to compare average values for a variable based on the mean of a number of subjects of different ages. This method, known as the cross-sectional method, identifies *age differences* between various groups of subjects. This method cannot measure *age changes*. Since the essence of the science of gerontology is the identification of age changes within individuals, serial measurements must be made on the same individual as time progresses. This, the longitudinal method, is so difficult (and expensive, particularly in humans) to apply that few such studies have been conducted. It is, however, the "gold standard" for gerontological research. Parenthetically, it should be pointed out that the processes of aging are characteristics of a given species and therefore can be studied only in populations or groups of a given species. Aging, as a universal biological phenomena characteristic of a species, cannot be studied only in limited numbers of individuals of a species. The baseline reference for individual manifestations of aging processes is the comparison to the population as a whole.

COHORT AND PERIOD EFFECTS

The longitudinal method has its own limitations and potential pitfalls. One limitation, intrinsic to cross-sectional studies as well, is the concomitant increase in the prevalence of disease with the passage of time, thereby potentially confounding the processes of disease with those of aging. This problem can be circumvented by carefully excluding those subjects with identifiable diseases. Although the incidence of many diseases increases with advancing age, it must be remembered that aging and disease are not synonymous. Aging represents the underlying biological alterations that increase the susceptibility of the individual to disease and thus increase the probability of death with advancing age. Aging itself, however, is not a disease. It is a normal component of the life cycle of any metazoan species.

A second limitation of longitudinal studies is that in a single study *period* effects are confounded with chronological age effects. Period effects include those which may be due to events that influence some of the subjects in a particular study, but not all. True age effects influence all members of the species. Examples of period effects include economic depressions, wars and natural disasters such as floods, tornadoes, etc. Such effects can be controlled for by including several different age *cohorts* in the same longitudinal study. Thus, one group of subjects would include those born in one decade while other groups would include subjects who reached the specified chronological age but were born in different decades.

Longitudinal studies also require testing of new groups of subjects of a specified age who have not been tested previously. Such controls are especially needed in testing performance when learning may improve performance on successive experimental trials. Creative and innovative research designs may be necessary to isolate the true effects of age changes even when the longitudinal method is applied.

While the above discussion obviously focuses primarily on the potential pitfalls of longitudinal studies on humans, one must be aware that the some of the same caveats are also present in research on experimental animals. This is particularly evident with regard to life expectancy in rodents, primarily caused by advances that have been made in animal husbandry over the last decades.

There are a number of crucial factors in any aging research protocol which must be controlled for. The first, particularly in animal studies, is the control of environmental factors from conception, i.e., temperature, housing conditions, lighting, humidity, dietary, behavioral artifacts, etc. If the environmental factors cannot be controlled for as they are in human studies, then the results must take into account the potential influences of cohort and period effects.

The ability to distinguish between processes of aging and the results of disease processes is crucial in both human and animal research. The screening of subjects human or animal, for disease must be rigorous throughout the life span. Detailed pathological and other clinical records should be compiled as part of any aging research protocol. In addition, periodic examination of other similar populations of the same species should be made in order to control for potential spurious events such as the presence of an ubiquitous virus.

DEFINITIONS IN GERONTOLOGY

Gerontology is a field of scientific inquiry, not a discipline. The term gerontology relates more to a subdiscipline or specialization within another identified area of expertise. An individual may be an architectural gerontologist or a zoological gerontologist. A good deal of current research activity in the field of gerontology is concerned with the problems of the "aged," i.e., geriatrics or socioeconomic problems, whereas fewer investigators are concerned with the processes of "aging."

We present some operational definitions of what we mean when we discuss terms within the field of gerontology. First is a general definition of *aging* as a biological process followed by that of the *aged*.

Aging is a universal phenomenon characterized by a series of irreversible biological and behavioral changes that occur at the molecular, biochemical, physiological, psychological and physical levels in all individuals of a given species. These changes render individuals more susceptible to the stresses of everyday living. The rates of aging for any species are governed by two major components.

The first, a genetic component imparts an intrinsic capability to the individual to manifest any number of species-specific biological processes. These intrinsic capabilities include, at least in part, life span and resistance to certain diseases.

The second governing component is the environment. Environmental influences are superimposed on the intrinsic genetic component and can affect the rate(s) of aging either positively or negatively. We are increasingly aware of the negative environmental influences on human health and longevity, i.e., various carcinogenic agents and risk factors for human diseases. We are less knowledgeable about the potential positive influences of environmental factors such as nutrition on the rates of biological aging processes particularly in humans.

The term "aged" is best defined as "as state of condition" wherein an individual becomes more vulnerable to multiple environmental stresses. Actually, a "state of agedness" is not necessarily a correlate of chronological age but rather a state of dependent versus independent lifestyle which could be caused by factors other than age, i.e., injury or disease. The manifestations of aging processes normally, however, include declines in various physiological functional capabilities and a general loss of adaptive or homeostatic capabilities, including an increased susceptibility to a number of disease states. Thus, an individual with advancing age is more likely to experience a period(s) of dependent status rather than an independent lifestyle.

The distinction between the term "aged" and "aging" is important because it directly impacts on one's approach to the phenomena under discussion. In terms of the potential advances in the field of gerontology researchers may expect to make, there are immense differences between the study of *aging* versus the study of the *aged*! The study of the *aged* will in all probability improve the immediate application of more effective clinical treatments to ameliorate the severity of various age-associated or related disease states or explain social phenomenon in a way which can affect change to improve the quality of life. Study of the *aged*, however, is not likely to tell us very much about the processes of aging. The study of the *aged*, regardless of how rigorous the experimental protocol, will give us information *only* as to end points in time. Indeed, the data give only the varied manifestations of an on-going phenomenon. Whereas the study of the processes of *aging*, whether psychosocial or biomedical, is more likely to have greater long term effects on the quality of life through the understanding of the processes of aging and thus the possibility of intervention in etiology of age-associated disease as well as psychosocial problems.

CRITERIA FOR BIOLOGICAL AGING

The definition of aging may be further characterized by the following criteria first proposed by B. L. Strehler (1962) and paraphrased here. If a phenomenon under study is truly an alteration due to the biological processes of aging, then the change should be progressive, irreversible and deleterious. There are those changes which are progressive such as those that occur during development and maturation, however, would not normally be considered as deleterious. On the other hand, there are events such as getting hit by a bus which will be deleterious and increase the probability of death, however, cannot specifically be considered a processes of aging. The intent of these criteria is to exclude those earlier progressive age-dependent changes which are part of the overall life cycle of the organism and cannot be considered deleterious in themselves.

Another criterion is that the phenomenon under study must be universal. By that, we mean that all members of the species under study must demonstrate that particular kind of change if it is representative of aging in that species. By this criterion, virtually all diseases cannot be considered a phenomenon of aging, although any number of age-associated diseases could fit the criteria of progressive and deleterious. For example, although many older individuals do have cancer or heart disease not all older individuals do. Conversely, any number of younger individuals also manifest these disease states.

The fourth criterion, and that which is most difficult for the researcher in biogerontology to control, is that of intrinsicality. By intrinsicality, we mean that if the parameter under study is truly a phenomenon of aging then the changes must be associated with the cellular processes of the organism under study and not due to *adverse* environmental influences. For example, there are many environmental factors which can negatively influence physiological performance and life span, such as exposure to ionizing radiation, toxins, carcinogens, and, as many papers contained in this volume illustrate, dietary factors which can not only increase/decrease the risks of certain age-associated diseases but conversely have been demonstrated to improve life span as well as physiological performance. The concept of intrinsicality is clear in the case of infectious diseases of radiation. However, it is not so clear when other less obvious environmental factors, such as nutrition, are involved. The rates of aging in any species are primarily determined by two major components—that of a genetic informational package which sets limits and that of environmental factors which can influence the expression of genetic information. For example, what are the optimal nutritional requirements for different stages of the life span? The answer is we simply do not know! Are there other environmental factors that can positively influence functional capacity and life span? Again, we have a paucity of scientifically validated research information!

AGING AS A MULTI-DIMENSIONAL PHENOMENON

Current research on aging shows clearly that there is probably no single aging process which modulates aging of all organ systems and processes. It is more probable that aging is a multidimensional process that involves interrelationships between many cellular processes and higher level integrated homeostatic mechanisms. Thus, gerontology must be a multiple disciplinary science which in fact is still in its infancy, but growing robustly. The goal of gerontologists is to reduce the dimensions of our ignorance about the basic mechanisms of aging by expanding knowledge about the interrelationships between variables and their relationships to the passage of time. This knowledge must be based on well-designed experiments that distinguish between aging as a biological process and the description of the characteristics of the aged. In this regard, perhaps the best axiom that the researcher in the basic sciences of aging research can follow, is to ask not "*How long does an individual of a given species live?*" but rather "*Why does an individual of a given species live so long?*" In other words, the researcher interested in understanding processes of aging should examine those biological mechanisms which allow an organism to live as long as it does, rather than concentrating on why the organism died.

AGING PHENOMENA: GENOTYPE-ENVIRONMENT INTERACTIONS

The marked differences in life span observed among different animal species support the notion that some genetic program influences the maximum longevity for each species. Thus, life spans for animals of different species can range from the one day of the adult may fly to more than a 150 years for the Galapagos tortoise. In this context, life span must be regarded as an evolved coadaptive trait of a life history strategy for a given species. Evidence for the genetic influences on species life span are self-evident in that no member of any metazoan species studied to date has lived beyond a finite point in time. In examining human genealogical studies, a good correlation between the life span of parents and their offspring is often reported. Thus, supporting a familial or genetic basis of longevity in man. In one of the better studies, there was demonstrated a positive correlation between 1,739 pairs of twins and parental longevity. Even more interesting and supportive of the genetic influences on longevity, it was found that the interval of death between identical twins (36.0 months) was less than half that of fraternal twins of the same sex

(74.6 months) or of separate sex (106.0 months). Simply stated, an identical genome results in more nearly identical life spans. While a number of these types of studies suffer from one or another statistical short-coming, they all point in the same direction that heredity does play a role in determining the course of the human life span.

Even more convincing of genetic influence on longevity are the studies done in cell culture or *in vitro*. Primarily, those conducted on fibroblasts that demonstrated that when cells are taken from a young human they have a finite life span as determined by so-called population doublings of 50 or so in culture. Other studies on the same cell type from various species have demonstrated a correlation between species longevity and the number of these population doublings. Similarly, with human subjects, there has been found a correlation between the age of donors and the number of population doublings. Again, simply stated this evidence offers strong evidence for the genetic influence on the rates and processes of aging—for even when the cells of a given species are removed from other *in vivo* factors and grown *in vitro* they manifest an intrinsic species-specific life span.

The second governing component on species life span is the environment. Environment influences are superimposed on the intrinsic genetic component and can affect the rates of aging either positively or negatively. As mentioned previously, we are increasingly aware of those environmental factors which have a deleterious effect on life span and physiological capability particularly with regard to carcinogens, toxins, and lifestyle risk factors such as diet and exercise. Conversely, we are much less knowledgeable about the potential positive environmental influences such as nutrition which will be further discussed in this book.

There is no question that environmental factors can and do introduce variations in life span within the individual genetic program as expressed in different species. For example, in poikilothermic species such as insects, rotifers, etc., an increase in environmental temperature will shorten life span whereas decreasing temperature will lengthen life span within limits.

Other environmental factors, such as exposure to ionizing radiation, will shorten the average life span in higher animal species. Conversely, the average life span of a number of animal species has been shown to increase with a reduction of food intake. Experiments showing the increase in life span in rats by reducing food intake was first demonstrated in the late 20's and early 30's by Clive McCay. These experiments have been repeated by a number of investigators since then, so that there is no doubt that caloric restriction can lengthen average life span. See Masoro (Chapter 8), Ingram (Chapter 18), Richardson and McCarter (Chapter 11), Merry and Holehan (Chapter 10), Harrison and Archer (Chapter 9) Nandy *et al.* (Chapter 22) and McNeill *et al.* (Chapter 19). Unfortunately, there is still no agreement among investigators (either nutritionist or gerontologist) on the mechanism(s) of the phenomenon. See Weindruch (Chapter 7). Nor has it been possible to conduct comparable comprehensive experiments in species above the rat in the phylogenic scale. Preliminary results, however, on caloric restriction in nonhuman primates being carried out at the Gerontological Research Center of the National Institute on Aging suggest that there may be positive effects. See Roth *et al.* (Chapter 12). Thus, dietary manipulations seem to provide a potential technique for manipulating life span even in higher animals.

In recent years epidemiological studies have given strong support for the concept that environmental factors play an important role in the etiology of disease such as hypertension, cardiovascular disease and cancer. The importance of saturated dietary fat in the genesis of coronary artery disease and atherosclerosis is now well established. Similarly, the intake of salt is now recognized as an important factor in the development of hypertension (See Kannel and Hatano for discussion of some of these issues). The role of fiber in the diet in reducing the incidence of cancer, especially in the gastrointestinal tract, is under investigation in a number of laboratories. The loss of calcium from the skeleton is an important problem among the elderly, particularly in post-menopausal women. Although there is some agreement that the problem is related to calcium metabolism that should yield to dietary manipulations, the problem is still unresolved. Thus, many studies point to the role of diet in developing a number of specific diseases that limit life span in humans.

The importance of good hygiene in maintaining health and vigor in old age is becoming more and more apparent. In addition to maintaining a varied balanced diet that keeps body weight at an optimal level, other factors such as elimination of cigarette smoking and maintaining a regular regimen of physical activity can contribute to the maintenance of health and vigor.

ONSET AND RATES OF AGING PROCESSES

The manifestation of the rates of aging processes can and do vary between species, within the different members of the same species as influenced by genotype-environment interactions, as well as between various physiological systems within the same individual with the passage of time. Three points should be emphasized: (1) Aging is not a single identifiable process within a species but rather a series of apparently unique processes which affect various physiological systems. (2) The onset of change for a given physiological system is a unique characteristic of that system within the life span. (3) The rate of change in a given physiological system is a relatively independent phenomenon. Figure 1.1 illustrates the varying time in onset of change as well as differential rates of change for selected physiological systems in humans.

As is observed in Fig. 1.1, some systems are optimum early in life, such as accommodation capacity of the eye and high frequency hearing. Others manifest measurable change only later in the life span, such as grip strength which does not show significant changes until the fourth and fifth decades of life (data not shown).

Other characteristics, such as personality, do not seem to demonstrate any significant change even in very old individuals.

The graph also clearly illustrates that the rates of change for the various systems are not identical. Some systems, such as accommodation capacity, exhibit a bimodal rate of change with a rather early rapid decline, while others manifest a relatively slow, almost linear, rate of change, such as nerve conduction velocity.

Most of the data presented above have been adapted from the Baltimore Longitudinal Study on Aging being conducted at the Gerontological Research Center of the National Institute on Aging/National Institutes of Health over the past 30 years.

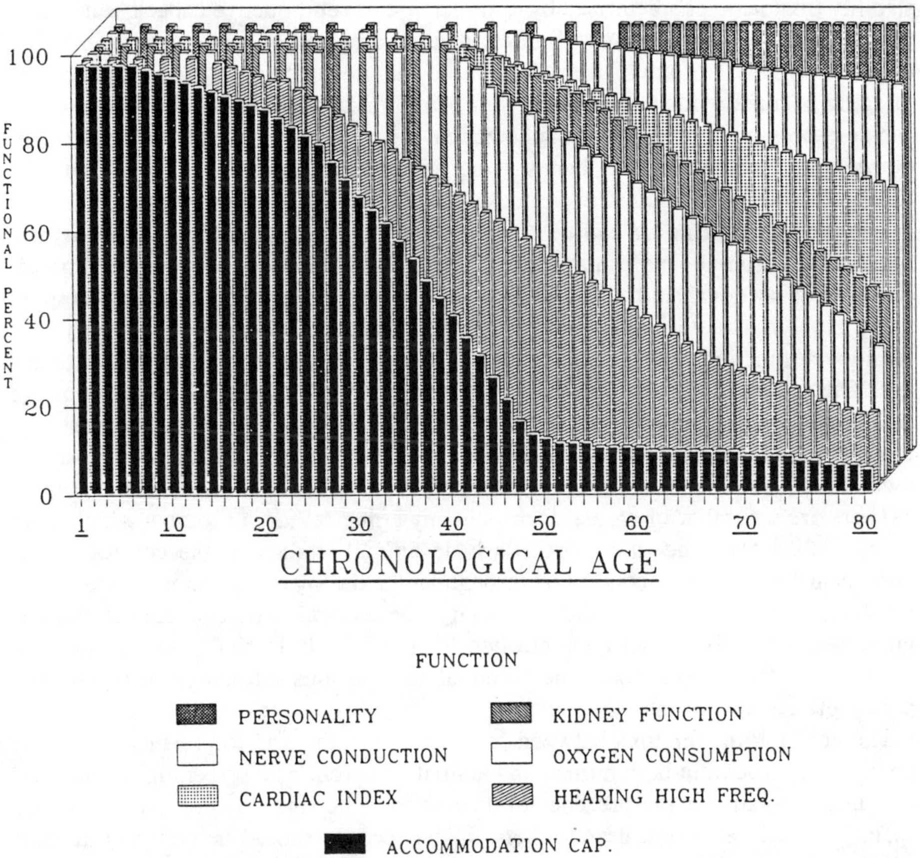

FIG. 1.1. TIME OF ONSET AND RATES OF CHANGE IN SELECTED HUMAN PHYSIOLOGICAL FUNCTIONS WITH ADVANCING AGE

All of the data presented have been adapted and interpolated from previously published reports most from the results of the Baltimore Longitudinal Study on Aging conducted at the Gerontology Research Center, National Institutes on Aging/National Institutes of Health.

METHODOLOGY AND CAVEATS IN AGING RESEARCH

Processes of aging can be studied only in relationship to populations of animals. Although the age-dependent changes occur in individuals they must be compared to the population as a whole. Therefore, survivorship curves and life tables need to be constructed to assure the researcher that they indeed are studying aging and not changes associated with other phases of the life span or spurious environmental artifacts. Generally speaking, the life span of most species can be described in three phases as follows: (1) a period of maturation and development characterized by increased growth and complexity of physiological systems; (2) a period of relative stability (maturity) characterized by optimization of reproductive capacity and other physiological or functional capabilities; and (3) a period of senescence, usually in the third trimester of adult life, wherein the manifestations of on-going processes of aging become evident, and the forces of mortality for populations increase and can be expressed in predictable mathematical terms. Given this operational description of aging, it is imperative, then, that any aging research protocol include a number of experimental time points to be measured throughout the life span.

The processes of aging can be studied at any level of biological or behavioral organization from the molecular-genetic to cognitive function. As mentioned previously, cross-sectional studies are the most commonly employed methodology to study aging phenomenon. Groups of individuals of the same age are experimentally tested for a given function or other variable and compared to another group of a different age. The results, however, can only characterize groups or age differences not age changes which may in fact be due to cohort or period effects. This is because age changes are a function of the individual and therefore, characterization of age changes requires measurement of the same parameter on the same individual over time.

There are a number of crucial factors in any aging research protocol which must be controlled for. The first, particularly in animal studies, is the control of environmental factors from conception throughout the life span, i.e., temperature, housing conditions, lighting, humidity, dietary, behavioral artifacts, etc. If the environmental factors cannot be controlled for (such as in human studies), then the results must take into account the potential for spurious influences of cohort and period effects as well as other factors.

The ability to distinguish between processes of aging and the results of disease processes is crucial in both human and animal research. The screening of subjects, human or animal, for the presence of disease must be rigorous throughout the life span. Detailed pathological and other clinical records should be compiled as part of any aging research protocol. In addition, periodic examination of other similar populations of the same species should be made in order to control for unusual events, such as the presence of an ubiquitous virus in an isolated population.

There is no "best" animal or plant system to study the biological mechanisms of aging. The single most critical mistake an investigator can make is to ask the wrong question of a given model system. There are many well-characterized rodent models for aging research bred and maintained under highly standardized environmental conditions which are readily available to researchers. The number of aging studies conducted on other mammalian species is comparatively limited and therefore extensive baseline data is often lacking. In addition, there are a number of well-characterized invertebrate models for aging research such as *Drosophila*, nematodes, etc. Again, there is no model system in which the processes of aging cannot be studied. The major caveat for the researcher would be to ascertain that the variable under study is intrinsic to the basic phenomenon of aging. For example, the life-history strategies of a number of species which are invariably linked to reproductive success can dramatically affect the mean life span. If these factors are not fully understood, the interpretation of experimental results could lead to erroneous conclusions. The Pacific salmon, on average, have a life span of three years, however, if they are prevented from spawning life span can be enhanced threefold. Similar scenarios can be demonstrated for any number of semiparous species, such as the octopus, which have one massive brood then undergo a rapid senescence and death. In species such as these, the biological phenomenon of aging must be understood in the context of these evolved life-history strategies.

Aside from the previously mentioned potential confounding variables such as life-history strategies, period and cohort effects, there are any number of potential methodological sources of error. For example, if a researcher is studying age-related changes in an enzyme system or virtually any other subcellular component, it is not enough to simply optimize the assay system for an animal of a given age. The enzyme assay must be optimal for all of the ages to be studied. Any number of parameters may have been changed with age including: pH, ionic, Km's, even temperature optimums. In addition, there could be inhibitors and/or activators at one age that are not present at another age that could effect enzyme activity. Furthermore, it is possible that extraction procedures which are optimal for one age are not the optimum for another age. Although age-dependent alterations in the primary sequence of a protein have not been conclusively demonstrated to date, post-translational modifications for a number of proteins have been.

There are numerous other examples were a methodology is optimal for the measurement or determination of a function or process in a younger animal but is inadequate as the animal ages. A number of investigations have demonstrated age-dependent alterations in the time course of enzyme induction either by substrate, hormones or environmental factors. Thus, the use of a time course established for a system in a younger animal would not be optimal at latter ages.

The question of how to express results of various measurements is another potential caveat in aging research. If, for example, a researcher expresses enzyme activity measurements as a function of protein concentration, as is standardly done, the researcher must be sure that the amount of protein is both qualitatively and quantitatively the same—even in purified preparations. If protein does demonstrate quantitative alterations, should the researcher then present such data as a function of number of cells or amount of DNA? Whichever alternative is chosen, any age-dependent alterations in those parameters must be established as independent variables with regard to what is being measured.

At the whole animal level, there are also any number of factors which can lead to misinterpretation of results, particularly when integrated physiological systems are measured. For example, by standard methodology the measurement of oxygen consumption in humans shows decreases with advancing age. If, however, the same results are expressed as a function of body water (an indicator of active cellular mass), no changes in oxygen consumption are observed. Similarly, albeit at a different level, if human subjects are screened for minute cardiac lesions, there is observed no significant age-dependent alterations in cardiac output even under moderate stress in very old individuals.

The interpretation of aging investigations on highly integrated physiological systems is often confounded by changes which occur in another system. Changes in some processes or functions may have wide-spread trophic effects on other systems. For example, if one wished to assess the causation of age-dependent changes in renal clearance, one would need to know the contribution to that change by a number of other factors, i.e., nephronal loss, cardiovascular alterations, glomerular changes, basement membrane alterations, etc., before one could say very much about causation. Indeed, there is still a great deal of necessary descriptive investigations to be done in many areas of aging research before a more comprehensive understanding of the processes of aging can be formulated.

SUMMARY

This short overview intends to present the reader with some of the features unique to aging research. Recognizing that each of the basic concept areas and tenets mentioned could justify a chapter unto itself for a full explanation and discussion, general references have been provided for the reader who wishes to pursue further study. Research in the field of aging is different from most other areas of scientific inquiry, primarily because of the added variable of time—chronological and biological. Indeed, gerontological or aging research presents a unique challenge to the scientific investigator through the variable of time! How and why do cells age?

ACKNOWLEDGMENTS

We would like to acknowledge the support of Dr. Richard Greulich, recent Scientific Director of the Gerontology Research Center of the National Institute on Aging, for providing working space. In addition, we are indebted to Dr. Richard Kriner for his invaluable technical assistance and to Dr. Donald Ingram for his most helpful insight and discussions in the preparation of this chapter. Finally, recognition must be given to the Food and Nutrition Council of the American Health Foundation, and in particular Dr. Guy Livingston, for their help in organizing and sponsoring the conference for which this chapter was prepared.

REFERENCES

BAKER, III, G. T. and SPROTT, R. L. 1988. Biomarkers of aging. Exp. Gerontol. *23*, (4/5), 223–239.

BIRREN, J. E. and SCHAIE, K. W. 1977. Handbook of the Psychology of Aging. Van Nostrand Reinhold, New York.

COMFORT, A. 1956. The Biology of Senescence. Rinehart, New York.

COWDRY, E. V. 1939. Problems of Ageing; Biological and Medical Aspects. Williams and Wilkens, Baltimore.

FINCH, C. E. and HAYFLICK, L. 1977. Handbook of the Biology of Aging. Van Nostrand Reinhold, New York.

FINCH, C. E. and SCHNEIDER, E. 1985. Handbook of the Biology of Aging, 2nd Edition. Van Nostrand Reinhold Co., New York.

LANSING, A. I. 1952. Cowdry's Problems of Ageing, 3rd Edition. Williams and Wilkins, Baltimore.

SHOCK, N. W. *et al.* 1984. Normal Human Aging: The Baltimore Longitudinal Study of Aging. NIH Publ. No. 84-2450. U.S. Govt. Printing Office, Washington, D.C.

STREHLER, B. L. 1962. Time, Cells and Aging. Academic Press, New York.

SECTION II

Age-Associated Effects of Nutrition on Human Morbidity and Mortality

CHAPTER 2

NUTRITIONAL CONSIDERATIONS IN OCCURRENCE AND PREVENTION OF CARDIOVASCULAR DISEASE IN THE ELDERLY

WILLIAM B. KANNEL, M.D.
Section of Preventive Medicine and Epidemiology
Boston University School of Medicine
Evans Research Foundation
Boston, Massachusetts

The elderly are the fastest growing segment of most affluent populations around the world. This poses major health and nutrition problems. In the United States this 11% of the population accounts for 29% of health costs and 34% of all short-stay hospitalizations (Brody and Brock 1985). Cardiovascular disease is a major cause of morbidity, mortality and disability in the elderly, and is responsible for 70% of all deaths beyond age 75 (Brody and Brock 1985; Kannel and McGee 1986). Atherosclerosis, hypertension and diabetes are responsible for most of the cardiovascular disease afflicting the elderly. Diet must be assigned a major role in atherogenesis because it influences atherogenic predisposing factors for cardiovascular disease, such as blood lipids, blood pressure and glucose tolerance. Unfortunately, nutrition data specific for the elderly are scarce, and there is scant direct evidence that this applies to atherogenesis in those who have already exceeded age 65. It is necessary to extrapolate from data on younger age groups to arrive at recommendations for the elderly who wish to reduce their risk of cardiovascular disease by modifying their diet.

At present, recommended daily allowances for nutrients in general for persons over age 65 yr are only tentative, chiefly because data are lacking on which to formulate such recommendations. However, some established facts are relevant. As people age, the rate at which energy is expended tends to decrease, food intake is reduced and lean body mass decreases. Intestinal changes may reduce absorption of vitamins, minerals, protein, fat and carbohydrate. Less exercise, decline in estrogen, and lack of calcium can promote osteoporosis. Fluid regulation is usually sluggish in the elderly. The elderly tend to become dehydrated more readily than the young and need to conserve fluid. Regulation of electrolyte balance is also less finely tuned. Especially relevant to atherogenesis in the elderly is the fact that lipid metabolism is not substantially altered in advanced age.

RISK FACTORS

It is widely believed that cardiovascular risk factors are no longer relevant in the elderly. However, epidemiologic evidence indicates that even in the elderly there are modifiable predisposing factors related to occurrence of cardiovascular events (Table 2.1). These are also quite prevalent in the elderly (Table 2.2).

TABLE 2.1
IMPACT OF RISK FACTORS ON CORONARY HEART DISEASE INCIDENCE
(30 YR FOLLOW-UP, FRAMINGHAM STUDY)

	Bivariate[1] Standardized Regression Coefficients			
	Age 35–64		Age 65–94	
Risk Factors	Men	Women	Men	Women
Systolic pressure	0.338[3]	0.418[3]	0.401[3]	0.286[3]
Diastolic pressure	0.321[3]	0.363[3]	0.296[3]	0.082 +
Serum cholesterol	0.322[3]	0.307[3]	0.121 +	0.213[3]
Cigarettes	0.259[3]	0.095 +	−0.107 +	−0.034 +
Blood glucose	0.043 +	0.206[3]	0.166[3]	0.209[3]
Vital capacity	−0.112[1]	−0.331[3]	−0.127 +	−0.253[3]
Relative weight	0.190[3]	0.264[3]	0.177[2]	0.1241[1]

[1]Age-adjusted coefficients +N.S.
[2]$P < 0.05$.
[3]$P < 0.01$.
[4]$P < 0.001$.

Risk of cardiovascular disease in general and of coronary disease in particular increases with age irrespective of risk factor level. However, a poor risk profile is associated with a substantial escalation of risk and tends to equalize the atherosclerotic disease potential in young and old. The high level of cardiovascular risk factors in the elderly is not a product of normal senescence since it is possible to reach advanced age without dangerous levels of any of the risk factors. When these factors are present, they continue to operate to promote cardiovascular events in old age.

TABLE 2.2
PERCENTAGE PREVALENCE CARDIOVASCULAR RISK FACTORS IN THE ELDERLY
(FRAMINGHAM STUDY, EXAM 16)

AGE	Definite Hypertension Men	Definite Hypertension Women	Hypercholesterolemia Men	Hypercholesterolemia Women	Glucose Intolerance Men	Glucose Intolerance Women	Obesity Men	Obesity Women	Cigarette Smoking Men	Cigarette Smoking Women
65–74	42.1	48.9	16.6	39.7	29.5	17.5	52.2	47.8	21.9	23.0
75–84	45.5	61.1	9.7	36.3	30.9	26.0	35.4	39.3	13.9	8.5
85–94	20.7	64.8	9.4	18.4	33.3	29.0	7.7	30.0	9.4	3.2

Obesity

Weight gain continuing on through middle age and on to old age is common. In very advanced age the average body weight then tends to slowly decline (Fig. 2.1). This decline in the senium is accompanied by a loss of water, lean body mass and some fat. As in younger adults men continue to take in more calories than women, but there is a fall in absolute calorie intake in both sexes in advanced old age. This is particularly true in institutionalized aged patients who often have surprisingly low energy intakes. However, even in the noninstitutionalized, energy intakes in affluent populations decline with age probably because of a decrease in physical activity.

Obesity worsens all the major cardiovascular risk factors in young and old and promotes cardiovascular disease (Intersociety Commission for Heart Disease Resources 1984; National Institutes of Health 1985). Obesity was found to be a major determinant of the incidence of hypertension in the Framingham Study with some 70% of newly acquired hypertension attributable to adiposity (Garrison *et al.* 1987). A 10 lb weight gain in men was found to be associated with a 4.3 mmHg rise in systolic blood pressure, 7.5 mg/dL rise in serum cholesterol, a 0.6 mg/dL rise in blood glucose and a 0.2 mg/dL increase in uric acid. In women the corresponding changes were respectively: 4.2, 5.8, 1.2 and 0.1 (Fig. 2.2). Much, but not all of the increased risk derives from the risk factors which obesity promotes. Abdominal obesity appears to be more of a contributor to cardiovascular morbidity and mortality than generalized obesity, its effect both independent of and mediated through promotion of other risk factors. Weight control is thus a means for improving most of the major risk factors which predispose to atherosclerotic cardiovascular disease (Intersociety Commission for Heart Disease Resources 1984; National Institutes of Health 1985). Weight reduction improves the entire cardiovascular risk profile (Intersociety Commission for Heart Disease Resources 1984).

There is nonetheless controversy about the health consequences of obesity in the elderly (Intersociety Commission for Heart Disease Resources 1984; National Institutes of Health 1985; Jarrett 1986; Andres 1984; Hubert *et al.* 1983; Bjorntorp 1985). An excess of mortality at both extremes of the distribution of body weight

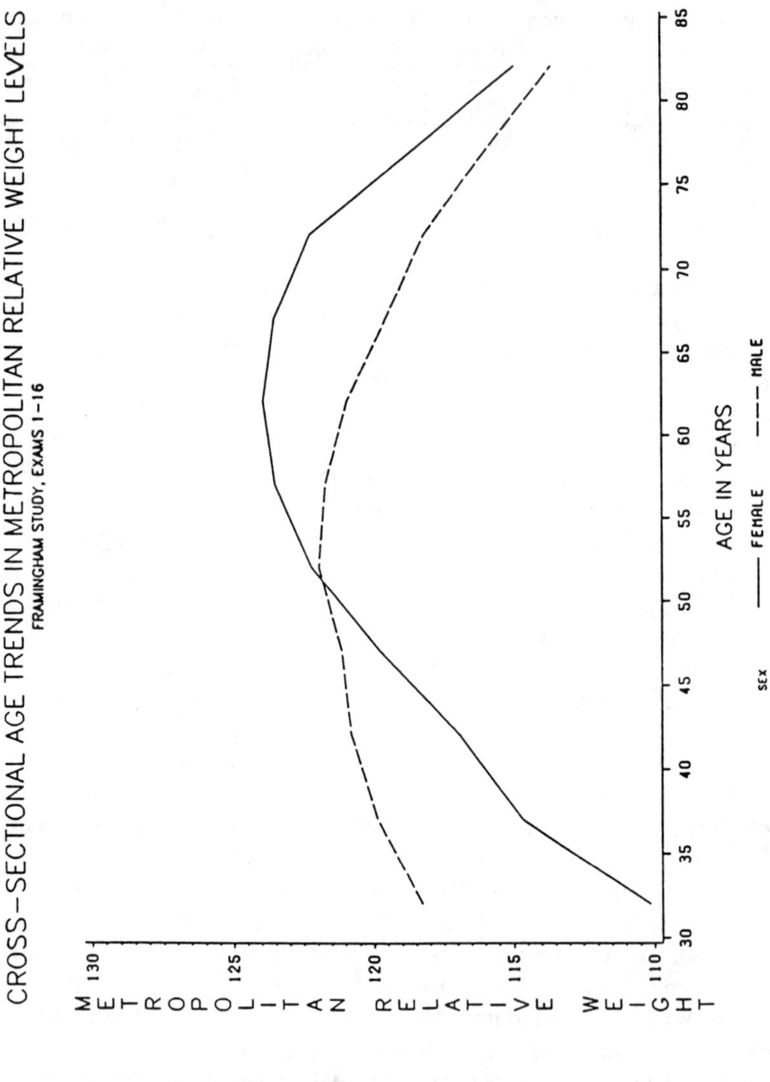

FIG. 2.1. CROSS-SECTIONAL AGE TRENDS IN METROPOLITAN RELATIVE WEIGHT LEVELS (FRAMINGHAM STUDY, EXAMS 1–16)

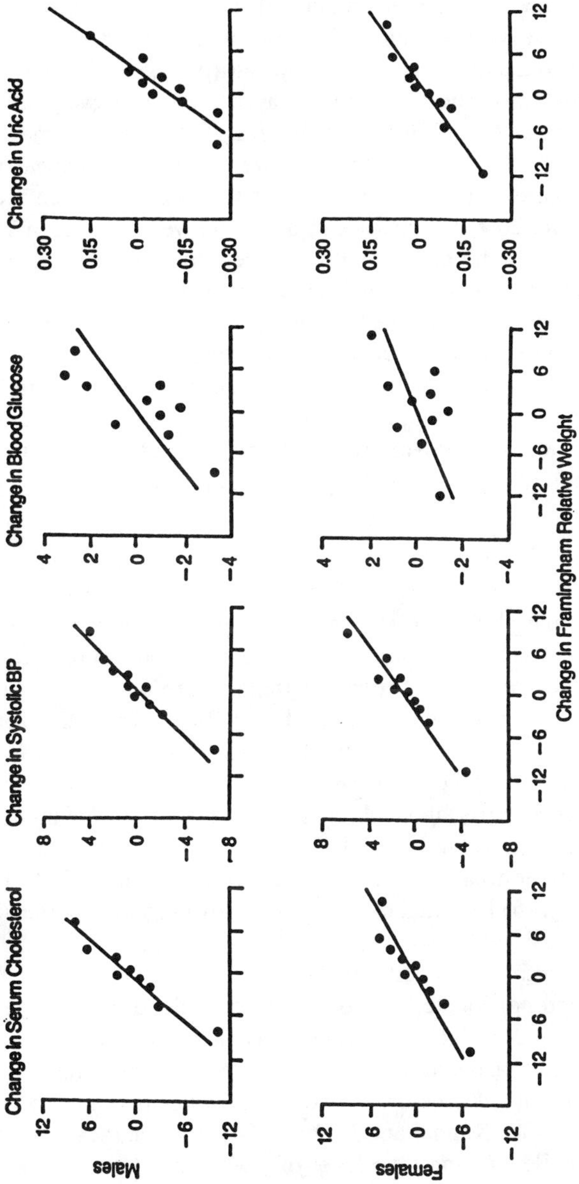

FIG 2.2. CHANGES IN CHARACTERISTIC VALUES WITH CHANGE IN FRAMINGHAM RELATIVE WEIGHT

has been noted. This is confounded by effects of smoking, coexistent subclinical disease and insufficient length of follow-up. Weight influences on cardiovascular disease are more apparent on long-term than on short-term follow-up. It is claimed that abdominal obesity may have more deleterious metabolic effects on atherogenesis than a more generalized pattern of obesity (Bjorntorp 1985). The elderly do appear to put on abdominal fat. There is general agreement that weights 20% above "desirable" constitute an established health hazard. Although there may be a penalty associated with substantial underweight, overweight does not appear to have any value for surviving cardiovascular events. Weight reduction can be recommended for the elderly who are 20% or more above desirable weight (BMI of 27.2 for men and 26.9 for women). In the elderly with diabetes, hypertension, dyslipidemia or gout even lesser degrees of overweight should be corrected.

Unfortunately, there are no acceptable data demonstrating that weight reduction actually improves the prognosis of the corpulent elderly. There is also no information on the prognosis associated with repeated unsuccessful attempts to lose weight. Weight control is a logical first approach to correction of dyslipidemia, glucose intolerance, hypertension and hyperuricemia. Correction of overweight should also improve exercise tolerance in the elderly with compromised cardiac function.

Hypertension

Hypertension in general, and isolated systolic hypertension in particular, are very common in the elderly and this accounts for a large percentage of their cardiovascular disease. The exact determinants of this hypertension are not known, but a number of predisposing factors have been identified: (1) Blacks are more susceptible to hypertension than whites. (2) Obesity predisposes to hypertension. Some believe this is related to insulin resistance, hyperinsulinemia, and the effect of this on sodium and potassium transport across all membranes and resorption of sodium by the kidney. (3) Alcohol raises blood pressure. (4) Those with hematocrits on the upper range of the normal distribution have twice as much hypertension as those in the lower ranges (Kaplan 1985). (5) Elevated blood lipids predispose to hypertension (Kaplan 1985).

In all but some primitive, unacculturated populations, blood pressure tends to rise with age with a disproportionate increase in systolic blood pressure resulting in a wide pulse pressure and a high prevalence of isolated systolic hypertension. The diastolic blood pressure peaks in middle age and then declines in both sexes in advanced age. Diastolic blood pressure in women is lower than that in men (Kannel 1985; Kannel *et al.* 1980; Kannel and Brand 1984). In men, systolic pressure also tends to peak in middle age and then level off, whereas in women pressures continue to rise, so that at advanced ages values converge on those found in men (Kannel 1985). As a result, the prevalence of hypertension in women continues to rise beyond age 80, whereas in men it declines substantially (Kannel 1985).

TABLE 2.3
RISK OF CARDIOVASCULAR DISEASE BY HYPERTENSIVE STATUS
ACCORDING TO AGE IN EACH SEX
(30 YR FOLLOW-UP, FRAMINGHAM STUDY)

	Annual Incidence Rate per 1,000		Age-adjusted Risk Ratio[1]	
Age	Men	Women	Men	Women
35–64	31	17	2.8[2]	3.4[2]
65–94	73	35	3.3[2]	1.8[2]

$$^{1}\text{HBP/NORMAL} = \frac{> 160/95\ \text{mmHg}}{< 149/90\ \text{mmHg}}$$

[2]$P < 0.001$.

Elevated blood pressure, which is influenced by nutrition in the elderly, continues unabated to influence risk of cardiovascular disease (Kannel and McGee 1986; Kannel and Gordon 1978; Kannel 1985; Harris *et al.* 1985; Kannel *et al.* 1980). The relative risk as judged by risk ratios are comparable in young and old and the absolute risk indicated by the incidence rate, is greater in the elderly (Table 2.3). Even isolated systolic hypertension, the dominant variety in the elderly, is hazardous in either sex (Kannel *et al.* 1980) (Fig. 2.3).

Weight reduction usually is accompanied by a fall in pressure in concert with reductions in cardiac output and plasma norepinephrine (Kaplan 1985; Reisen *et al.* 1983). Conversely, weight gain usually increases blood pressure. Several studies have

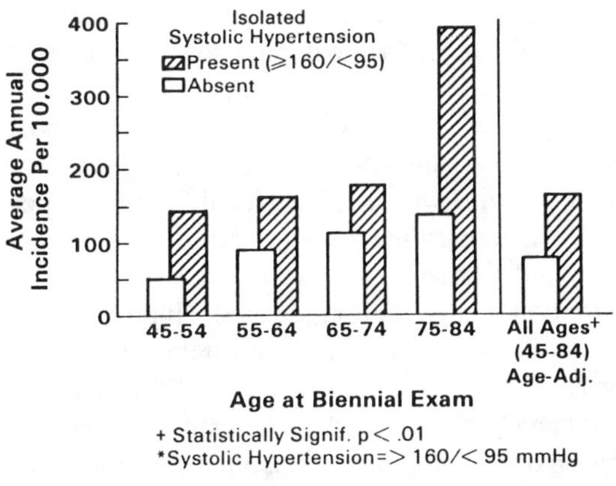

FIG. 2.3. RISK OF MYOCARDIAL INFARCTION WITH ISOLATED SYSTOLIC HYPERTENSION* AMONG MEN 45–84 (24-YR FOLLOW-UP, FRAMINGHAM STUDY)

demonstrated the efficacy of weight reduction in reducing blood pressure independent of dietary sodium restriction (Kaplan 1985; Reisen *et al.* 1983). Weight loss is apparently also antihypertensive without sodium restriction (Reisen *et al.* 1978). Even small amounts of weight loss usually will lower blood pressure. However, better means for achieving sustained weight reduction are sorely needed.

There is evidence that moderate sodium restriction may prevent or delay development of hypertension, particularly in susceptible persons (Kaplan 1985). There is a greater responsiveness to sodium restriction in the elderly, particularly those with higher pressures and those with low renin values (Kaplan 1985).

It has been postulated that the higher ratio of sodium to potassium in the diet of acculturated peoples is a factor in hypertension and that adjustment back to the ratio consumed by primitives could help control hypertension (Treasure and Bloth 1980). There is some evidence for this in humans as well as in animals, and the lower pressures found in vegetarians have been ascribed to their high intake of potassium. A modest antihypertensive effect of potassium supplements has been shown in some controlled trials (Stamler *et al.* 1980). This may be a result of potassium-induced natriuresis, neural effects, vasodilation, renin suppression, natriuretic hormone, and antagonism or inhibition of cellular transport mechanisms (Kaplan 1985).

Increased intravascular tone induced by raising intracellular calcium is postulated as a contributor to essential hypertension. On the other hand, intake of too little dietary calcium seems to be associated with hypertension, and calcium supplements may lower blood pressure (Belizan *et al.* 1983).

Administration of magnesium also may lower blood pressure (Dykner and Wester 1983). Dietary deficiency of magnesium raises the blood pressure of rats by enhancing calcium influx into cells causing vasconstriction. Recent data suggest that decreased fat intake and increased polyunsaturated fatty acids will reduce blood pressure. This is in accord with a modest association between serum cholesterol and blood pressure (Kaplan 1985). Animal data are inconsistent on this, and the mechanism for an effect is unclear.

Vegetarian diets appear to be associated with lower blood pressures, possibly because of the increased potassium content or increased fiber (Anderson and Tietyen-Clark 1986). Dietary protein, which affects renal function, appears to be unrelated to blood pressure. Variations in the amount and type of carbohydrate have only a transient effect on blood pressure.

Excessive consumption of alcohol is associated with increased rates of stroke, cardiac failure, cardiomyopathy and hypertension (Klatsky *et al.* 1986; Hennekens *et al.* 1978; Klatsky *et al.* 1981a,b; Colditz *et al.* 1985). Epidemiologic evidence strongly links alcohol and hypertension even adjusting for age, obesity, coffee, smoking and administration of alcohol under controlled conditions raises blood pressure. About 10% of hypertension in men and 1% in women may be attributable to alcohol (Kaplan 1985).

Caffeine in coffee can raise the blood pressure transiently, but there is no evidence that it causes sustained hypertension possibly because of the development of tolerance (Lang *et al.* 1983). Thus, the evidence for dietary contributions to hypertension is not as extensive as for atherosclerosis. Excessive weight, alcohol, fat and sodium may contribute. Deficiencies of potassium, calcium and magnesium may promote hypertension. The dietary strategy to prevent and control hypertension consists of weight loss, fat and sodium restriction, along with increased amounts of calcium, potassium, magnesium and fiber. This is consistent with that proposed to prevent atherosclerotic cardiovascular disease.

Total Cholesterol

Serum Cholesterol in Advanced Age. High blood cholesterol values, like many other risk factors, are more common in older patients. By National Cholesterol Education Program criteria they occur in 32% of men and 52% of women aged 65–74 yr. Despite the high prevalence of hypercholesterolemia in the elderly and the lipid-induced coronary disease rates they engender, the expert panel was cautious about extending their recommendations beyond age 60. This caution is based on the lack of controlled trial data demonstrating the efficacy of cholesterol-lowering in older patients and on the fact that epidemiologic data indicate that cholesterol is less strongly predictive of coronary heart disease with increasing age.

With the aging of the Framingham Study cohort and the acquisition of additional data on the oldest age groups, it is now evident that blood cholesterol continues to predict coronary heart disease events although the strength of the relationship diminishes with age (Table 2.1). In the Framingham Study the relation of total cholesterol to coronary heart disease incidence after age 65 remains weaker after adjusting for HDL-cholesterol (Castelli *et al.* 1986). In advanced age, plaque ruptures and thrombosis may become more important features of clinical events. Selective survival may also be responsible for attenuating the cholesterol-coronary heart disease relationship in the elderly.

The declining impact of cholesterol on coronary heart disease incidence and mortality cannot be taken to mean that there is necessarily less to be gained by treating hypercholesterolemia in older persons. By treating 1,000 persons with serum cholesterol values above 285 mg/dL to reduce their cholesterol to 200 mg/dL at age 35–44, we might prevent 11.8 coronary heart disease events per year in men and 3.2 in women. At age 65–84 yr we would prevent 20.4 events in men and 11.4 in women. Thus, despite the diminishing strength of the cholesterol-coronary heart disease relationship with increasing age, the short-term preventive potential of cholesterol reduction appears to be at least as great after age 65 as before that age.

Most of the benefit of lowering cholesterol in younger people accrues from events in later life. Hence, cholesterol is more important at an early age if the goal is to reach advanced age free of coronary heart disease. However, the short-term risk is also important for the elderly who would like to live their remaining years free of disabling disease.

The possible benefits of reducing cholesterol in the elderly are based on observational rather than experimental data. Randomized cholesterol-lowering trials have, with the exception of the Los Angeles Veterans Domiciliary Trial (Dayton *et al.* 1969), been confined to middle-aged men. Any speculation about benefits for the elderly requires extrapolation from studies of middle-aged men. However, the attenuated cholesterol-coronary heart disease relationship in advanced age is not sufficient reason *per se* to neglect cholesterol in the elderly. Continuing treatment into advanced age would appear justified unless life expectancy or quality of life is so poor as to result in no useful gains.

Lipids, which are fundamental to the atherosclerotic process, continue to influence risk in the elderly, although the strength of the serum total cholesterol effect wanes with advancing age (Table 2.1). A potent predictive capacity of lipids is restored in the elderly when the serum total cholesterol is partitioned into its atherogenic LDL and protective HDL-cholesterol components (Kannel 1983) (Fig. 2.4).

Cholesterol-Lipoprotein Ratios

The proportion of the total blood cholesterol in the LDL and HDL fractions is an important consideration in determining the risk associated with high serum cholesterol values. A total serum cholesterol rise is accompanied by a predominant increase in the LDL component, with only a slight change in HDL and hence the total to HDL ratio deteriorates as the total serum cholesterol rises.

The total/HDL-cholesterol ratio is a practical and efficient predictor of coronary heart disease, particularly in the elderly. This ratio is an accurate predictor at both high and low cholesterol and LDL values (Kannel 1983; Castelli *et al.* 1977). The optimal total/HDL-cholesterol ratio is about 3.5 which corresponds to about half the high average American risk (Kannel 1983). The average risk corresponds to a ratio of 5, a ratio of 10 doubles the risk and ratio of 20 triples the risk. Both at high and low cholesterol values, HDL exerts a powerful influence on coronary heart disease susceptibility (Castelli *et al.* 1986).

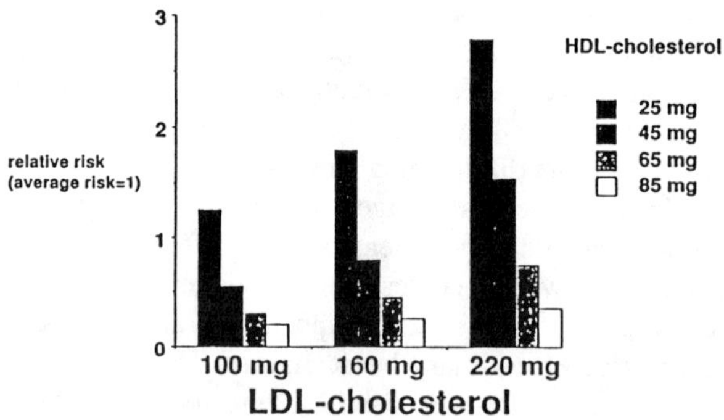

FIG. 2.4. RISK OF DEVELOPING CHD IN 4 YR
BY HDL AND LDL CHOLESTEROL
(FRAMINGHAM MEN AGED 50–70)

TABLE 2.4
RATIO OF TOTAL SERUM CHOLESTEROL/HDL CHOLESTEROL
BY AGE AND SEX
(FRAMINGHAM STUDY)

	Men		Women	
Age	Mean	S.D.	Mean	S.D.
15–24	3.9	1.1	3.4	0.9
25–34	4.6	1.7	3.4	1.1
35–44	5.1	1.7	3.6	1.2
45–54	5.2	1.6	4.0	1.5
55–64	5.1	1.8	4.5	1.5
65–74	5.1	1.7	4.6	1.5
75–79	4.8	1.6	4.7	1.4

The total to HDL-cholesterol ratio which is highly predictive of coronary heart disease in the elderly, rises with age in women up to age 80 yr, indicating an increasing lipid-derived vulnerability to coronary heart disease. In men this atherogenic lipid ratio plateaus at age 54, but remains higher in men than in women (Table 2.4).

Thus, all of the atherogenic lipids rise with age in men up to age 60, but in general they rise no further, and even decline some in advanced age (Castelli *et al.* 1977). In women the lipid increase with age is steeper and more prolonged, so that in advanced age they exceed those in men. However, even in women no further increase occurs in old age. But in both sexes atherogenic serum lipids are substantially higher later in life than in youth. This is not necessarily an intrinsic biologic consequence of aging *per se*.

In comparing the LDL/HDL ratio with the total/HDL ratio, both appear to predict coronary heart disease risk equally well because there is a fairly high correlation between LDL and total cholesterol. This is fortunate because this ratio is much easier to obtain than that using LDL. Women have a relative immunity to coronary heart disease compared to men, but lose that advantage when their total to HDL-cholesterol reaches 7.5 (Fig. 2.5). Optimal management of the blood lipids requires not only improvement in the serum total cholesterol, but also in the total/HDL-cholesterol ratio and in the entire cardiovascular risk profile.

New recommendations issued by the National Cholesterol Education Program have indicated that total blood cholesterols below 200 mg/dL are desirable, 200–239 are borderline and 240 mg/dL or greater are to be regarded as high. By these criteria an estimated 58% of the adult population are abnormal. Those with borderline cholesterol values are recommended for treatment if they have two or more other risk factors.

The average serum total cholesterol of coronary heart disease cases in the Framingham Study was only 225 mg/dL in men and 248 mg/dL in women. For HDL-cholesterol ratios averages are 5.6 and 5.0 for men and women, respectively. At the 240 mg/dL total cholesterol recommended for treatment, coronary heart disease risk varies over a 2–3 fold range depending on the associated HDL-cholesterol. Thus,

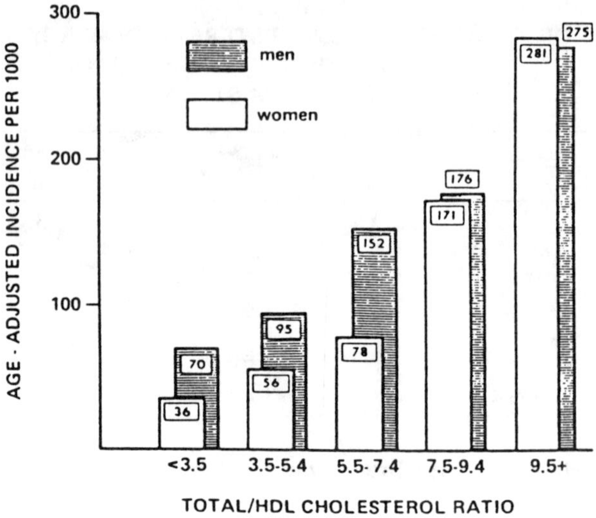

FIG. 2.5. RISK OF CORONARY HEART DISEASE BY TOTAL/HDL CHOLESTEROL AMONG MEN AND WOMEN 50–90 YR OLD (26-YR FOLLOW-UP, FRAMINGHAM STUDY)

persons at truly high risk because of elevated cholesterol can be identified by their HDL-cholesterol avoiding needlessly alarming or falsely reassuring large segments of the asymptomatic population.

Blood Lipid Trends

In contrast to some other cardiovascular risk factors, the serum total cholesterol and its atherogenic LDL fraction tend not to rise further with age beyond age 60 in men (Fig. 2.6). In women, however, the serum total cholesterol continues to rise to age 70 yr; and, in contrast to the situation at younger ages, cholesterol values in the aged are higher in women than men. A similar pattern of age trends occurs for LDL-cholesterol (Fig. 2.7). Elderly women in the 70's and 80's have LDL-cholesterol values 16–17 mg/dL higher than that in men of advanced age. In contrast to the foregoing, triglycerides in men tend to *decline* slightly after age 50, and women have *lower* values than men up to about age 60, after which they are higher (Castelli *et al.* 1977).

The proportion of the serum total cholesterol as HDL-cholesterol falls preciptiously after birth and is substantially lower in persons who have sustained coronary events. Mean levels of protective HDL-cholesterol do not decline in men as they go through the geriatric age range (Fig. 2.7). They do, however, decline in women, but even in elderly women HDL-cholesterol averages 10 mg/dL higher than in men. Also,

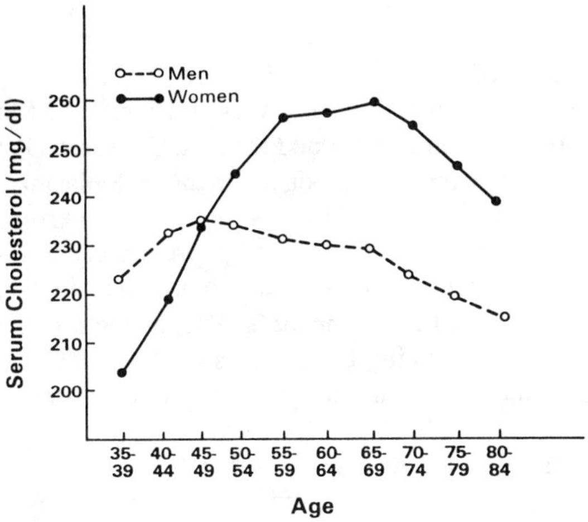

FIG. 2.6. MEAN SERUM CHOLESTEROL AGE TRENDS
IN EACH SEX
(26-YR FOLLOW-UP, FRAMINGHAM STUDY)

for reasons that are not clear, HDL-cholesterol values in blacks are uniformly higher than those in whites, even in old age (Castelli *et al.* 1977).

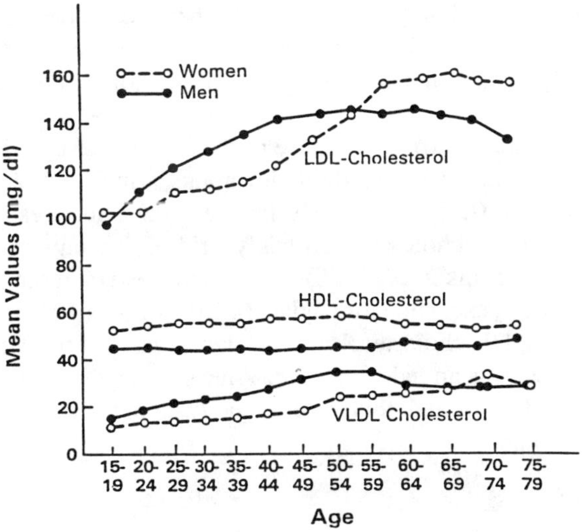

FIG. 2.7. AGE TRENDS
IN LIPOPROTEIN-CHOLESTEROL FRACTIONS
(FRAMINGHAM STUDY)

Triglyceride

Despite three decades of research, the relevance of plasma triglyceride as a coronary heart disease risk factor remains controversial (Kannel and McGee 1986; Hulley *et al.* 1980; National Heart, Lung and Blood Institute Consensus Panel 1985; Wallace and Anderson 1987). Triglyceride is produced in the endoplasmic reticulum of liver cells and cells of the small intestine (Havel *et al.* 1980; Jackson *et al.* 1977). This triglyceride is assembled into triglyceride-rich lipoprotein in association with specific apoproteins. These lipoproteins are degraded into remnants in the peripheral tissues by lipoprotein lipases. The VLDL remnant is IDL, a fraction of which is taken up by the liver, the remainder forming LDL (Jackson *et al.* 1977). In this process the core triglyceride is removed leaving a cholesterol-rich particle and only apolipoprotein B present.

Case-control studies have indicated an association between triglyceride and development of coronary heart disease (Albrink and Man 1959; Antonis and Bershon 1960; Carlson 1960; Gustafson 1972; Patterson and Slack 1972; Goldstein *et al.* 1973; Thind and Sandhu 1981; Lewis *et al.* 1974; Brunner *et al.* 1977). Also angiographic studies have shown an association of the extent of coronary artery disease and triglyceride (Barboriak *et al.* 1974; Cohn *et al.* 1976; Berenson *et al.* 1975; Gotto *et al.* 1977, Wieland *et al.* 1980; Holmes *et al.* 1980). A univariate relationship of triglyceride with development of coronary heart disease is seen less consistently in prospective studies (Kannel and McGee 1986; Brown *et al.* 1965; Bottiger and Carlson 1980; Criqui *et al.* 1987; Cambien *et al.* 1986). Also, they have been equivocal regarding triglyceride as an independent predictor of coronary heart disease controlling for LDL and HDL-cholesterol and other risk factors. Findings from recent ecological study based on international data are consistent with the epidemiologic appraisal that triglyceride is not an independent risk factor for coronary heart disease (Simons 1986).

Study of triglyceride is difficult because of the larger interindividual variation of the measurement resulting in standard deviations which are 2–3 times that of cholesterol distributions (U.S. Dept. of Health and Human Services 1980). The strong inverse relation of HDL-cholesterol to triglyceride is an important consideration (Davis *et al.* 1980; Albrink *et al.* 1980). Cholesterol esters in the core of HDL are transferred to VLDL in exchange for triglyceride (Eisenberg 1974). Thus, the strong inverse relation to HDL-cholesterol and the large variability of triglyceride may preclude its emergence as an independent risk factor. Triglyceride occurs under different clinical conditions and this heterogeneity could explain the variation in epidemiologic findings.

Dietary Influences on Blood Lipids

Although inborn errors of lipid metabolism are not uncommon, international comparisons, migrant studies, secular trends and experimental investigations indicate that there are powerful environmental influences on serum total cholesterol. Among these environmental factors none have been shown to influence the serum total cholesterol and its LDL atherogenic component more than the nutrient composition of the diet. The serum total cholesterol and LDL-cholesterol are raised by excess calories, saturated fat, dietary cholesterol and possibly by animal protein (Intersociety Commission for Heart Disease Resources 1984). They can be reduced by weight reduction, PUFA substitution, dietary fiber and possibly vegetable protein (Intersociety Commission for Heart Disease Resources 1984; Gustafson *et al.* 1972). Data on the influence of the nutrients on lipids in the elderly are, however, sparse.

There is good evidence that diets low in saturated fat and cholesterol are antiatherogenic permitting the serum lipids to return to normal and causing lesions to involute. Experimental evidence in animals, including nonhuman primates, indicates that diet-induced reduction in serum cholesterol directly leads to stabilization or reversal of either natural or induced lesions (Intersociety Commission for Heart Disease Resources 1984; Grundy *et al.* 1982).

Coronary heart disease mortality rates vary internationally in correspondence with differences in average serum total cholesterol levels (Intersociety Commission for Heart Disease Resources 1984; Keys *et al.* 1958). The average serum total cholesterol value within a population tends to correlate with the intake of saturated fat and cholesterol (Intersociety Commission for Heart Disease Resources 1984; Keys *et al.* 1958). These international epidemiologic data further support the inference that there is a strong relationship between dietary fat intake, dietary cholesterol and coronary heart disease rates among populations.

The dietary factors that influence the serum total cholesterol similarly raise and lower the atherogenic LDL-cholesterol component. The influence of diet on protective HDL-cholesterol and on the LDL/HDL-cholesterol ratio is currently under intensive investigation. Recommendations for reducing LDL or total serum cholesterol include weight reduction and exercise (which raises HDL) and restriction of saturated fat and cholesterol, which do not adversely affect the LDL/HDL-cholesterol ratio (Intersociety Commission for Heart Disease Resources 1984; Grundy *et al.* 1982). Metabolic studies in humans have clearly and consistently established the effect of dietary saturated fat, PUFA's and cholesterol on the serum total cholesterol under controlled isocaloric conditions (Intersociety Commission for Heart Disease Resources 1984; Grundy *et al.* 1982). Predictable reductions in serum total cholesterol are achieved by decreasing the percentage of calories obtained from saturated fat, increasing the proportion from PUFA's and decreasing the amount of dietary cholesterol (Intersociety Commission for Heart Disease Resources 1984).

Dietary Saturated Fatty Acids and Blood Cholesterol

Not all saturated fatty acids have the same potential to raise blood cholesterol. Diets high in stearic acid, for example, do not elevate plasma LDL-cholesterol in contrast to a diet high in palmitic acid (Rosenberg and Schaefer 1988; Bonanome and Grundy 1988). However, experiments to date have been confined to liquid formula diets, and its is not demonstrated that the finding applies to nonformula diets. An advantage of diets high in oleic or stearic acid over those rich in linoleic acid (e.g., corn oil) is that they do not appear to reduce HDL.

Saturated fatty acids such as palmitic acid down-regulate receptor-mediated clearance of LDL-cholesterol. Whereas monounsaturated fatty acids such as oleic acid (to which stearic acid is converted), PUFA's and high-carbohydrate diets do not have this effect. The data on acceptability of stearic acid do not mean that it is permissible to consume food such as beef fat and cocoa butter rich in stearic acid, as these foods are also high in palmitic acid.

Recommendations to reduce total fat in our diets continues to be sound. This reduces calorie intake, cholesterol intake and saturated fat intake. Data specific to the elderly on the effects of dietary manipulations are sparse, but there is no reason to believe that they react differently. There is also no reason to believe that the elderly are less willing to alter their diet than the young in response to medical advice.

Fish Oils

Western Greenland Eskimos have been noted to have a very low cardiovascular morbidity and mortality rate despite a high total fat intake (Glomset 1985). These Eskimos were found to have low LDL and triglyceride values and an increased HDL. However, these lipid changes and the P/S ratio of their diet were deemed insufficient to account for the extremely low coronary heart disease rate. The benefit appears to derive from the high ratio of omega-3 and omega-6 fatty acids and less linoleic acid, features which retard thrombogenesis (Glomset 1985). Supporting this hypothesis, Greenland Eskimos have been found to have a bleeding tendency. Eicosapentanoic acid competes with arachidonic acid for cyclooxygenase, inhibiting platelet aggregation (Glomset 1985).

Antithrombogenic influences may be especially important in the elderly in whom prevention of thrombotic occlusion of advanced lesions may be a more realistic objective than attempts to regress or retard fibrocalcific atherosclerotic disease. Fish consumption could also favorably influence atherosclerosis by improving the plasma lipids, by inhibiting platelet aggregation, or by producing beneficial effects on the endothelium and smooth muscle cells (Glomset 1985). Trials of diets rich in fish, fish oil and omega-3 fatty acid concentrates in normal volunteers indicate that they favorably alter lipoproteins, fatty acids. prostaglandins, platelet function and blood pressure (Glomset 1985; Fehily *et al.* 1985; Lorenz *et al.* 1983). VLDL and triglycerides are consistently reduced (Fehily *et al.* 1985; Lorenz *et al.* 1983), but effects on total cholesterol and HDL have been inconsistent. However, the majority of studies show an improvement in the ratio of total/HDL-cholesterol after a fish product enriched diet. Decreased blood pressure responses to norepinephrine and angiotensin have been reported. Perhaps as a result of all these effects, recent reports have noted a significant inverse relation between fish consumption and coronary heart disease mortality (Kromhout *et al.* 1985; Norell *et al.* 1976; Shekelle *et al.* 1985).

Fiber

Countries consuming high fiber diets have low coronary heart disease mortality rates. Fiber (other than cellulose and wheat bran) reduces serum cholesterol and has been shown to inhibit experimental atherosclerosis (Anderson and Tietyen-Clark 1986). Dietary fiber appears to improve each of the atherogenic risk factors including blood lipids. Whereas the American Heart Association diet has been shown to lower the serum total cholesterol only 3–7%, diets rich in soluble fiber have been found to reduce cholesterol by more than 20% and sustain this lowering for 2 yr; even in hypercholesterolemic men (Anderson and Tietyen-Clark 1986). LDL-cholesterol values are sustained at 25% lower values and HDL-cholesterol is raised more than 10%, producing a more favorable lipid profile.

High fiber diets generous in complex carbohydrate and limited in fat, lower triglycerides. Although the specific role of dietary fiber in triglyceride metabolism is not established, fiber intake, along with avoidance of alcohol, weight reduction and restricted fat intake appears beneficial. Dietary fiber is another nutrient factor which affects blood pressure.

Coronary heart disease prevalence and mortality rates also appear to be related to dietary fiber intake. Several epidemiologic studies have shown an inverse relationship between dietary fiber intake and the incidence of coronary heart disease (Kromhout *et al.* 1982; Kushi *et al.* 1986; Anderson and Tietyen-Clark 1986). The apparent protective effect of fiber may not only operate by reducing blood pressure, but by other mechanisms as well (Anderson and Tietyen-Clark 1986). However, no definitive clinical trials or intervention studies are available to document the apparent protective effect against coronary heart disease.

Beverages and Coronary Disease

Coffee, tea and alcohol are consumed in abundance both in the general population and by the elderly. Consumption of coffee has been suspected of contributing to coronary heart disease, but strong independent effects of coffee drinking have not been consistently documented in well-designed prospective studies (Intersociety Commission for Heart Disease Resources 1984), despite recent claims to the contrary (LaCroix *et al.* 1986). Paul was the first to suggest that generous intakes of coffee might be associated with excessive coronary attack rates (Paul *et al.* 1963). Accumulation of more data convinced these investigators that associated cigarette smoking was the culprit. The Framingham Study concluded that coffee consumption was not a significant independent risk factor, although victims of coronary attacks tended to drink more coffee (Intersociety Commission for Heart Disease Resources 1984). The Kaiser-Permanente Study recently found that hospitalizations for coronary heart disease were independently but weakly related to coffee intake (Klatsky *et al.* 1986). Investigators in Paris found coffee intake weakly related to systolic blood pressure (Lang *et al.* 1983). On reviewing the literature, it is concluded that coffee consumption is of no clinical importance in cholesterol metabolism despite some claims to the contrary. Coffee drinking is often associated with atherogenic food habits, smoking and low levels of physical activity, and these seem more fundamental risk factors. There would appear to be little reason to prohibit moderate (less than 5 cups) coffee intake for the purpose of avoiding coronary heart disease.

The role of alcohol in cardiovascular disease is complex. Depending on the amount consumed, it may be beneficial or harmful and while protecting against some disease it promotes others. There appears to be a beneficial effect, at moderate intakes, for coronary heart disease, and as a result, for cardiovascular disease in general. On the other hand, there are adverse effects on stroke, cancer, accidents and violence.

Hospital data suggest a protective effect of alcohol for coronary heart disease, but indicate an excessive occurrence of hypertension, stroke, cardiomyopathy and cardiac failure in association with alcohol intake (Klatsky *et al.* 1981a, 1981b, 1986; Hennekins *et al.* 1978; Colditz *et al.* 1985). Prospective studies have generally, but not without exception, shown an inverse relationship. A review of most of the major prospective epidemiologic studies, including the Framingham Study, the Hawaii Heart Study and the Kaiser-Permanente Study, have indicated a protective effect (Klatsky *et al.* 1981a; Paul *et al.* 1963; Gordon and Kannel 1983). There is, however, some diversity as to the coronary heart disease endpoint affected. Data on alcoholics and problem drinkers show a consistent and substantial *adverse* effect on coronary heart disease mortality. Framingham Study data on moderate intakes indicate a protective effect of all forms of alcoholic beverages against coronary heart disease, especially in nonsmokers (Gordon and Kannell 1983). Data on quitting alcohol have generally shown ex-drinkers to be at very high risk of mortality. This is generally attributed to poor health as the reason for quitting.

The pathogenetic mechanism whereby alcohol protects against coronary heart disease is uncertain. Alcohol alters the blood lipid composition raising triglyceride and its VLDL carrier at both moderate and high intakes. It tends, however, to lower the more atherogenic cholesterol-rich lipoproteins and raises HDL-cholesterol values producing a more favorable lipid profile. Social drinkers have HDL-cholesterol values 33% higher than abstainers. This may be irrelevant if, as some claim, it is only the HDL-3 subfraction which is raised. However, some claim that the antiatherogenic HDL-2 fraction is also raised and in any event, APO-A and A-2 lipoproteins are higher in those consuming alcohol.

Any beneficial effect of alcohol on coronary heart disease incidence occurs despite an adverse effect on blood pressure. The protective effect of alcohol seems to be independent of all associated risk factors for coronary heart disease, with the possible exception of HDL.

Heavy alcohol consumption is associated with a number of cardiovascular effects which enhance risk of stroke. These include: arrhythmias, impaired ventricular function, increased blood pressure and coagulation and platelet disorders. Prospective epidemiologic studies have generally linked alcohol intake to occurrence of stroke. However, they are inconsistent as to whether this is confined to hemorrhagic stroke and whether largely mediated through effects of alcohol on blood pressure.

There is evidence of a direct toxic effect of alcohol or its metabolites on the myocardium which can induce cardiomyopathy, rhythm disturbances and cardiac failure (Klatsky *et al.* 1981a). There is little evidence to connect alcohol with aortic or peripheral arterial disease. A more precise determination is needed regarding the amounts of alcohol that are beneficial or harmful, and more data are needed on the cardiovascular effects of alcohol in women. However, in moderation alcohol appears to be harmless and may be beneficial against coronary heart disease despite possible adverse effects on blood pressure, triglyceride and rhythm. In excess it may increase coronary heart disease mortality, raise blood pressure, cause arrhythmia, promote thrombogenesis and damage the myocardium. Since these effects are more likely to occur in the presence of already existent cardiovascular disease, alcohol abuse can be dangerous in the elderly. It may promote hemorrhagic strokes to which the elderly are more prone.

The data available do not allow firm conclusions about protective effects of alcohol in the elderly. They do not indicate a need to restrict alcohol if intakes are truly moderate unless there is hypertension, hypertriglyceridemia, cardiac dysrhythmia or impaired ventricular function. Unfortunately, these conditions are quite common in the elderly so it is not often possible to recommend alcohol for elderly persons who want to avoid coronary disease.

Some living habits predispose to atherosclerotic cardiovascular disease in the elderly as well as the young. Physical inactivity predisposes to coronary heart disease as much in elderly men as in the young (Kannel *et al.* 1985). Alcohol and coffee in moderation do not appear to promote coronary heart disease. Cigarette smoking appears to have a diminished impact on coronary heart disease events beyond age 65, but continues to predispose to peripheral arterial disease. Unfortunately, evidence that quitting smoking after age 65 reduces risk as it does prior to that age is lacking (Kannel *et al.* 1986; Kannel and Gordon 1978). ECG abnormalities continue to identify persons beyond age 65 with a compromised coronary circulation at high risk of atherosclerotic cardiovascular events (Kannel *et al.* 1986; Kannel and Gordon 1978; Kannel and Brand 1984).

Cardiovascular risk profiles incorporating the standard risk factors can predict atherosclerotic cardiovascular events in the elderly, defining risk over a wide range. These profiles can identify susceptibles at high risk because of multiple marginal abnormalities who might be overlooked (Kannel *et al.* 1986; Kannel and Gordon 1978). Despite a lesser impact of some risk factors in advanced age, these risk factor profiles are just as efficient in predicting cardiovascular events in the elderly as in younger persons (Table 2.5). Profiles which include the lipoprotein-cholesterol fractions, vital capacity and heart rate are likely to be even more efficient. This suggests that a multivariate risk reduction program may have a substantial impact in the elderly.

The increased incidence of atherosclerotic cardiovascular disease in advanced age probably reflects both altered tissue response to risk factors and the time-dose product of noxious environmental influences. This is not inevitable and occurs in

TABLE 2.5
PERCENTAGE OF CARDIOVASCULAR EVENTS IN UPPER DECLINE OF MUTIVARIATE RISK[1]
(16 YEAR FOLLOW-UP, FRAMINGHAM STUDY)

Age	Coronary Disease		Brain Infarction		Peripheral Vascular Disease	
	Men	Women	Men	Women	Men	Women
45–54	26	20	55	44	30	60
55–64	27	26	52	43	47	43
65–74	21	41	57	46	27	50

[1]Based on systolic blood pressure, serum cholesterol, number of cigarettes, glucose tolerance, ECG-LVH.

relation to modifiable risk factors including faulty nutrition. Despite a paucity of controlled trial data specific to the elderly, optimism about the efficacy of controlling risk factors seems justified. The dramatic decline in cardiovascular mortality which has occurred in the United States has included the elderly (Thom *et al.* 1985).

CLINICAL TRIALS

Controlled trials are now providing concrete evidence connecting nutrients to serum lipids and ultimately to coronary heart disease incidence. Three recently complete controlled trials have shown that reduction of serum cholesterol by diet and lipid-lowering drugs can reduce coronary heart disease morbidity and mortality (Hjermann *et al.* 1981; Lipid Research Clinics 1981; Frick *et al.* 1987). The Lipid Research Clinic's Coronary Primary Prevention Trial convincingly showed the efficacy of reducing elevated serum total cholesterol by drug and diet therapy in middle-aged men (Lipid Research Clinics 1981). A 19% reduction in coronary attacks and a 24% reduction in mortality from coronary heart disease was achieved by a fat-modified diet and cholestyramine (Fig. 2.8). Improvement in risk with the combined therapy over diet alone was correlated with the degree of reduction in serum cholesterol achieved. The Helsinki Study has recently shown the efficacy of lowering triglyceride and raising HDL-cholesterol with gemfibrozil (Frick *et al.* 1987) (Fig. 2.9).

The Oslo Study demonstrated the efficacy of dietary modification, without concommitant drug therapy, in reducing coronary heart disease events in hypercholesterolemic, but normotensive persons (Hjermann *et al.* 1981). Reduced intake of saturated fat and cholesterol were undertaken with 60% of the benefit demonstrated against coronary heart disease attributed to a 13% reduction in serum cholesterol achieved. Coronary heart disease morbidity and mortality were reduced an impressive 47% (Fig. 2.10).

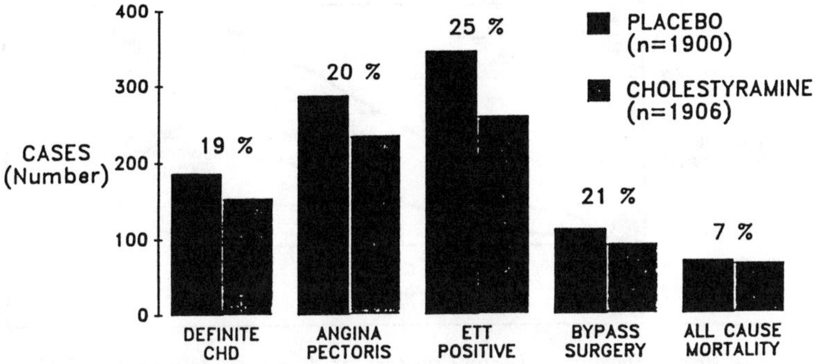

FIG. 2.8. RESULTS FROM THE LIPID RESEARCH CLINIC'S CORONARY PRIMARY PREVENTION TRIAL (CPPT)

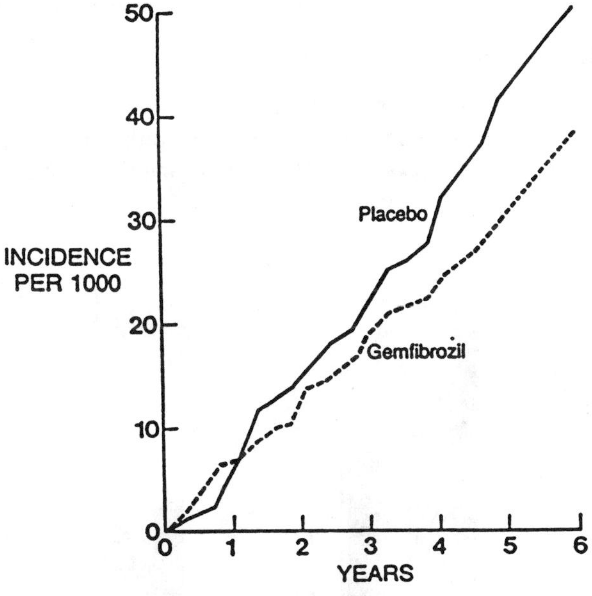

		0	1	2	3	4	5	6
Gemfibrozil	N =	2051	14	13	12	10	6	1☆
Placebo	N =	2030	13	15	16	19	18	3☆

From Frick et al. (1987)
Courtesy of the New England Journal of Medicine

FIG. 2.9. KAPLAN-MEIER CUMULATIVE INCIDENCE (PER 1000) AND ANNUAL NUMBER OF CARDIAC END POINTS, ACCORDING TO TREATMENT GROUP AND TIME

Data for the sixth year (stars) were derived from 305 persons-years of observation for gemfibrozil and from 316 person-years observation for placebo.

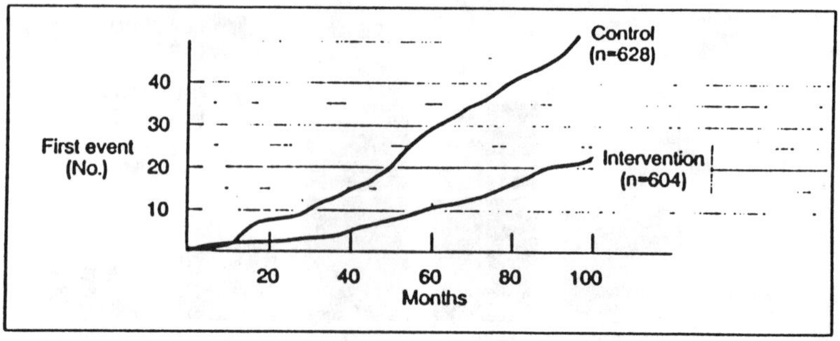

From Hjermann (1986) Courtesy of American Journal of Medicine

FIG. 2.10. OSLO STUDY DIET AND ANTISMOKING TRIAL

Cumulative incidence of coronary events (i.e., fatal and nonfatal myocardial infarction and sudden death) at the 102-month follow-up shows the same trend as at 60 months. Three participants were lost to follow-up but were alive.

Lipid Modification and Atherosclerotic Plaques

Intervention studies have shown that rates of coronary heart disease events can be reduced by lowering blood cholesterol. Five investigations designed to lower LDL-cholesterol have also shown associations between changes in serum total cholesterol,

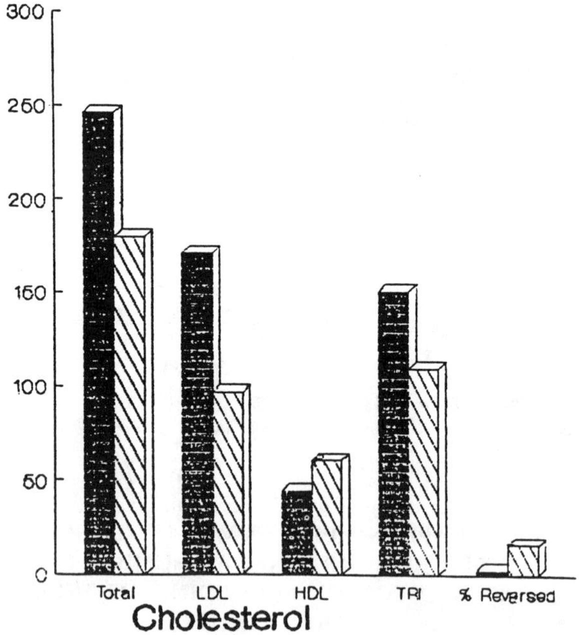

From Blankenhorn et al. (1987)
© 1987, American Medical Association

FIG. 2.11. COLESTIPOL-NIACIN THERAPY: REDUCING CORONARY ATHEROSCLEROSIS ratio of total/HDL-cholesterol and HDL-cholesterol itself and atherosclerotic lesion growth as assessed by repeated angiography (Berenson *et al.* 1985; Cohn *et al.* 1976; Gotto *et al.* 1977; Wieland *et al.* 1980; Holmes *et al.* 1981). Although regression was uncommon, failure to progress was a frequent beneficial finding, providing encouragement that dietary or drug treatments to lower lipids can actually slow the progression of lesions (Fig. 2.11).

It is not reasonable to expect that treatment begun in advanced age, when fibrocalcific lesions abound, will cause significant regression. However, it is distinctly possible that progression can be slowed so that occurrence of critical narrowing of the lumen, enough to interfere with flow and cause symptoms, can be significantly delayed. Also, since many myocardial infarctions are produced by thrombus formation on advanced lesions, it is reasonable to expect that diets rich in fish may be beneficial by providing omega-3 fatty acids which can retard thrombogenesis.

Nutritional Adequacy and Safety

Antiatherogenic, fat-modified diets are adequate in protein, minerals, vitamins and need not be deficient in any nutrient. The level of fat intake proposed is higher than the 10–15% of calories eaten by the Japanese whose life expectancy exceeds that of United States citizens. Italians who eat less saturated fat and cholesterol than North Americans are also long-lived. Since there is no evidence that such diets are deleterious to growing children and adolescents, they should not be harmful to the elderly whose nutrient needs are unlikely to exceed those of active children.

Low serum cholesterol values have been found to be associated with cancer. Data from 325,348 MRFIT screenees allows a precise evaluation of the relation of concentrations of total cholesterol in serum to causes of mortality (Stamler *et al.* 1986; Kannell *et al.* 1986). In contrast to mortality from coronary heart disease, overall mortality shows a quadratic relationship to total cholesterol in serum. Despite a progressive rise in mortality in relation to the serum cholesterol value, all-cause mortality appears to occur in excess at cholesterol values below 160 mg/dL. This increased overall mortality at the lowest concentrations of serum cholesterol has also been noted elsewhere (Kark *et al.* 1986; Peterson and Trell 1983).

The increased mortality at low cholesterol values has been found to be related to colon cancer in particular. This is paradoxical because high fat intake, likely to increase cholesterol in serum, has been related to the occurrence of colon cancer (Andres 1981; Hubert *et al.* 1983; Bjorntorp 1985; Kannell *et al.* 1985; Thom *et al.* 1985). Analysis of the time course of the cholesterol-cancer relationship suggests a cholesterol-lowering effect of subclinical cancer (Sorlie and Feinleib 1982; Rose and Shipley 1980). Data from the International Collaborative Group on 81,567 men support this contention (International Collaborative Group 1982). This inference has been recently strengthened by data from a long-term Swedish cohort study, which demonstrated a *direct* relationship between colorectal cancer and the concentration of cholesterol in serum on long-term follow-up (Thornberg 1986). Furthermore, serum cholesterol has been recently shown to be positively related to colorectal adenoma, a possible precursor of cancer (Mannes *et al.* 1986).

Preventive Implications

Among the various factors contributing to occurrence of cardiovascular disease in the elderly, the dominant remediable predisposing influences include hypertension, dyslipidemia, and impaired glucose tolerance. These risk factors are prevalent in the elderly and can be favorably influenced by dietary changes, weight control and exercise.

An optimal preventive approach to cardiovascular disease in the elderly requires a strategy that includes public health measures to alter the ecology, personal hygiene to avoid or correct risk factors, and preventive measures to correct them in high risk persons. If cardiovascular disease is to be minimized, it will be necessary to change the national diet, engineer physical activity back into daily living, and eliminate the cigarette. Community control of predisposing risk factors for cardiovascular disease requires not only that high risk persons be identified and treated but also that population-oriented measures be implemented to shift the entire distribution of the various risk factors to lower, less atherogenic average levels.

The decline in cardiovascular mortality, which has accelerated since 1968 in the United States, indicates that these major killers of the elderly are controllable since the aged have shared in the reduced mortality (Fig. 2.12). Although there is evidence from this declining mortality in advanced age that preventive measures implemented beyond age 65 may be effective, the earlier in life such measures are undertaken, the more beneficial they are likely to be. Some countries that have not emphasized risk factor control to the extent accomplished in the United States, Australia, Canada and New Zealand have not shared in the decline in cardiovascular mortality; some with equally sophisticated medical care even have rising death rates (Thom *et al.* 1985).

Ideally, preventive measures should be continued from early in life to reduce the burden of atherosclerotic cardiovascular disease in advanced age. However, measures instituted in advanced age should not be considered without value. The incidence of cardiovascular disease in the elderly is not uniform and varies widely in relation to modifiable risk factors, many of which respond to nutritional alterations. Because cardiovascular disease incidence rates are so high in the elderly, preventive measures could have a substantial impact in the old. The secular trends in cardiovascular mortality which have included the elderly are correlated with corresponding changes in known risk factors for cardiovascular disease in both young and old. Comprehensive risk factor modification seems a reasonable option in the elderly as well as the young.

Most cardiovascular disease risk factors that are highly prevalent in the elderly are subject to modification by dietary measures. Dietary change and weight control along with treatment of hypertension and avoidance of cigarettes, can favorably influence the cardiovascular risk profile of the elderly. Although randomized controlled trials to test the efficacy of modification of risk factors in the elderly are lacking, optimism is justified. Serum total and atherogenic LDL-cholesterol can be reduced by acceptable dietary changes. Recently complete controlled trials in middle-aged

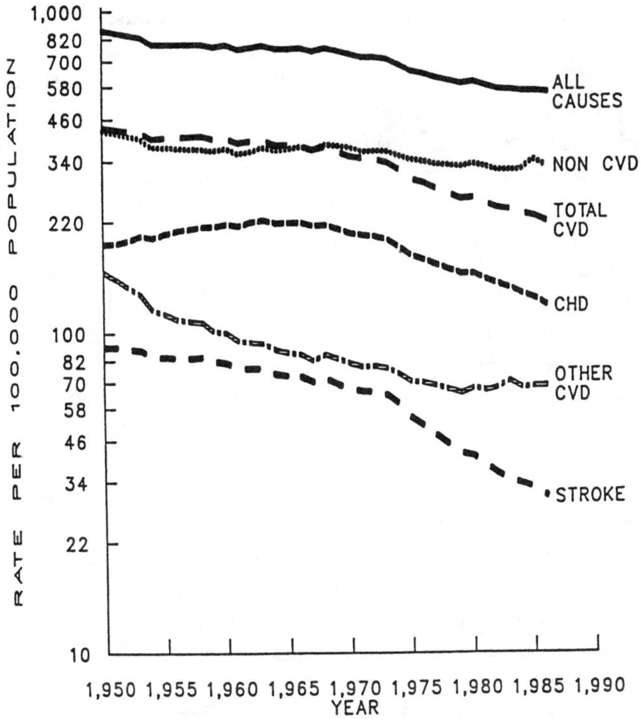

FIG. 2.12. AGE-ADJUSTED DEATH RATES FOR SELECTED CAUSES OF DEATH (UNITED STATES 1950–1986)

populations have convincingly shown that reducing elevated serum cholesterol by diet or drugs can lower coronary morbidity and mortality (Kannel 1986) and the fat-modified diets required to achieve more favorable lipid values are safe, convenient, palatable and nutritionally adequate.

Although there is no great enthusiasm for them, nondrug therapies can reduce blood pressure in mild to moderate hypertension (Kaplan 1985). When weight is reduced, blood pressure usually falls proportionally. Reduction in sodium intake has been shown to control some hypertension, so there is no harm in encouraging all hypertensive persons to reduce the excessively high intakes habitually consumed. This may be a problem in the elderly who suffer a decrease in perception of taste and smell. Although the response is variable, recent carefully controlled trials have shown significant reduction in blood pressure on 60–100 mg daily sodium intakes (Kaplan 1985). Sodium restriction can reduce dependence on antihypertensive drugs.

There is generally a greater response of the elderly to sodium restriction particularly in those with higher pressures and in those who exhibit less rise in renin-angiotensin when salt is restricted. The addition of potassium is reported to reduce the hypertensive effect of a high sodium intake and also its hypertensive sequelae (Castelli *et al.* 1980). Hence, increased intake of high potassium foods, along with avoidance of high sodium intake would seem sensible for the hypertensive elderly. In attempting to reduce dietary sodium, fat and cholesterol in the elderly, care should be taken not to drastically restrict calcium-containing foods. Hypo-magnesemia is also regularly induced by diuretics and should be avoided or corrected. Since some controlled studies suggest that decreased fat intake coupled with increased PUFA's will lower blood pressure, there is reason to modify fat intake and increase linoleic acid and fish oil intake to achieve an antihypertensive effect.

Vegetarian diets are helpful because they tend to lower blood pressure by increasing potassium, fiber, calcium, magnesium and P/S ratios. A recent randomized crossover trial showed a 5 mmHg fall in systolic blood pressure during vegetarian diet periods in untreated mild hypertensives (Margetts *et al.* 1986). Eating less, in general, may be helpful because a 40% reduction in calorie intake was found to increase the life span of spontaneously hypertensive rats (Lloyd 1984). Regular exercise seems to lower blood pressure (Boyer and Kasch 1970).

The aforementioned dietary and other measures are meritorious for the atherosclerosis-prone, elderly, hypertensive person since they favorably influence blood lipids and diabetic control and counter diuretic metabolic side effects. These measures are reasonable in elderly hypertensives as an adjunct to drug therapy and in the mild hypertensive should be considered as a possible alternative to drugs. A sensible non-drug regimen for the hypertensive elderly should include: weight control, sodium restriction to 2 g, maintenance of calcium intake, more fiber and less saturated fat, more fish, avoidance of alcohol in excess (no more than 2 drinks per day) and supplemental magnesium for those on diuretics.

Since obesity aggravates all the atherogenic traits in both young and old, weight control is an important means for improving the atherogenic risk profile of the elderly. This would appear especially important for the elderly with central or abdominal obesity. Weight control is also an effective means for improving glucose tolerance in the late-onset diabetes of the elderly. We need a greater sense of urgency about moderate obesity lest it reach intractible proportions. Assurance of a fall in pressure, lipids and glucose without drugs may be used to motivate the obese to keep their weight down.

Nutrition should influence the rate of occurrence of cardiovascular disease in advanced age as it is one of the chief contributors to cardiovascular risk factors. However, once advanced age is reached, there is deficient knowledge on how much nutrition affects these risk factors, advanced fibrocalcific lesions, or the occurrence of clinical events. Clearly, more research is needed to support recommendations on optimal nutrition for avoiding cardiovascular disease in advanced age. However, the inclusion of the elderly in the recent decline in cardiovascular mortality in the United States suggests that even in advanced age nutritional factors may continue to influence cardiovascular mortality rates.

The dietary modifications needed are met by Oriental or Mediterranean eating patterns that are eminently palatable. To achieve the optimal dietary specifications, it is necessary to de-emphasize red meats, dairy products and baked goods. Fish and poultry are preferred over red meats. Whole grain, fruit, cereal, vegetable and legume intake should be increased and egg yolk, and sugar intake decreased. These required changes in diet can be achieved without a radical change in personal eating habits. The level of exercise and food intake should be adjusted to achieve and maintain a lean body weight. Dietary cholesterol intakes should not exceed 250 mg/day. An intake of less than 30% of calories from all fats is recommended to help achieve calorie control, reduce intake of saturated fat and cholesterol and to possibly reduce thrombogenesis. Less than 8% of calories from saturated fat is required if an optimal serum cholesterol is to be achieved. Polyunsaturated or monounsaturated fats may be used in moderation to replace part of the saturated fats. Regular weekly intake of fish (at least 30 g/day), especially fatty fish, may provide additional protection by inhibiting thrombogenesis. Increased vegetable food intake appears to also provide benefits in addition to those of calorie control and fat modification. These dietary principles meet the requirements for optimal nutrition for both older persons and other subgroups of the population.

There are a number of impediments to preventive programs for cardiovascular disease in the elderly, including nutritional measures. Foremost is the propriety of modifying lifestyles which have already been compatible with longevity. In the very old, a conservative, individualized approach is indicated. However, there is no justification for regarding cardiovascular disease in the elderly as inevitable. Nor is it acceptable to believe that their habits are too ingrained to be changed. The elderly are actually good consumers of health education, and they comply with medical advice as enthusiastically as younger adults. Hence, physicians should be encouraged to give nutrition advice to the elderly and aid them in improving their living habits in general.

Nutrition in the elderly is influenced by many factors including ignorance about a balanced nonatherogenic diet, poverty, social isolation, physical disability, mental deterioration, illness, immobility, depression, malabsorption, poor teeth, diminished taste and smell, alcoholism and various drugs taken for illnesses. Some subgroups need special attention including those living alone, the disabled and the enfeebled. It is important to dissuade patients and their families from regarding the infirmities of old age as an inevitable burden to be suffered.

SUMMARY

Cardiovascular disease in the elderly is a growing public health concern in most affluent parts of the world. As in the young, the major established cardiovascular risk factors also apply in the elderly, including hypertension, dyslipidemia, impaired glucose tolerance, physical indolence and cigarette smoking. Diet plays a major role by its influence on many of these atherogenic risk factors. As in the young, blood lipids, blood pressure and glucose tolerance can be improved by alterations in the nutrient and calorie content of the diet. However, direct evidence that dietary changes can reduce risk of cardiovascular disease in the elderly is lacking and assertions of efficacy require extrapolation from data collected on younger adults.

Most cardiovascular risk factors are highly prevalent in the elderly, but the rise in blood pressure, blood lipids and blood glucose with advancing age is not inevitable. Diet can contribute to hypertension through excessive intakes of calories, sodium and saturated fat coupled with deficiencies of potassium, magnesium, calcium and fish oils. Serum lipids tend to be normalized by diets low in saturated fat and cholesterol, and abundant in polyunsaturated fatty acids and fish. Emphasis on intakes of vegetable protein and fiber-rich food has merit because these foods also provide increased intakes of polyunsaturated fatty acids, magnesium, selenium, complex carbohydrate, potassium and copper, as well as reduce cholesterol, saturated fat and sodium intakes.

Fat-modified diets need not be unpalatable, deficient in any other nutrient or too costly. Ideally, such diets should be implemented early in life and continued into advanced age. The substantial decline in cardiovascular mortality in the United States, Canada and Australia has included elderly. This indicates that cardiovascular disease is controllable and not inevitable in the elderly and that nutrition may play a role.

ACKNOWLEDGMENTS

This work was supported by Charles A. Dana Foundation and Merck, Sharp and Dohme.

REFERENCES

ALBRINK, M. J. *et al.* 1980. Intercorrelations amongst HDL, obesity and triglycerides in a normal population. Lipids *14*, 668–676.

ALBRINK, M. J. and MAN, E. B. 1959. Serum triglycerides in coronary artery disease. Arch. Intern. Med. *103*, 4–8.

ALDERMAN, E. and COLTANT, D. 1982 Alcohol and the heart. Br. Med. Bull. *38*, 77.

ANDERSON, J. W. and TIETYEN-CLARK, J. 1986. Dietary fiber: Hyperlipidemia, hypertension and coronary heart disease. Am. J. Gastroenterology *81*, 907–919.

ANDRES, R. 1981. Influence of obesity on longevity in the aged. *In* Aging: A Challenge to Science and Society, D. Danon, N. W. Schode and N. Marois (eds.) Oxford University Press, Oxford.

ANTONIS, A. and BERSHON, I. 1960. Serum triglyceride levels in South African Europeans and Bantu in ischemic heart disease. Lancet *1*, 998–1002.

BARBORIAK, J. J. *et al.* 1974. Coronary artery occlusion and blood lipids. Am. Heart J. *87*, 716–721.

BELIZAN, J. M. *et al.* 1983. Reduction of blood pressure with calcium supplementation in young adults. JAMA *249*, 1161–1165.

BERENSON, G. S. *et al.* 1975. A Study of serum lipoproteins and angiographic evidence of coronary artery disease. South. Med. J. *68*, 1513–1519.

BJORNTORP, P. 1985. Regional patterns of fat distribution. Ann. Intern. Med. *103*, 994–995.

BLANKENHORN, D. H. *et al.* 1987. JAMA *257*, 3233.

BONANOME, A. and GRUNDY, S. M. 1988. Effect of dietary stearic acid on plasma cholesterol and lipoprotein levels. N. Engl. J. Med. *318*, 1248.

BORDIA, A. 1980. The effect of vitamin C on blood lipids, fibrinolytic and platelet adhesiveness in patients with coronary artery disease. Atherosclerosis *35*, 181–187.

BOTTIGER, L. E. and CARLSON, L. A. 1980. Risk factors for ischemic vascular death for men in Stockholm Prospective Study. Atherosclerosis *36*, 389–408.

BOYER, J. L. and KASCH, F. W. 1970. Exercise therapy in hypertensive men. JAMA *211*, 1668–1671.

BRODY, J. A., BROCK, D. B. 1985. Epidemiologic and statistical characteristics of the United States elderly population. *In* Handbook of the Biology of Aging, 2nd Edition. C. E. Finch and E. L Schneider (eds.). Van Nostrand Reinhold, New York.

BROWN, D. F., KINCH, S. H. and DOYLE, J. T. 1965. Serum triglycerides in health and in ischemic heart disease. N. Engl. J. Med. *273*, 947–952.

BRUNNER, D. *et al.* 1977. Serum cholesterol and triglyceride in patients suffering from ischemic heart disease and in healthy subjects. Atherosclerosis *28*, 197–204.

CAMBIEN, F. *et al.* 1986. Is the level of serum triglyceride a significant predictor of coronary death in "normocholesterolemic" subjects? Am. J. Epidemiol. *124*, 624–632.

CARLSON, L. A. 1960. Serum lipid in men with myocardial infarction. Acta Med. Scand. *167*, 399–414.

CASTELLI, W. P. *et al.* 1977. HDL-cholesterol and other lipids in CHD. The Cooperative Lipoprotein Phenotyping Study. Circulation. *55*, 767.

CASTELLI, W. P. *et al.* 1986. Incidence of coronary heart disease and lipoprotein cholesterol levels. JAMA *256*, 2835–2838.

COHN, P. E., GABBAY, S. I. and WEGLICKI, W. B. 1976. Serum lipid levels in angiographically defined coronary artery disease. Ann. Intern. Med. *84*, 241–245.

COLDITZ, G. A. *et al.* 1985. Moderate alcohol intake and decreased C-V mortality in an elderly cohort. Am. Heart J. *109*, 886–889.

CONNOR, W. E. *et al.* 1978. The plasma lipids, lipoproteins and the diet of Tarahmara Indians of Mexico. Am. J. Clin. Nutr. *31*, 1131.

CRIQUI, M. H. *et al.* 1987. Triglycerides and coronary heart disease mortality. The Lipid Research Clinics follow-up study. Presented at the American Heart Association 27th Conference of Cardiovascular Epidemiology. C V Dis. Epidemiology Newsletter *41*, 13.

DAVIS, C. E. *et al.* 1980. Correlations of plasma high density lipoprotein cholesterol levels with other plasma lipid and lipoprotein concentrations. Circulation *62* (Suppl IV), 24–30.

DAYTON, S. *et al.* 1969. A controlled clinical trial of a diet high in unsaturated fat in preventing complications of atherosclerosis. Circulation *40*, 1–63.

DYCKNER, T. and WESTER, P. O. 1983. Effect of magnesium of blood pressure. Br. Med. J. (Clin. Res.) *286*, 1847–1849.

EASTY, D. L. 1970. The relationship of diet to serum cholesterol levels in young men in Antarctica. Br. Nutr. *24*, 307.

EISENBERG, S. 1984. High density lipoprotein metabolism. J. Lipid Res. *25*, 1017–1058.

FEHILY, A. M., BURR, M. L., PHILLIPS, K. M. and DEADOM, N. M. 1985. The effect of fatty fish on plasma lipid and lipoprotein concentrations. Am. J. Clin. Nutr. *38*, 349–351.

FRICK, M. H. *et al.* 1987. Helsinki Heart Study: Primary prevention trial with gemfibrozil in middle-aged men with dyslipidemia: Safety of treatment, changes in risk factors and incidence of CHD. N. Engl. J. Med. *317*, 1237–1245.

GARRISON, R. J., KANNEL, W. B., STOKES, III, J. and CASTELLI, W. P. 1987. Incidence and precursors of hypertension in young adults: The Framingham Offspring Study. Prev. Med. *16*, 235–251.

GLOMSET, J. A. 1985. Fish, fatty acids and human health. N. Engl. J. Med. *312*, 1253–1254.

GOLDSTEIN, J. L. *et al.* 1973. Hyperlipidemia in coronary heart disease. I. Lipid levels in 500 survivors of myocardial infarction. J. Clin. Invest. *52*, 1533–1543.

GORDON, T. and KANNEL, W. B. 1983. Drinking habits and cardiovascular disease: The Framingham Study. Am. Heart J. *105*, 667–673.

GOTTO, A. M. *et al.* 1977. Relationship between plasma lipid concentrations and coronary artery disease in 496 patients. Circulation *56*, 875–883.

GRUNDY, S. M. *et al.* 1982. Rationale of the diet-heart statement of the American Heart Association. Report of Nutrition Committee. Circulation *65*, 839A.

GUSTAFSON, A. *et al.* 1972. Serum lipids and lipoproteins in men after myocardial infarction compared with representative population sample. Circulation *46*, 709–716.

HARRIS, T. B. *et al.* 1985. Blood pressure experience and risk of cardiovascular disease in the elderly. Hypertension *7*, 118–124.

HAVEL, R. J., GOLDSTEIN, J. L. and BROWN, M. S. 1980. Lipoproteins and lipid transport. *In* Metabolic Control and Disease, 8th Edition, P. K. Brandy and L. E. Rosenberg (eds.). W. B. Saunders Co. Philadelphia.

HENNEKENS, C. H., ROSNER, B. and COLE, D. S. 1978. Daily alcohol consumption and fatal CHD. Am. J. Epidemiol. *107*, 196–200.

HJERMANN, I. *et al.* 1981. Effect of diet and smoking intervention on the incidence of CHD. Lancet *2*, 1303.

HOLMES, D. R. *et al.* 1981. Association of risk factor variables and coronary artery disease documented by angiography. Circulation *63*, 293–299.

HUBERT, H. B., FEINLEIB, M., McNAMARE, P. M. and CASTELLI, W. P. 1983. Obesity as an independent risk factor for cardiovascular disease: A 26-year follow-up of participants in the Framingham Heart Study. Circulation *67*, 968–977.

HULLEY, S. B., ROSENMAN, R. H., BAWOL, R. D. and BRAND, R. J. 1980. Epidemiology as a guide to clinical decisions. The association between triglyceride and coronary heart disease. N. Engl. J. Med. *302*, 1383–1389.

International Collaborative Group. 1982. Circulating cholesterol level and risk of death from cancer in men and 40–69 years: Experience of an international collaborative group. JAMA *248*, 2853–2859.

Intersociety Commission for Heart Disease Resources. 1984. Optimal resources for primary prevention of atherosclerotic disease. Circulation *70*, 155A–205A.

JACKSON, R. L., MORRISETT, J. D. and GOTTO, A. M. JR. 1977. Lipoproteins and lipid transport. Structural and functional concepts. *In* Hyperlipidemia. Diagnosis and Treatment. B. M. Rifkind and R. I. Levy (eds.). Grune and Statton, New York.

JARRETT, R. J. 1986. Is there an ideal body weight? Br. Med. J. *293*, 493–495.

KANNEL, W. B. 1983. High-density lipoproteins: Epidemiologic profile and risks of coronary artery disease. Am. J. Cardiol. *52*, 9A–12A.

KANNEL, W. B. 1985a. Lipids, diabetes and coronary heart disease: Insights from the Framingham Study. Am. Heart J. *110*, 1100–1107.

KANNEL, W. B. 1985b. Hypertension and aging. *In* Biology of Aging 2nd Edition. C. E. Finch, E. L. Schneider (eds.). Van Nostrand Reinhold, New York.

KANNEL, W. B. 1986. Nutritional contributors to cardiovascular disease in the elderly. J. Am. Geriatric Soc. *34*, 27–36.

KANNEL, W. B. and BRAND, F. N. 1984. Cardiovascular risk factors in the elderly. *In* Principles of Geriatric Medicine. R. Andres, E. L. Birman and N. R. Hezzard (eds.). McGraw Hill, New York.

KANNEL, W. B., DAWBER, T. R. and McGEE, D. L. 1980. Perspectives on Systolic Hypertension: The Framingham Study. Circulation *61*, 1179–1182.

KANNEL, W. B., GORDON, T. 1978. Evaluation of cardiovascular disease in the elderly: The Framingham Study. Bull. N.Y. Acad. Med. *45*, 573.

KANNEL, W. B. and McGEE, D. L. 1986. Evaluation of cardiovascular risk. *In* Geriatric Anesthesia, C. A. Stephen and R. C. E. Assaf (eds.). Butterworth Publishers, Reading, MA.

KANNEL, W. B., WILSON, P. W. F. and BLAIR, S. N. 1985. Epidemiological assessment of the role of physical activity and fitness in development of cardiovascular disease. Am. Heart J. *109*, 876–884.

KANNEL, W. B. *et al.* 1986. Overall and coronary heart disease mortality rates in relation to major risk factors in 325,348 men screened for the MRFIT. Am. Heart J. *112*, 825–836.

KAPLAN, N. 1985. Non-drug treatment of hypertension. Ann. Intern. Med. *102*, 359–373.

KARK, J. D., SMITH, A. H. and HAMES, C. G. 1980. The relationship of serum cholesterol to the incidence of cancer in Evans County, Georgia. J. Chron. Dis. *33*, 311–322.

KEYS, A. *et al.* 1958. Lessons from serum cholesterol studies in Japan, Hawaii and Los Angeles. Ann. Intern. Med. *48*, 83.

KLATSKY, A. L., ARMSTRONG, M. A. and FRIEDMAN, G. D. 1986. Relations of alcohol beverages to subsequent CHD hospitalization. Am. J. Cardiol. *58*, 710.

KLATSKY, A. L., FRIEDMAN, G. D. and SIEGALAUB, A. B. 1981a. Alcohol and cardiovascular disease: The Kaiser-Permanente experience. Circulation *64* (Suppl. III), 32–41.

KLATSKY, A. L., FRIEDMAN, G. D. and SIEGALAUB, A. B. 1981b. Alcohol and mortality: A ten-year Kaiser-Permanente experience. Ann. Intern. Med. *95*, 139–145.

KLEVAY, L. 1983. Copper and ischemic heart disease. Biol. Trace Element Res. *5*, 245.

KROMHOUT, D., BOSSCHIETER, E. B. and DE LEZANNE COULANDRE, C. 1982. Dietary fiber and 10 year mortality for coronary heart disease, cancer and all causes. Lancet *2*, 518–522.

KROMHOUT, D., BOSSCHIETER, E. B. and COULANDRE, C. 1985. The inverse relation between fish consumption and 20-year mortality from coronary heart disease. N. Engl. J. Med. *312*, 1205–1209.

KUSHI, L. H. *et al.* 1986. Diet and 20 year mortality from coronary heart disease. The Ireland-Boston Diet Heart Study. N. Engl. J. Med. *312*, 811–818.

LA CROIX, A. Z. *et al.* 1986. Coffee consumption and the incidence of CHD. N. Engl. J. Med. *315*, 977–982.

LANG, T. *et al.* 1983. Relation between coffee drinking and blood pressure analysis of 6,321 subjects in the Paris region. Am. J. Cardiol. *52*, 1238.

LEWIS, B. *et al.* 1974. Serum lipoprotein abnormalities in patients with ischaemic heart disease. Comparisons with a control population. Br. Med. J. *3*, 489–492.

Lipid Research Clinics. 1981. The Lipid Research Clinics coronary primary prevention trial results. I. Reduction in incidence of CHD. JAMA *251*, 351.

LIPPEL, K. *et al.* 1981. Relationship of hypertriglyceridemia to atherosclerosis. Arteriosclerosis *1*, 406–417.

LLOYD, T. 1984. Food restriction increases life span of hypertensive animals. Life Sci. *34*, 401–407.

LORENZ, R. *et al.* Platelet function, thromboxane formation and blood pressure control during supplementation of the western diet with cod liver oil. Circulation *67*, 504–511.

MANNES, G. A. *et al.* 1986. Relation between the frequency of cholesterol adenoma and the serum cholesterol level. N. Engl. J. Med. *315*, 1634–1638.

MARGETTS, B. M., BEILIN, L. J., VANDONGEN, R. and ARMSTRONG, B. K. 1986. Vegetarian diet in mild hypertension: A randomized controlled trial. Br. Med. J. *293*, 1468–1471.

National Heart, Lung and Blood Institute Concensus Development Panel. 1985. Treatment of hypertriglyceridemia. JAMA *253*, 2080–2086.

National Institutes of Health. 1985. Health implications of obesity. NIH Consensum Development Conference Statement. Ann. Intern. Med. *103*,6 (pt. 2), 1073–1077.

NORELL, S. E., ALHBOM, A., FEYCHTING, M. and PEDERSON, N. 1986. Fish consumption and mortality from coronary heart disease. Br. Med. J. *293*, 426.

PATTERSON, D. and SLACK, J. 1972. Lipid abnormalities in male and female survivors of myocardial infarction and their first degree relatives. Lancet *1*, 393–399.

PAUL, O. *et al.* 1963. Longitudinal study of coronary heart disease. Circulation *28*, 20.

PETERSON, B. and TRELL, E. 1983. Premature mortality in middle-aged men: Serum cholesterol as a risk factor. Klin. Wochenschr. *61*, 795–801.

REISEN, E. *et al.* 1978. Effect of Weight loss without salt restriction in the reduction of blood pressure in overweight hypertensive persons. N. Eng. J. Med. *298*, 1–6.

REISEN, E. *et al.* 1978. Effect of weight loss without salt restriction in the reduction of blood pressure in overweight hypertensive persons. N. Eng. J. Med. *298*, 1–6.

REISEN, E. *et al.* 1983. Cardiovascular changes after weight reduction in obese hypertensives. Ann. Intern. Med. *98*, 315–319.

ROSE, G. and SHIPLEY, M. J. 1980. Plasma lipids and mortality: A source of error. The Lancet *1*, 523–526.

ROSENBERG, I. H. and SCHAEFER, E. J. 1988. Dietary saturated fatty acids and blood cholesterol. N. Engl. J. Med. *318*, 1270–1271.

SALONEN, J. *et al.* 1982. Association between cardiovascular death and myocardial infarction and serum selenium in a matched pair longitudinal study. Lancet *2*, 175.

SHEKELLE, R. B., OGELSBY, P., MacMILLAN, S. A. and STAMLER, J. 1985. Fish consumption and mortality from coronary heart disease. N. Engl. J. Med. *313*, 820.

SHEKELLE, R. B. *et al.* 1981. Diet serum cholesterol and death from CHD. The Western Electric Study. N. Engl. J. Med. *34*, 65.

SINGH, R. *et al.* 1981. Magnesium in atherosclerotic cardiovascular disease and sudden death. Acta Cardiol. *36*, 441.

SIMONS, L. A. 1986. Interrelations of lipid and lipoproteins with coronary mortality in 19 countries. Am. J. Cardiol. *57*, 5G–10G.

SORLIE, P. D. and FEINLEIB, M. 1982. The serum cholesterol-cancer relationship: An analysis of time-trends in the Framingham Study. J. Natl. Cancer Inst. *69*, 989–996.

STAMLER, J., WENTWORTH, D. and NEATON, J. D. 1986. Is the relationship between serum cholesterol and risk of premature death from coronary heart disease continuous and graded? Findings in 356,222 primary screenees of MRFIT. JAMA *256*, 2823–2826.

STAMLER, J. *et al.* 1980. Prevention and control of hypertension by nutritional-hygienic measures: Long-term experience of the Chicago Coronary Prevention Evaluation Program. JAMA *243*, 1819–1823.

THIND, I. S. and SANDHU, R. S. 1981. Signification of high density and total cholesterol and triglycerides in acute myocardial infarction—A case-control study. Clin. Biochem. *14*, 57–60.

THOM, T., KANNEL, W. B., and FEINLEIB, M. 1985. Factors in the decline of coronary heart disease mortality. *In* Coronary Heart Disease, W. E. Connor and J. D. Bristow (eds.). J. B. Lippencott Co., Philadelphia.

THORNBERG, S. A. *et al.* 1986. Risk of cancer of the colon and rectum in relation to serum cholesterol and beta-lipoprotein. N. Engl. J. Med. *315*, 1629–1633.

TREASURE, J. and BLOTH, D. 1983. Role of dietary potassium in the treatment of hypertension. Hypertension *5*, 864–872.

U.S. Dept. of Health and Human Services, Public Health Service. 1980. The Lipid Research Clinics Population Studies Data Book, Vol. I. The Prevalence Study. National Institutes of Health Publ. No. 80-1527.

WALLACE, R. B. and ANDERSON, R. A. 1987. Blood lipids, lipid-related measures, and risk of atherosclerotic cardiovascular disease. Epidemiol. Rev. *9*, 95–119.

WARD, P. *et al.* 1982. Isolation of an inhibitor of hepatic cholesterologenesis from human milk. Atherosclerosis *41*, 185–192.

WIELAND, H. *et al.* 1980. Serum lipoproteins and coronary artery disease (CAD). Atherosclerosis *36*, 269–280.

CHAPTER 3

AGING AND CANCER

JOHN P. RICHIE, JR., Ph.D., and GARY M. WILLIAMS, M.D.
American Health Foundation
Valhalla, New York

INTRODUCTION

It is well-documented that the incidence and mortality rates from cancer increase progressively with age (Anisimov 1987; Newell 1985; Yancic 1983). With the exception of those cancers that occur predominantly in children and young adults, such as nephroblastomas, retinoblastomas, bone and testicular tumors, and lymphoid leukemia, the incidences of most neoplasms increase exponentially with age, reaching a maximum between 50 and 70 yr of age. Indeed, a 50-fold increase in cancer incidence is observed from 25–65 yr of age (Doll *et al.* 1970). The magnitude of this problem will likely grow as the percentage of elderly is expected to increase from about 11% of the current U.S. population to near 20% by the year 2000 (Brody and Brock 1985). A similar aging-related pattern in tumor incidence is also observed in experimental animals (Tannenbaum 1942; Sass *et al.* 1975).

In order to understand the basis for this aging effect, it is necessary to consider the mechanisms involved in both carcinogenesis as well as senescence. Despite the universality of biological aging, and extensive research in gerontology, much of the current knowledge in this area is descriptive and little is known of the cellular or molecular mechanisms involved. The present status of aging research is discussed by others in these proceedings and has been thoroughly reviewed elsewhere (Finch and Schneider 1985; Comfort 1979; Strehler 1982).

MECHANISMS OF CARCINOGENESIS

Cancer is not a single disease entity, and most cancers appear to arise from interaction of multiple causes (Weisburger and Williams 1982), many of which may not yet be understood. Nevertheless, despite the multiplicity of originating factors the production of neoplasms by chemical carcinogens can be conceived to involve two distinct processes, neoplastic conversion and neoplastic development (Williams and Weisburger 1986). During neoplastic conversion or initiation in the terminology of Berenblum (1974), irreversible changes occur in the genome of a normal cell resulting in transformation to a neoplastic cell. The subsequent sequence involves the steps that lead to the growth and further development of the neoplastic population, commonly called promotion (Berenblum 1974), and progression of the neoplastic population to form a tumor. Chemical carcinogens can act in either sequence.

Chemical carcinogens are of two basic types, those that react with DNA, called genotoxic, and those that operate by other indirect mechanisms, designated epigenetic carcinogens (Weisburger and Williams 1981). The majority of genotoxic or DNA-reactive carcinogens are not active in their parent form, but are activated by cellular enzymes of the host organisms to the ultimate carcinogens (Miller and Miller 1976). These activated products are chemically reactive species, most often electrophiles or free radicals, which can react with sites in target cells, including nucleic acids and proteins. Considerable evidence supports the hypothesis that DNA is the critical target in carcinogenesis (Magee *et al.* 1975; Williams and Weisburger 1986). For this reason, carcinogens with the ability to damage DNA through formation of covalent adducts are referred to as genotoxic or DNA-reactive carcinogens (Williams and Weisburger 1986). The enzyme systems responsible for the metabolic activation of chemical carcinogens belong mainly to the group of microsomal hydroxylases or mixed-function oxidases that require oxygen and reduced pyridine nucleotides and are dependent on cytochrome P-450 for their activity. Cocarcinogens can enhance the carcinogenicity of chemicals by inducing these activation systems.

Metabolic activation of precarcinogens is only one of the biotransformation pathways; other routes of metabolism lead to deactivation of carcinogens. These detoxification reactions often involve adduct formation with compounds such as glutathione, sulfate, or glucuronic acid, resulting in a product which is more water soluble and easily excreted (Williams and Weisburger 1986).

The efficacy of most DNA-reactive carcinogens is dependent on the balance between their metabolic activation and detoxification. Under normal circumstances, detoxification predominates. However, the small amount of activated product which is produced causes cumulative damage over time. Also, when changes occur in the activity of either of the metabolic systems involved, the carcinogenic effect will be altered accordingly.

Carcinogen-induced DNA damage can be repaired by a variety of processes (Lindahl 1982). Repair occurs at varying rates and if the cell divides before the chemical damage is corrected, then a permanent mutation will occur. Cocarcinogens function in part at this stage by enhancing cellular proliferation in tissues in which carcinogen damage is present.

The production of mutations in the cell by a genotoxic carcinogen may result directly in neoplastic conversion if the alterations are sufficient. This appears to involve activation of oncogenes or inactivation of antioncogenes (Bishop 1983; Stanbridge 1985). However, altered populations of cells which are considered to be "preneoplastic" often precede the appearance of tumors. This suggests that the normal cell may pass through a series of stages before reaching full neoplastic potential (Farber 1982). From that point, the progression of a neoplastic cell to form a tumor requires its sustained proliferation. Tumor promoters act to enable the proliferation and clonal expansion of neoplastic cells so that they can form tumors.

After neoplastic cells have proliferated to acquire a certain mass, they are no longer dependent upon promoters and can express their abnormal genotype through further progressive growth. During the continued growth of tumors, the cells may acquire new permanent, abnormal characteristics resulting in further deviation from the normal phenotype of the cell of origin. This phenomenon is known as progression (Foulds 1969; Nowell 1986).

MECHANISMS OF THE AGING-INCREASE IN TUMOR INCIDENCE

At the present time, there is no consensus on the nature of the relationship between aging and the development of neoplasms or on the causes of the aging-related increase of tumor incidence (Anisimov 1987; Pitot 1977; Magee 1978). Some have suggested that the underlying mechanisms of aging and carcinogenesis are closely related (Anisimov 1985; Dilman 1978, 1985; Dix *et al.* 1980). Indeed, a number of similarities have been noted between many theories of aging and current concepts of oncology (Anisimov 1987). For example, several aging hypotheses are based on the assumption that an accumulation of nonrepairable lesions occur in cells over time, a notion which is analogous to theories developed to explain the occurrence of cryptogenic tumors.

Others have argued that there is no relation between aging and cancer and cite inconsistencies such as the loss of replicative capacity of senescent cells (Doll 1973; Peto *et al.* 1975, 1985). This view attributes the aging-associated increase in cancer to the well-known relationship between the dose of carcinogen and time required for tumor development. Cancer incidence is held to be determined by the accumulation of carcinogenic doses and/or an increased exposure to carcinogen action and not to intrinsic, aging-specific alterations within the host. Thus, all lesions induced by exogenous and endogenous factors causing malignant transformation are summed up independently of the host age, and the probability of developing tumors is greater with increased life span because of these factors. However, spontaneous tumor incidence does not correlate with life span of a species (Anisimov 1976; Dix *et al.* 1980; Staats 1980; Stukonis 1979). For example the tumor incidence of humans who live to be 69–77 yr of age is 30%, the same as found in noninbred rats which live about 3 yr (Anisimov 1986). Also, no positive correlations were observed in tumor incidence and mean life span in inbred mice (Storer 1966) and hamsters (Pour *et al.* 1979) or in 12 different groups of noninbred rats (Anisimov 1983) with different life spans. Thus, although the dose/time of exposure relationship certainly is an important factor in the aging-related increase in cancer incidence, it seems likely that other factors are also involved.

Another hypothesis for the relationship of aging and cancer is that changes which occur in the organism during natural aging increase the probability of tumor occurrence and facilitate tumor growth and progression. This notion is consistent with a classical definition of senescence as "an increased vulnerability occurring with advance age" (Comfort 1979). Based on current knowledge of the mechanisms of chemical carcinogenesis, there are a number of factors which, if altered in senescence, could result in an increase in susceptibility to carcinogens. These include either increases in carcinogen activation, DNA susceptibility to chemical damage, and cell proliferation or impairments in carcinogen detoxification, DNA repair, and immunological surveillance.

Aging and Factors Regulating Carcinogenesis

Carcinogen Activation. Since the efficacy of most chemical carcinogens is dependent on the balance between their metabolic activation and detoxification, changes in the activities of these systems could alter their carcinogenic effects. The dominant mechanism for carcinogen-activation involves the microsomal mixed-function oxidase system and its component, cytochrome P-450. Numerous studies have demonstrated that the levels and activities of the cytochrome P-450 system are decreased in aging rats (McMartin *et al.* 1980; Schmucker and Wang 1981). Studies with several activation-dependent carcinogens have revealed evidence for unchanged or even reduced susceptibility of aged rats (Stenbäck *et al.* 1981a, 1981b, 1981c; Kroes *et al.* 1975). Finally, in humans, the biological half-lives of a number of activation-dependent drugs are increased with old age (Gillette 1979). Thus, it is unlikely that an increase in carcinogen activation is responsible for the aging-increase in cancer incidence. Nevertheless, there could be a role for those carcinogens which are detoxified by cytochrome P-450 oxidation.

Carcinogen Detoxification Involving Glutathione. The detoxification of many carcinogenic agents involves the cysteine-containing tripeptide, glutathione (GSH). This endogenous antioxidant is found in high concentrations (0.5–8.0 mM) in nearly all living cells and has many important functional roles including the detoxification of many exogenous compounds, such as a wide variety of peroxides and free radicals, xenobiotics, and carcinogens (Sakamoto *et al.* 1983; Meister and Anderson 1983; Reed and Beatty 1980). For example, GSH protects against benzo(a)pyrene by conjugating with its ultimate carcinogen, 7,8-dihydro-9,10-epoxy-7,8,9,10-tetrahydrobenzo(a)pyrene (BPDE) and a depletion of GSH leads to an increase in BPDE binding to DNA (Cooper *et al.* 1980).

Studies by Lang and coworkers on a variety of aging models have indicated that a GSH reduction is a general phenomenon of aging tissues: lower GSH levels were found in a number of experimental aging organisms and tissues (Abraham *et al.* 1978; Hazelton and Lang 1980, 1983, 1984; Naryshkin *et al.* 1984; Schneider *et al.* 1982; Chen *et al.* 1989). Indeed, recent results in human subjects suggest that elderly individuals with high blood GSH levels are physically, psychologically and sociologically healthier than those with lower GSH levels (Julius and Lang 1988).

The importance of the GSH deficiency in the aging process was demonstrated in studies by Richie *et al.* (1987) where the cysteine and GSH precursor, thiazolidine-4-carboxylic acid, was fed to mosquitoes of different ages (Richie and Lang 1988). The GSH levels increased 50–100% regardless of the age when feeding was initiated or whether the feeding period was 2 days or the entire life span. This suggested that the GSH deficiency was due to a lack of cysteine and not to an enzymatic impairment or other factor. Most importantly, the median life span of the life-long fed mosquitoes was increased about 40% over control fed adults.

The GSH deficiency of aging could have a number of important consequences due to the essential roles of GSH in a variety of metabolic reactions. One possible sequelum could be a decrease in the detoxification capacity for carcinogens leading to increased risk for cancer induction. In this regard, studies were conducted using the drug acetaminophen (APAP), which is activated to a reactive electrophile by the mixed-function oxidase system, and is subsequently detoxified by conjugation with GSH (Potter *et al.* 1973, 1974; Jollow *et al.* 1973). These studies demonstrated, in an aging mosquito model, that the toxicity of APAP was 7-fold higher in the very old compared to the mature adult (Richie and Lang 1985). Further, the observed aging-decrease in APAP LD_{50} values was highly correlated with the aging-specific decrease in GSH concentration ($r = 0.99$). Recently, these results were verified in aging C57BL/6 mice by determining the loss of ability to recover GSH levels after depletion by APAP (Chen *et al.* 1987, 1988a). Detoxification capacity in the mouse was regained after tissue levels of GSH were replenished by administering GSH-monoethylester (Chen *et al.* 1988b). Collectively these results support the hypothesis that a GSH deficiency leading to a loss in detoxification capacity is an important factor in the aging-increase observed in cancer incidence.

Other Detoxification Mechanisms. Two other common detoxification reactions involve conjugation of carcinogen with glucuronic acid or sulfate. These reactions are carried out with the enzymes UDP-glucuronyl transferase and sulfotransferase respectively. As with GSH, these conjugation reactions increase the water solubility of carcinogens, allowing for ready excretion. Very little is known on the effects of aging on these enzyme systems. Both slight increases and decreases have been observed in UDP-glucuronyl transferase activity in aging F-344 rats (Kitahara *et al.* 1982). Further investigation is needed in this area.

DNA Susceptibility to Chemical Damage. The interaction between the chemical carcinogen and DNA could be altered during the processes of aging, resulting in an enhanced sensitivity of the cell to DNA damage. Few valid aging studies have addressed this aspect. However, recent studies have demonstrated that cells from older humans are more susceptible to chromosomal damage by ^{3}H-thymidine than those from younger subjects (Staiano-Coico *et al.* 1982, 1983; Dutkowski *et al.* 1985). These results suggest that old cells are more vulnerable to chromosomal rearrangement and to the toxic effects of irradiation. Research is needed in this area to determine the relationship of this age-related change to carcinogenesis.

DNA Repair. The DNA repair systems that eliminate carcinogen-induced damage in DNA structure are thought to play a critical role in maintaining gene integrity. Thus, an impairment in DNA repair may contribute both to the mechanisms of aging and of carcinogenesis. There have been a number of studies which investigated the relationship between aging and DNA repair and these have been recently reviewed (Anisimov 1987; Setlow 1982). The results have been quite varied as both increases and decreases in DNA repair have been observed in aging, while in the majority of studies, no changes were found. This disparity is likely due to variation in methodological approaches in measuring DNA repair, as well as differences in animal models (Anisimov 1987).

The results of two studies involving a differentiated epithelial cell type representative of an *in vivo* population suggest that a decline in DNA repair activity is an important factor in the aging process. In hepatocytes isolated from 6–32 month-old rats, Plesko and Richardson (1984) observed that repair of UV-induced DNA damage was significantly impaired in cells from animals of more than 14 months of age. In a related study, it was found that UV light-induced DNA repair synthesis in hepatocytes from 5 different mammalian species was positively correlated with life span potential (Maslansky and Williams 1985). These studies merit extension to other types of DNA damage.

The overall conclusion from these results, taking into account methodological differences and limitations, is unclear. Nevertheless, it does seem likely that DNA repair may play a permissive rather than a leading role in the mechanism of the age-related increase in tissue sensitivity to carcinogens (Anisimov 1987; Setlow 1982).

Cell Proliferation. The level of proliferative activity of tissues is an important factor in determining susceptibility to chemical carcinogenesis. An enhancement in proliferation of tissues in which DNA damage has occurred will decrease the effectiveness of DNA repair mechanisms. Damaged DNA is repaired by a number of processes, but if the cell divides before repair takes place, then the damage can be translated into a permanent change in the base sequence and a mutation occurs. Thus, the efficiency of DNA repair is dependant upon the level of proliferative activity of the damaged tissue. The available data indicate that the proliferative activity of the majority of growing and renewing tissues is decreased in senescence (Cameron and Thrasher 1976) and, therefore, cannot explain the aging-increase in cancer incidence.

Promotion of Carcinogenesis. It has been proposed that tumor promotion is enhanced in aging organisms leading to an increase in cancer incidence (Burnet 1971; Dilman 1978, 1985). However, contrary to this notion, Stenbäck *et al.* (1981b) found that skin tumor promotion susceptibility was actually decreased in aging mice.

To assess the influence of age on growth of neoplasms, a number of studies have been carried out involving the transplantation of tumors to animals of different ages. In these experiments, the efficiency of transplantability reflected immunological vigor, whereas, tumor growth rate and survival time of the animals were considered to serve as an index of tumor promoting activity. The results of these studies, which have been reviewed by Anisimov (1987), vary greatly due to differences in methodologies and animal models used. Again, in many reports, growth and maturational changes, rather than aging effects, were described. Another major source of variation was the tumor type used for transplantation. For example, hematopoietic neoplasms appeared to develop at the same rate or faster in younger animals (Rodriguez *et al.* 1976; Anisimov and Zhukovskaya 1981), whereas, squamous cell epidermal cancer and lung adenocarcinomas grew faster in old organisms (Anisimov and Zhukovskaya 1981; Stjernwärd, 1966; Yuhas and Ullrich 1976). More research of this type is needed using well-defined model systems before any conclusions can be drawn.

Immunological function is an important factor involved in tumor promotion and a decline in the effectiveness of the immune system may contribute to the increased incidence of cancer in older age groups. This notion is based on the immunological surveillance hypothesis of Burnet (1971) which assumes that cancer cells carry surface antigens that differ from those of the host, and, thus, immunological defense mechanisms can be mobilized against the tumor cells. Indeed a number of dramatic changes in immune structure and function have been described in aging organisms (Makinodan and Hirayama 1985). Central to these changes is the involution of the thymus resulting in a loss of 90% of its cellular mass by the age of 50 yr (Boyd 1932). As a result of this loss, a dramatic depletion of thymic hormone is observed between 30 and 60 yr (Lewis *et al.* 1978), as well as a redistribution of T-lymphocyte subpopulations in which the percentage of immature T-cells in the blood greatly increases (Schwab *et al.* 1983). Although the importance of immunological surveillance was widely accepted at first, subsequently this hypothesis has been challenged (Baldwin 1973; Kripke and Borsos 1974; Currie 1976). A particular point of importance is that nude mice, which have virtually no T-lymphocytes, have a very low incidence of cryptogenic tumors and do not have increased sensitivity to chemical carcinogens (Rygaard and Povlsen 1976).

Experimentally Induced Carcinogenesis and Aging

To test the importance of the aging changes described previously on host sensitivity, a number of studies have been performed in which the efficacy of chemical carcinogens administered to organisms of different ages were determined. These studies, which have been extensively reviewed by Anisimov (1987), have yielded inconsistent and controversial results. In some studies, the sensitivity of old organisms to carcinogens was increased, while in others there was a decrease or no change in carcinogen sensitivity. The variability in results could be caused by several factors. Variations between target tissues have been implicated by Anisimov (1981) as, in the same experiment, aging-related increases (cervix, uteri, and vagina), decreases (mammary gland and kidney) and no change (hemopoietic system) were found in tissue sensitivity to N-nitrosomethylurea in rats. Other factors include differences in the type of carcinogen used, dosage regimen and mode of administration. The species and strain of the test organism is also of major importance due to differences in life span potential. Finally, a major source of variation in many of these studies is the use of animals that are too young, so that the effects observed were indicative of growth or maturation rather than aging.

More research is needed in this area before any conclusions can be drawn. It is important that well-characterized, long-lived species and strains are used as well as truly old animals. The type of carcinogen and its mode of administration should be chosen carefully so that comparisons can be made to determine those aging changes which are most important in tumor production. Finally, carcinogens which are of known or suspected importance in the production of human cancer should be preferentially used.

Nutritional Aspects of Cancer and Aging

The importance of nutrition and diet on cancer incidence and mortality is well known and has been subject to many reviews (Weisburger *et al.* 1980; Miller 1983; National Academy of Sciences 1982; Willett and MacMahon 1984). Indeed, the wide international variation in cancer incidence has been attributed in large part to differences in diet and nutrition between cultures. The nutritional basis of a large number of cancers has been elucidated, including cancers of the esophagus, stomach, colon, rectum, liver, lung and breast. Also, the roles of many specific nutrients and food constituents such as fat, fiber, alcohol, vitamins and nitrates, to name a few, have been studied extensively.

The involvement of nutrition in the aging process also has been subject to much recent interest (Hutchinson and Munro 1986; Kohrs and Kamath 1981; Albanese 1980), although less is known of this relationship than with cancer. Many nutrients and food constituents have been implicated as factors involved in the aging process, including such compounds as fats, vitamins and protein. However, to date, very little is known of the involvement of specific nutrients in the aging process.

The role of nutrition in both the biochemistry of cancer and the biological aging process has been reviewed recently (Mills 1986). Although promising areas in protection against cancer formation and aging decrements were discussed, an enormous amount of research is still needed to elucidate the relationships and mechanisms involved.

A very exciting area of research involves the beneficial effects of caloric restriction of the diet on both cancer and aging (Weindruch and Walford 1988). The pioneering work of McCay (1947) demonstrated that an increase in life span could be obtained by restricting the caloric intake of rats and mice throughout their life spans. Later, it was shown that this effect is due to a retardation of the aging process as caloric restriction started at maturity was also effective (Weindruch and Walford 1982). It has been well established that caloric restriction delays the development and reduces the incidence of spontaneous tumors characteristic of the strain or species of animals used (Tannenbaum 1942; Weindruch and Walford 1988). This important phenomenon has generated a great deal of interest and research, and the results are reviewed and discussed elsewhere in these proceedings. However, the mechanisms involved in the effects of caloric restriction remain elusive.

Dietary antioxidants have been described to have both geroprotective and antitumor effects. A number of antimutagenic properties of antioxidants have been described (Wattenberg 1985; Renner 1984). It appears that most exert their effects on carcinogen initiation reactions by altering the activities of enzymes involved in their activation and detoxification (Anisimov 1983; Wattenberg 1980; McKee and Tometsko 1979; Griffin and Lane 1981; Kahl 1980). It should be noted that antioxidants which decrease the activity of carcinogen-activating enzymes in some cases could lead to an enhancement of carcinogenesis by carcinogens that are detoxified by the same enzymes (Balanski 1978).

The use of antioxidants as geroprotectors is based on the free radical theory of aging (Harman 1962, 1981; Leibovitz and Siegel 1980). This theory suggests that oxidative processes involved in normal metabolism generate free radical by-products which cause molecular damage over time leading to the decrements observed in senescence. This theory is based on the positive correlation between the activity of antioxidant systems and species-specific life span. An important aspect of this theory is the notion that antioxidant administration should delay the aging process and consequentially increase life span. A number of experiments have been performed along these lines and have been reviewed (Schneider and Reed 1985; Weber and Miquel 1986). The overall conclusion from these studies is that antioxidant administration has little effect on life span and cryptogenic tumor incidence in mammals. Indeed, in the majority of studies, no changes were found in either parameter. For example, in studies by Stenbäck *et al.* (1987, 1988) the antioxidants hydroxylamine and dimethylaminoethanol had no effect on longevity when administered to C3H mice. Although increases were observed in some studies, most were complicated by the use of poorly defined experimental organisms. In several instances, suboptimal conditions for maximal life span resulted in shorter than expected control life spans. Thus, the beneficial effect of the antioxidant probably was due to the correction of an abnormal condition prevalent in the animals rather than a decrease in the rate of aging.

Recently, the antioxidant nordihydroguaiaretic acid (NDGA) was shown to increase the life span about 50% in the well-characterized aging mosquito (*Aedes aegypti*) model (Richie *et al.* 1986). This antioxidant was also found effective at delaying aging-changes and increasing life span in *Neurospora crassa* (Munkres and Missen 1976) and *Drosophila melanogaster* (Miquel and Johnson 1975). Although a dietary supplement of NDGA apparently caused an increase in rat survival, vague methodology and insufficient numbers of animals made the results inconclusive (Buu-Hoi and Ratsunamanga 1959). There is teleological support for the importance of

NDGA for longevity, as it is the major chemical component of the cresote bush, one of the longest lived organisms known (Oliveto 1972; Mabry *et al.* 1977). Studies are needed to determine if NDGA has similar longevity-enhancing properties in mammalian aging models.

SUMMARY

The incidence of most types of cancers increases greatly in senescence. Theories on the underlying causes of the aging-enhancement of tumor incidence have encompassed two basic views. Some investigators propose that this phenomena is intricately related to the actual biological aging process while others believe that it is merely due to the passage of time, regardless of the age of the individual. This latter view is supported by the well-known relationship between carcinogen dose and time required for tumor development. However, a good deal of evidence exists to suggest that an increase in carcinogen sensitivity of the host is also an important factor.

There are several systems which, if altered in senescence, could result in an increase in susceptibility of the host to carcinogens. One promising area of research involves the loss of carcinogen detoxification capacity involving glutathione, as a deficiency in glutathione appears to be a general phenomenon of aging cells and tissues. More work in this area is needed to elucidate the importance of this mechanism on cryptogenic tumor production.

Nutrition and diet have also been involved in the prevention of carcinogenesis and the postponement of aging changes. The important findings of increased life span and reduced cancer incidence by caloric restriction should provide new and important information on the mechanisms of spontaneous tumor production in aging organisms. However, further research is needed to determine the causal factors involved in this phenomena.

Finally, the effects of aging on susceptibility to chemical carcinogens need to be elucidated. It is essential in these studies to use well-characterized organisms with known and verified life spans and to sample systematically over the entire adult life span.

REFERENCES

ABRAHAM, E. C., TAYLOR, J. F. and LANG, C. A. 1978. Influence of mouse age and erythrocyte age on glutathione metabolism. Biochem. J. *174*, 819–825.

ALBANESE, A. A. 1980. Nutrition for the Elderly. Current Topics in Nutrition and Disease, Vol. 3. Alan R. Liss, Inc., New York.

ANISIMOV, V. N. 1976. Spontaneous tumors in rats of different strains. Vopr. Oncol. *22*, 98–110.

ANISIMOV, V. N. 1981. Carcinogenesis and aging. I. Modifying effect of aging on N-methyl-N-nitrosourea-induced carcinogenesis in female rats. Exp. Pathol. *19*, 81–90.

ANISIMOV, V. N. 1983. Carcinogenesis and aging. Adv. Cancer Res. *40*, 265–424.

ANISIMOV, V. N. 1985. Relevance of age to some aspects of carcinogenesis. *In* Age-Related Factors in Carcinogenesis. (IARC Sci. Publ. No. 58), A. Likhachev, V. Anisimov and R. Montesano (eds.). IARC (Int. Agency for Research on Cancer), Lyon.

ANISIMOV, V. N. 1987. Carcinogenesis and Aging. CRC Press, Inc., Boca Raton.

ANISIMOV, V. N. and ZHUKOVSKAYA, N. V. 1981. Effect of host age on transplantable tumor development in mice. Vopr. Onkol. *27*, 52–59.

BALANSKI, R. M. 1978. Metabolism of chemical blastomogenic agents and carcinogenesis. Vopr. Onkol. *24*, 100–106.

BALDWIN, R. W. 1973. Immunological aspects of chemical carcinogenesis. Adv. Cancer Res. *18*, 1–75.

BERENBLUM, I. 1974. Carcinogenesis as a Biological Problem. Elsevier Science Publishing, New York.

BISHOP, J. M. 1983. Cellular oncogenes and retroviruses. Annu. Rev. Biochem. *52*, 301–354.

BOYD, E. 1932. Progress in pediatrics: the weight of the thymus gland in health and in disease. Am. J. Dis. Child. *43*, 1162.

BRODY, J. A. and BROCK, D. W. 1985. Epidemiologic and statistical characterizations of the United States elderly population. *In* Handbook of the Biology of Aging, 2nd Edition. C. E. Finch and E. L. Schneider (eds.). Van Nostrand Reinhold, Princeton, NJ.

BURNET, F. M. 1971. Immunological surveillance in neoplasia. Transplant. Rev. *7*, 3–25.

BUU-HOI, N. P. and RATSUNAMANGA, A. R. 1959. Action retardante de lácide nordihydroguaiaretique sur le vieillissement chez le rat. C.R. Soc. Biol. *153*, 1180–1182.

CAMERON, I. and THRASHER, J. D. 1976. Cell renewal and cell loss in the tissues of aging animals. Interdiscip. Top. Gerontol. *10*, 108–129.

CHEN, T. S., RICHIE, JR., J. P. and LANG, C. A. 1987. The aging decrease in acetaminophen detoxification by glutathione in the mouse. Presented at the 10th International Congress of Pharmacology, Aug. 23–28, Sidney, Australia.

CHEN, T. S., RICHIE, JR., J. P. and LANG, C. A. 1988a. A glutathione and cysteine deficiency in the aging mouse kidney leads to impaired acetaminophen detoxification. Fed. Am. Soc. Exp. Biol. J. *2*, A804.

CHEN, T. S., RICHIE, JR., J. P. and LANG, C. A. 1988b. Glutathione ester protects against glutathione deficiencies due to aging and acetaminophen. Pharmacologist *30*, A78.

CHEN, T. S. , RICHIE, JR., J. P. and LANG. C. A. 1989. The effects of aging on glutathione and cysteine levels in different regions of the mouse brain. Proc. Soc. Exp. Biol. Med. *190*, 399–402.

COMFORT, A. 1979. The Biology of Senescence, 3rd Edition. Elsevier Science Publishing, New York.

COOPER, C. S. *et al.* 1980. The enzyme-catalysed conversion of *anti*-benzo(a)pyrene-7,8-diol-9,10-oxide into a glutathione conjugate. Carcinogenesis (London) *1*, 1075–1080.

CURRIE, G. 1976. Immunological aspects of host resistance to the development and growth of cancer. Biochim. Biophys. Acta *458*, 135–165.

DILMAN, V. M. 1978. Aging, metabolic immunodepression and carcinogenesis. Mech. Aging Dev. *8*, 153–173.

DILMAN, V. M. 1985. Aging and cancer in the light of the ontogenetic model of medicine. *In* Age-Related Factors in Carcinogenesis (IARC Sci. Publ. No. 58), A. Likhachev, V. Anisimov and R. Montesano (eds.). IARC (Int. Agency for Research on Cancer), Lyon.

DIX, D., COHEN, P. and FLANNERY, J. 1980. On the role of aging in cancer incidence. J. Theor. Biol. *83*, 163–173.

DOLL, R. 1973. Age. *In* Host Environment Interactions in the Etiology of Cancer in Man (IARC Sci. Publ. No. 7), R. Doll and I. Vodopija (eds.). IARC (Int. Agency for Research on Cancer), Lyon.

DOLL, R., MUIR, C. and WATERHOUSE, J. 1970. Cancer Incidence in Five Continents. UICC (Union Int. Contre Cancer), Geneva.

DUTKOWSKI, R. T. *et al.* 1985. Increased chromosomal instability in lymphocytes from elderly humans. Mutat. Res. *149*, 505–512.

FARBER, E. 1982. Sequential events in chemical carcinogenesis. *In* Cancer: A Comprehensive Treatise, 2nd Edition, F. F. Becker (ed.). Plenum Press, New York.

FINCH, C. E. and SCHNEIDER, E. L. 1985 Handbook of the Biology of Aging, 2nd Edition. Van Nostrand Reinhold Co., Princeton, NJ.

FOULDS, L. 1969. Neoplastic Development. Academic Press, Inc., New York.

GILLETTE, J. R. 1979. Biotransformation of drugs during aging. Fed. Proc. *38*, 1900–1909.

GRIFFIN, A. C. and LANE, H. W. 1981. Selenium chemoprevention of cancer in animals and possible implication. *In* Selenium in Biology and Medicine, J. E. Spallholz, J. L. Martin and H. E. Ganther (eds.). AVI/Van Nostrand Reinhold, New York.

HARMAN, D. 1962. Role of free radicals in mutation, cancer, aging and maintenance of life. Radiat. Res. *16*, 753.

HARMAN, D. 1981. The aging process. Proc. Natl. Acad. Sci. USA *78*, 7124–7128.

HAZELTON, G. A. and LANG, C. A. 1980. Glutathione contents of tissues in the aging mouse. Biochem. J. *188*, 25–30.

HAZELTON, G. A. and LANG, C. A. 1983. Glutathione biosynthesis in the aging adult yellow fever mosquito. Biochem. J. *210*, 289–295.

HAZELTON, G. A. and LANG, C. A. 1984. Glutathione levels during the mosquito life span with emphasis on senescence. Proc. Soc. Exp. Biol. Med. *176*, 249–256.

HUTCHINSON, M. L. and MUNRO, H. N. 1986. Nutrition and Aging. Bristol-Meyers Nutrition Symposium, Vol. 5, Academic Press, Orlando.

JOLLOW, D. J. *et al.* 1973. Acetaminophen-induced hepatic necrosis. II. The role of covalent binding *in vivo*. J. Pharmacol. Exp. Ther. *187*, 195–202.

JULIUS, M. and LANG, C. A. 1988. Blood glutathione levels reflect subjective and objective health status in the Southfield elderly. Gerontologist *28*, 228A.

KAHL, R. 1980. Enhancement of epoxide hydratase activity in rat lung, kidney and liver by dietary antioxidants. Cancer Lett. *8*, 323–328.

KITAHARA, A. *et al.* 1982. Changes in activities and molecular forms of rat hepatic drug metabolizing enzymes during aging. *In* Liver and Aging—1982. Liver and Drugs, H. Katani (ed.). Elsevier, Amsterdam.

KOHRS, M. B. and KAMATH, S. K. 1981. Symposium on nutrition and aging. Am. J. Clin. Nutr. *36*, 734–822.

KRIPKE, M. C. and BORSOS, T. 1974. Immune surveillance revisited. J. Natl. Cancer Inst. *52*, 1393–1395.

KROES, R. *et al.* 1975. Elevated concentrations of serum α-fetoprotein in rats with chemically induced liver tumors. Cancer Res. *35*, 1214–1217.

LEIBOVITZ, B. E. and SIEGEL, B. V. 1980. Aspects of free radical reactions in biological systems. Aging J. Gerontol. *35*, 45–56.

LEWIS, V. M. *et al.* 1978. Age, thymic involution and circulating thymic hormone activity. J. Clin. Endocrinol. Metab. *48*, 145–150.

LINDAHL, T. 1982. DNA repair enzymes. Ann. Rev. Biochem. *51*, 61–87.

MABRY, T. J., HUNZIKER, J. H. and DIFEO, JR., D. R. 1977. Creosote Bush, Biology and Chemistry of Larrea in New World Deserts. Hutchinson and Ross, Stroudsburg, PA.

MAGEE, P. N. 1978. Carcinogenesis and aging. *In* Pharmacological Intervention in the Aging Process, J. Roberts, R. C. Adelman and V. J. Christofolo (eds.). Plenum Publishing Corp., New York.

MAGEE, P. N., PEGG, A. E. and SWANN, P. F. 1975. Molecular Mechanisms of Chemical Carcinogenesis. Springer-Verlag, Berlin.

MAKINODAN, T. and HIRAYAMA, R. 1985. Age-related changes in immunologic and hormonal activities. *In* Age-Related Factors in Carcinogenesis (IARC Sci. Publ. No. 58), A. Likhachev, V. Anisimov and R. Montesano (eds.). IARC (Int. Agency for Research on Cancer), Lyon.

MASLANSKY, C. J. and WILLIAMS, G. M. 1985. Ultra-violet light-induced DNA repair synthesis in hepatocytes from species of differing longevities. Mech. Aging Dev. *29*, 191–203.

McCAY, C. M. 1947. Effect of restricted feeding upon aging and chronic diseases in rats and dogs. Am. J. Publ. Health *37*, 521.

McKEE, R. H. and TOMETSKO, A. M. 1979. Inhibition of promutagen activation by the antioxidants butylated hydroxyanisole and butylated hydroxytoluene. J. Natl. Cancer Inst. *63*, 473–477.

McMARTIN, D. N., O'CONNOR, J. A., FASCO, M. J. and KAMINSKY, L. S. 1980. Influence of aging and induction on rat liver and kidney microsomal mixed function oxidase systems. Toxicol. Appl. Pharmacol. *54*, 411–419.

MEISTER, A. and ANDERSON, M. E. 1983. Glutathione. Ann. Rev. Biochem. *52*, 711, 760.

MILLER, A. B. 1983. Nutrition and cancer—an overview. *In* Environmental Aspects of Cancer. The Role of Macro and Micro Components of Foods. E. L. Wynder *et al.* (eds.). Food and Nutrition Press, Trumbull, CT.

MILLER, E. C. and MILLER, J. A. 1976. The metabolism of chemical carcinogens to reactive electrophiles and their possible mechanisms of action in carcinogenesis. *In* Chemical Carcinogenesis, C. E. Searle (ed.). ACS Monograph.

MILLS, B. J. 1986. Nutritional biochemistry of cancer. *In* Nutritional Aspects of Aging, Vol II, L. H. Chen (ed.). CRC Press, Inc. Boca Raton.

MIQUEL, J. and JOHNSON, JR., J. E. 1975. Effects of various antioxidants and radiation protectants on the life span and lipofuscin of *Drosophila* and of C57BL/6J mice. Gerontologist *15*, 25.

MUNKRES, K. D. and MISSEN, M. 1976. Aging of *Neurospora crassa*. I. Evidence for the free radical theory of aging from studies of a natural death mutant. Mech. Aging Dev. *5*, 79–98.

NARYSHKIN, S., MILLER, L., LINDEMAN, R. and LANG, C. A. 1981. Blood glutathione: a biochemical index of human aging. Fed. Proc. *40*, 3179.

National Academy of Sciences. 1982. Diet, Nutrition and Cancer. National Academy Press, Washington, D.C.

NEWELL, G. R. 1985. Epidemiology of cancer. *In* Cancer: Principals and Practice of Oncology, T. DeVita, Jr., S. Hellman and S. A. Rosenberg (eds). Lippincott, Philadelphia.

NOWELL, P. C. 1986. Mechanisms of tumor progression. Cancer Res. *46*, 2203–2207.

OLIVETO, E. P. 1972. Nordihydroguaiaretic acid: A naturally occurring antioxidant. Chem. Ind. (Dekker) *17*, 677–679.

PETO, R., PARISH, S. E. and GRAY, R. G. 1985. There is no such thing as aging, and cancer is not related to it. *In* Age-Related Factors in Carcinogenesis (IARC Sci. Publ. No. 58), A. Likhachev, V. Anisimov and R. Montesano (eds.). IARC (Int. Agency for Research on Cancer), Lyon.

PETO, R. *et al.* 1975. Cancer and aging in mice and man. Br. J. Cancer *32*, 411–426.

PITOT, H. C. 1977. Carcinogenesis and aging: Two related phenomena? Am. J. Pathol. *87*, 444–472.

PLESKO, M. M. and RICHARDSON, A. 1984. Age-related changes in unscheduled DNA synthesis by rat hepatocytes. Biochem. Biophys. Res. Commun. *118*, 730–735.

POTTER, W. Z., THORGEIRSSON, S. S., JOLLOW, D. J. and MITCHELL, J. R. 1974. Acetaminophen-induced hepatic necrosis, covalent binding and glutathione depletion in hamsters. Pharmacology *12*, 129–143.

POTTER, W. Z. *et al.* 1973. Acetaminophen-induced hepatic necrosis. III. Cytochrome P-450 mediated covalent binding *in vitro*. J. Pharmacol. Exp. Ther. *187*, 203–210.

POUR, P., ALTHOFF, J., SALMASIS, Z. and STEPAN, K. 1979. Spontaneous tumors and common diseases in three types of hamsters. J. Natl. Cancer Inst. *63*, 797–811.

REED, D. and BEATTY, P. W. 1980. Biosynthesis and regulation of glutathione: toxicological implications. *In* Review of Biochemical Toxicology, Vol. 2, E. Hodgson, J. Bend and R. Philpot (eds.). Elsevier Science Publishing, New York.

RENNER, H. W. 1984. Antimutagenic effect of an antioxidant in mammals. Mutat. Res. *135*, 125–129.

RICHIE, JR., J. P. and LANG, C. A. 1985. Aging effects on acetaminophen toxicity and glutathione status in the mosquito. Drug. Metabol. Dispos. *13*, 14–17.

RICHIE, JR., J. P. and LANG, C. A. 1988. Cysteine loss is the cause of glutathione deficiency in the aging mosquito. Proc. Soc. Exp. Biol. Med. *187*, 235–240.

RICHIE, JR., J. P., MILLS, B. J. and LANG, C. A. 1986. Dietary nordihydroguaiaretic acid increases life span of the mosquito. Proc. Soc. Exp. Biol. Med. *183*, 81–85.

RICHIE, JR., J. P., MILLS, B. J. and LANG, C. A. 1987. Correction of a glutathione deficiency in the aging mosquito increases its longevity. Proc. Soc. Exp. Biol. Med. *184*, 113–117.

RODRIGUEZ, P. E., DEBONAPARTE, Y. P., D'ELIA, I. and KLEIN, D. 1976. Studies on NZB mice. III. Failure of growth of isogeneic tumors transplanted to old NZB mice. Sangre *21*, 805.

RYGAARD, J. and POVLSEN, C. O. 1976. The nude mouse vs. the hypothesis of immunological surveillance. Transplant. Rev. *28*, 43–61.

SAKAMOTO, Y., HIGASHI, T. and TATEISHI, N. 1983. Glutathione. VNU Science Press, Utrecht, The Netherlands.

SASS, B. *et al.* 1975. Incidence of spontaneous neoplasms in F344 rats throughout the natural lifespan. J. Natl. Cancer Inst. *54*, 1449–1456.

SCHMUCKER, D. L. and WANG, R. K. 1981. Effects of aging and phenobarbital on the rat liver microsomal drug-metabolizing system. Mech. Aging Dev. *15*, 189–202.

SCHNEIDER, D., NARYSHKIN, S. and LANG, C. A. 1982. Blood glutathione: a biochemical index of aging women. Fed. Proc. *41*, 7671.

SCHNEIDER, E. L. and REED, J. D. 1985. Modulation of the aging process. *In* Handbook of Biology of Aging, 2nd Edition, C. E. Finch and E. L. Schneider (eds.). Van Nostrand Reinhold, New York.

SCHWAB, R., STAIANO-COICO, L. and WEKSLER, M. E. 1983. Immunological studies in aging: IX. Quantitative differences in T lymphocyte subsets in young and old individuals. Diagn. Immunol. *1*, 195–198.

SETLOW, R. B. 1982. DNA repair, aging and cancer. Natl. Cancer Inst. Monogr. *60*, 249–255.

STAATS, J. 1980. Standardized nomenclature for inbred strains of mice: Seventh listing. Cancer Res. *40*, 2083–2185.

STAIANO-COICO, L. *et al.* 1983. Increased sensitivity of lymphocytes from people over 65 to cell cycle arrest and chomosomal changes. Science *219*, 1335–1337.

STAIANO-COICO, L., DANZYNKIEWICZ, Z., MELAMED, M. R. and WEKSLER, M. E. 1982. Changes in DNA content of human blood mononuclear cells with senescence. Cytometry *3*, 79–83.

STANBRIDGE, E. J. 1985. A case for human tumor-suppressor genes. Bioessays *3*, 252–256.

STENBÄCK, F., PETO, R. and SHUBIK, P. 1981a. Initiation and promotion at different ages and doses in 2200 mice. I. Methods and the apparent persistence of initiated cells. Br. J. Cancer *44*, 1–14.

STENBÄCK, F., PETO, R. and SHUBIK, P. 1981b. Initiation and promotion at different ages and doses in 2200 mice. II. Decrease in promotion by TPA with aging. Br. J. Cancer *44*, 15–23.

STENBÄCK, F., PETO, R. and SHUBIK, P. 1981c. Initiation and promotion at different ages and doses in 2200 mice. III. Linear extrapolation from high doses may underestimate low-dose tumor risks. Br. J. Cancer *44*, 24–34.

STENBÄCK, F., WEISBURGER, J. H. and WILLIAMS, G. M. 1987. Hydroxylamine effects on cryptogenic neoplasm development in C3H mice. Cancer Letter. *38*, 73–85

STENBÄCK, F., WEISBURGER, J. H. and WILLIAMS, G. M. 1988. Effect of lifetime administration of dimethylaminoethanol on longevity, aging changes and cryptogenic neoplasms in C3H mice. Mech. Aging Dev. *42*, 129–138.

STJERNWÄRD, T. 1966. Age-dependent tumor-host barrier and effect of carcinogen-induced immunodepression on rejection of isografted methylcholanthrene-induced sarcoma cells. J. Natl. Cancer Inst. *37*, 505–512.

STORER, J. B. 1966. Longevity and gross pathology at death in 22 inbred mouse strains. J. Gerontol. *21*, 404–409.

STREHLER, B. L. 1982. Aging: concepts and theories. *In* Lectures on Gerontology, Vol 1: On Biology of Aging, Part A, A. Viidik (ed.). Academic Press, London.

STUKONIS, M. K. 1979. Cancer Cumulative Risk (IARC Int. Tech. Rept. No. 79/004). IARC (Int. Agency for Research on Cancer), Lyon.

TANNENBAUM, A. 1942. The genesis and growth of tumors. II. Effects of caloric restriction *per se*. Cancer Res. *2*, 460.

WATTENBERG, L. W. 1980. Inhibitors of chemical carcinogens. J. Environ. Pathol. Toxicol. *3*, 35–52.

WATTENBERG, L. W. 1985. Chemoprevention of cancer. Cancer Res. *45*, 1–8.

WEBER, H. V. and MIQUEL, J. 1986. Antioxidant supplementation and longevity. *In* Nutritional Aspects of Aging, L. H. Chen (ed.). CRC Press, Boca Raton, FL.

WEINDRUCH, R. and WALFORD, R. L. 1982. Dietary restrictions in mice beginning at 1 year of age: effect on lifespan and spontaneous cancer incidence. Science *215*, 1415–1418.

WEINDRUCH, R. and WALFORD, R. L. 1988. The Retardation of Aging and Disease by Dietary Restriction. Charles C. Thomas, Springfield, IL.

WEISBURGER, J. H. and WILLIAMS, G. M. 1981. Carcinogen testing. Current problems and new approaches. Science *214*, 401–407.

WEISBURGER, J. H. and WILLIAMS, G. M. 1982. Chemical carcinogenesis. *In* Cancer Medicine, 2nd Edition, J. F. Holland and E. Frei, III, (eds.). Lea & Febiger, Philadelphia.

WEISBURGER, J. H. *et al.* 1980. Dietary factors in the causation and prevention of neoplasia. *In* Challenges and Prospects for the 1980's, Vol. 1, J. Burchenal and H. Oettgen (eds.). Grune & Stratton, Inc., New York.

WILLETT, W. and MACMAHON, B. 1984. Diet and cancer: An overview. N. Engl. J. Med. *310*, 633–638, 697–703.

WILLIAMS, G. M. and WEISBURGER, J. H. 1986. Chemical carcinogenesis. *In* Toxicology, the Basic Science of Poisons, 3rd Edition, J. Doull, E. D. Klaassen and M. O. Amdur (eds.). Macmillan Publishing Co., New York.

YANCIC, R. 1983. Frames of reference: Old age as the context for prevention and treatment of cancer. *In* Perspectives on Prevention and Treatment of Cancer in the Elderly, R. Yancic (ed.). Raven Press, New York.

YUHAS, J. M. and ULLRICH, R. L. 1976. Responsiveness of senescent mice to the antitumor properties of *Corynebacte panvum*. Cancer Res. *36*, 162.

CHAPTER 4

THE RELATIONSHIP OF NUTRITIONAL VARIABLES TO AGING: RESULTS FROM THE BALTIMORE LONGITUDINAL STUDY OF AGING

JUDITH HALLFRISCH, Ph.D.
Gerontology Research Center
National Institute on Aging
Baltimore, Maryland

For centuries, the connection between a prudent diet and a long, healthy life has been known:

. . .If thou well observe
The rule of not too much, by temperance taught
In what thou eat and drink, seeking from thence
Due nourishment, not gluttonous delight,
Till many years over thy head return:
So may thou live, till like ripe Fruit thou drop
Into thy Mother's lap, or be with ease
Gathered, not harshly plucked, for death mature.
John Milton
Paradise Lost, Book XI (1667)

This quote from *Paradise Lost* prefaced the Nutrition and Aging Chapter of the recent Surgeon General's Report on Nutrition and Health (USDHHS 1988). The report suggests that over two-thirds of the deaths in this country are due to diseases which are affected by diet (coronary heart disease, stroke, diabetes, atherosclerosis, and some forms of cancer). If one includes excessive alcohol intake as a nutritional problem, 3 more of the 10 leading causes of death (accident, suicide, and liver disease) would be considered to be affected by diet. By stretching one's imagination, the other causes of death in the top ten (chronic obstructive lung disease and pneumonia or influenza) could also be considered to be related to diet. Dietary vitamin A is reported to be a protective factor in maintenance of epithelial cells, including lung (DeLuca *et al.* 1972), and relationships between immune function, infection and malnutrition are well established (Chandra and Puri 1985). Specific nutrients are now being examined (Beisel 1982). Thus diet can affect all 10 leading causes of death in this country (Table 4.1).

TABLE 4.1
10 LEADING CAUSES OF DEATH: UNITED STATES 1987

Rank	Cause of Death	Number	%Total
1	Heart diseases[1]	759,400	35.7
2	Cancers[1]	476,700	22.4
3	Strokes[1]	148,700	7.0
4	Unintentional[2]	92,500	4.4
5	COPD	78,000	3.7
6	Pneumonia and influenza	68,600	3.2
7	Diabetes mellitus[1]	37,800	1.8
8	Suicide[2]	29,600	1.4
9	Liver disease/cirrhosis[2]	26,000	1.2
10	Atherosclerosis[1]	23,100	1.1
		2,125,100	100.0

Source: National Center for Health Statistics (1988).
[1]Diet a factor.
[2]Excessive alcohol a factor.

The prevalence of coronary heart disease, the leading cause of death in this county, increases with age from about one person in a thousand under age 45 to well over 100 per thousand in both men and women over 75 (Table 4.2) (National Center for Health Statistics 1988). There are a variety of nutritional factors in addition to the well-established relationship of saturated fat and cholesterol that might affect cor-

TABLE 4.2
PREVALENCE OF CORONARY HEART DISEASE BY AGE, RACE, AND SEX, UNITED STATES, 1985
(Prevalence per 1000 persons)

Age	Men	Women	White	Black
Total	32.9	24.7	31.8	11.3
Under 45	0.9	1.6	1.3	1.1
45–64	80.9	44.4	65.1	46.3
65–74	175.6	107.0	143.9	62.2
75+	169.0	124.6	154.7	NR

Source: National Center for Health Statistics (1985).

onary heart disease (Table 4.3) (USDHHS 1988). Some of these are secondary effects. For example, obesity promotes hypertension, hyperlipidemia, and hyperglycemia—all risk factors for coronary disease. Some effects are secondary to deficiency syndromes, such as beriberi and scurvy. The fact that a deficiency of a specific nutrient causes coronary abnormalities does not mean that excessive or pharmacologic amounts will prevent or cure heart disease.

TABLE 4.3
DIETARY FACTORS IN CHD

Factor	Mechanism
Obesity	Promotes hypertension, hyperglycemia, hyperlipidemia
Alcohol	Light/moderate—increases HDL. Heavy—cardiomyopathy, hypertension
Carbohydrate	Complex lowers risk, sugars may increase lipids, glucose, blood pressure
Protein	High levels animal protein may increase risk
Coffee	Mixed reviews. > 4 cups may increase cholesterol
Vitamin E	No controlled studies
Vitamin C	Conflicting results, scurvy associated with abnormalities
Thiamin	Beriberi associated with congestive heart failure
Niacin	Pharmacologic doses ↑HDL and ↓VLDL; with colestipol and cholesterol-lowering diet, slow progression of lesions
Calcium	Reduces cholesterol levels
Magnesium	May correct arrhythmias; may protect against excessive calcium
Copper	Deficiency increases cholesterol
Zinc	Possibly high doses decrease HDL
Selenium	Deficiency results in cardiomyopathy

Source: U.S. DHHS (1988)

Cancers are the second leading cause of death in the United States. They cause 22% of total deaths. A number of these cancers may be modified by diet (Table 4.4). However, some of these effects may also be secondary to obesity. Breast, colon, prostate, endometrial, kidney, cervical, and thyroid cancers have all been reported to be positively correlated with body weight (Sondik *et al.* 1987). Fat intake is also correlated with a number of these cancers. Fiber and fruit and vegetable intakes are inversely related to a number of cancers (cervix, prostate, and digestive tract). Many of these relationships are based on epidemiological data. In view of the covariability of nutrient factors, it is difficult to separate out one as a cause. For example, a diet high in fruits and vegetables is automatically high in fiber and low in fat. It also is probably low in calories and therefore would be unlikely to promote obesity. Many animal studies and some controlled human studies are now examining the effects of specific nutrients either on tumor growth or on the removal of carcinogenic substances from the body (Hebert and Miller 1988).

TABLE 4.4
RELATIONSHIP BETWEEN DIET AND CANCER

Type/Rate[1]	Diet Components
Lung/55	(−)Fruits, vegetables. (+)alcohol
Breast/51	(+)Fat, body weight, calories, alcohol
Colon/36	(+)Fat, body weight, calories, (−)fiber, fruits, vegetables
Prostate/34	(+)Fat, body weight, calories, (−)fruits, vegetables
Bladder/16	(−)Fruits, vegetables
Rectum/15	(+)Fat, alcohol
Endometrium/13	(+)Fat, body weight, calories
Oral cavity/11	(−)Fruits, vegetables, (+)alcohol
Stomach/8	(−)Fruits, vegetables, (+)smoked, salted, pickled foods
Kidney/8	(+)Body weight, calories
Cervix/5	(+)Body weight, calories, (−)fruits, vegetables
Thyroid/4	(+)Body weight, calories
Esophagus/4	(+)Alcohol, smoked, salted, pickled foods

Source: Sondik (1987).
[1]Rate per 100,000 population.

Stroke is the third leading cause of death in the United States. Hypertension is one of the most prevalent conditions affecting older Americans (Table 4.5). Prevalence rates as percentage based on either an average of 3 blood pressure measurements over 140/90 mm Hg or reported treatment with antihypertensive medication show a steady increase with age in both sexes (Subcommittee 1985). Blacks have higher rates of hypertension than observed among whites. While sodium restriction is the major dietary intervention used to control hypertension, many nutrients can raise or lower blood pressure (Table 4.6) (McCarron *et al.* 1982). There are a number of other minerals including K, Ca, P, Mg, and Mn that may affect

TABLE 4.5
HYPERTENSION PREVALENCE RATES(%) BY SEX, RACE, AND AGE IN THE CIVILIAN, NONINSTITUTIONALIZED POPULATION, 1976–80

	Men		Women	
Age	Whites	Blacks	Whites	Blacks
All	32.6	37.9	25.3	38.6
18–24	16.2	10.9	2.3	9.6
25–34	21.1	23.2	5.7	15.3
35–44	26.4	44.2	16.6	37.0
45–54	42.6	55.2	36.3	67.4
55–64	51.4	66.3	50.0	74.3
65–74	59.2	67.1	66.2	82.9

Source: Subcommittee of the 1984 Joint National Committee (1985).

TABLE 4.6
NUTRIENTS WHICH MAY AFFECT BLOOD PRESSURE

Nutrient	Mechanisms
Total calories	Obesity, energy generation
Carbohydrates/alcohol	Membrane synthesis, insulin regulation/sodium excretion Catecholamine regulation—vascular tone
Proteins	Protein/peptide synthesis cellular function membrane transport
Lipids	Prostaglandin synthesis
Sodium	Intravascular volume, hormone regulation, membrane potential
Potassium	Vascular tone, hormone regulation, cation transport
Calcium	Receptor-ligand binding, hormone regulation, vascular tone, contractile protein interactions
Magnesium	Regulation of Ca^{++} channels, ATP production, contractile protein interaction
Phosphorus	ATP—energy metabolism, cAMP
Copper	Vascular integrity
Manganese	Energy metabolism
Chromium	Lipid metabolism
Vanadium	Sodium/potassium, ATP-ase

Source: McCarron *et al.* (1982).

blood pressure through a variety of mechanisms. Lipids, especially certain fatty acids, may affect production of prostaglandins, thereby altering blood pressure. Sucrose and fructose may increase blood pressure by increasing sodium retention. Total calorie intake may secondarily increase blood pressure by encouraging obesity.

The Baltimore Longitudinal Study of Aging (BLSA) is one of the few in which detailed diet intake information has been collected over a long enough period of time to relate specific nutrient intakes to outcome variables such as risk factors for, development of, and mortality from specific diseases. Since this population also provides detailed medical, physiological and biochemical data along with diet information, it is possible to distinguish changes which occur as a natural consequence of aging from changes resulting from the development of disease. Over the 30 years the study has been progressing, a number of studies involving nutritional factors and their relationship to aging have been reported. This review will attempt to cover those reports and present future projects in the BLSA involving the effects of nutrition on aging.

Dietary information collected from the BLSA is unusual in two respects. First, it consists of 7-day dietary records which are considered much more reliable than the more commonly used 24-h recall, and, second, it is longitudinal with the same men providing multiple records for over more than a 25-year span. From 1961–1975 detailed 7-day diet records were collected from men of the longitudinal study between their periodical visits. The men were instructed by dietitians during their regular visits to the Gerontology Research Center. Records were reviewed, corrected, and coded for computer analysis. Analysis of intake was based on U.S. Department of Agriculture Handbook 8 (Watt and Merrill 1975). A longitudinal analysis of these data was published in 1983 (Elahi *et al.* 1983).

One hundred eighty men provided diet records in each of three 5-year time periods (1961–5, 1966–70, 1971–5). Age distribution over the life span was reasonably well balanced (Table 4.7). To attempt to separate aging, cohort, and secular effects, a series of cross-sectional, longitudinal, and time-series analyses were conducted. The effect of age on a number of dietary variables was measured. Age was considered to affect the variable if the cross-sectional and longitudinal analyses detected differences. For example, older men ate more fiber within time periods, and men ate more fiber as time progressed. Cohort was considered significant if cross-sectional and time series effects were significant. For example, men born from 1910–20 drank less alcohol throughout their lives than other age groups. A secular effect was noted if longitudinal and time-series analyses were significant. For example, P/S (polyunsaturated to saturated fatty acid) ratio increased as time progressed, and men of similar ages had higher P/S ratios in the later than in the earlier time periods.

Nutritional variables for which there were significant effects include calories, carbohydrate, fat, polyunsaturated to saturated fatty acid (P/S) ratio, and cholesterol intake. Generally, protein intake was stable across the age span while fat declined and carbohydrate increased (Table 4.8). The proportion of fat in the diet decreased

TABLE 4.7
DESIGN OF ELAHI ANALYSIS

	Time		
Age	1961–5	1966–70	1971–5
80–84	—	—	14
75–79	—	14	18
70–74	14	18	20
65–69	18	20	23
60–64	20	23	40
55–59	23	40	24
50–54	40	24	23
45–49	24	23	18
40–44	23	18	—
35–39	18	—	—

Effect		Significant
Aging	=	Cross-sectional Longitudinal
Cohort	=	Cross-sectional Time
Secular	=	Longitudinal Time

TABLE 4.8
SUMMARY OF RESULTS FROM 1961–75

Factor	Effects
Calories	Aging decrease
Kcal/kg	None
% Protein	None
% CHO	None
% Fat	Aging decrease
P/S ratio	Secular increase
Cholesterol	Aging, secular, some cohort decreases

Source: Elahi *et al.* (1983).

longitudinally and cross-sectionally with age, but not with time which indicated an aging effect on fat intake. However, analyses of cholesterol intake and P/S ratio show a secular change in the character of the fat the men consumed.

Longitudinal analysis of cholesterol intake shows a marked longitudinal decline in all age groups. There was an overall cross-sectional decline in intake with increasing age. Comparison of similar age groups during the three time periods reveal an overall decline with time and some significant cohort decreases. Therefore, secular and aging effects are significantly reflecting both a greater concern with health as men advance into middle and later age, public promotion of low cholesterol diets, as well as availability of more low-cholesterol products in the food supply. The increase in P/S ratio seen longitudinally and over time, but not cross-sectionally reflects a secular change in the types of fat the men were consuming regardless of age. This change also reflects a greater awareness of the impact of diet on development of heart disease and the change in lipids in the food supply.

In 1984 after a 9-year hiatus, collection of diet records resumed. A similar analysis was conducted on intake data from 79 men who provided diet records in 3 decades (1960s, 1970s, 1980s). Preliminary results of this analysis were presented earlier (Hallfrisch *et al.* 1988a). These men initially ranged in age from 27–65 years and, finally, from 39–93 years. Analysis of intake since 1984 was based on updated information from the USDA from 1976–87 (U.S. Dept of Agriculture 1988). Only nutrients for which adequate data were available in the 1960s were included in the longitudinal analysis. Over the 25-year span the diets of these 79 men changed dramatically (Table 4.9). As their average age increased from 47 to 69 years, body mass index (BMI), % carbohydrate, % ethanol, fiber, and P/S ratio increased while kcal, kcal/kg, % fat, and cholesterol intake all decreased. Within individual decades some significant effects of age were noted. In the 1960s older men consumed a higher proportion of their calories as protein than younger men, while the total intake and kcal/kg were both lower in older than in younger men. There were no significant cross-sectional differences attributed to age in the 1970s, but in the 1980s both % carbohydrate and fiber intake were higher in older men than younger men. These changes in the 1980s could reflect the fact that the whole group of 79 men is older.

TABLE 4.9
LONGITUDINAL AND CROSS-SECTIONAL ANALYSES OF DIET INTAKE IN 79 MEN OF THE BALTIMORE STUDY

	1960s	1970s	1980s	LC[1]
Age	46	57	69	↑
BMI	24.7	25.3	25.7	↑
Kcal	2544↓[2]	2289	2195	↓
Kcal/Kg	33.4↓[2]	29.5	28.0↑[3]	x
% Protein	15.4↑[3]	15.9	15.7	—
% Fat	42.4	40.9	35.3	↓
% Carbohydrate	39.0	38.3	43.9↑[3]	↑
% Et OH	3.2	4.9	5.2	↑
Cholesterol (mg)	609	489	388	↓
Fiber (g)	4.3	4.9	5.7↑[3]	↑
P/S ratio	0.33	0.46	0.57	↑

[1]LC Longitudinal change, $P < 0.05$.
[2]Inversely correlated with age, $P < 0.05$.
[3]Positively correlated with age, $P < 0.05$.

Elahi *et al.* (1983) found a cross-sectional effect of age on % carbohydrate at three different times from 1961–1975.

By dividing these 79 men into purely arbitrary age groups labeled young, middle, and old, it is possible to examine cohort differences and secular trends of similar age groups (Table 4.10). BMI increased in the two younger groups while kcal/kg decreased. Total calories decreased in all groups. Protein intake increased only in the middle-aged group. Percentage of calories from fat and cholesterol intake decreased in all age groups while P/S ratio increased, indicating both a reduction in overall fat and an improvement in the type of fat consumed (Table 4.11). These changes reflect secular change in diet. Fiber and % calories from carbohydrate increases in the two older age groups indicated a change also in the type of carbohydrate consumed, with the greater emphasis recently on complex rather than simple sources. Ethanol intake was lower throughout in older men, highest in the middle-aged group, and increased with time in the young men. These are examples of cohort differences. The diet trends reported by Elahi *et al.* (1983) and continued into the 1980s to reflect the growing awareness of the importance of diet to health and suggest that beneficial changes in diet can be made at any age.

B_6 intakes in many older Americans are below RDA standards, even though changes with age in the metabolism of this vitamin may actually result in higher requirements than present RDA levels (Suter and Russell 1987). Rose *et al.* (1976) examined the B_6 status of 617 men of the BLSA. This group of men ranged in age from 18–90 (Table 4.12). Detailed vitamin intake information was collected to determine the level of B_6 supplementation. Plasma pyridoxal phosphate (PLP) determined by a radioimmunoassay using tyrosine decarboxylase was used as a measure of B_6 status.

TABLE 4.10
LONGITUDINAL ANALYSIS BY AGE GROUPS

	1960	1970	1980	LC[1]
Age				
Young (17)	37	48	59	↑
Middle (39)	47	57	69	↑
Old (19)	54	66	77	↑
BMI				
Young	24.4	25.6	26.0	↑
Middle	24.7	25.3	25.7	↑
Old	24.7	24.9	25.3	—
Kcal				
Young	2787	2333	2243	↓
Middle	2479	2312	2192	↓
Old	2391	2213	2193	↓
Kcal/kg				
Young	36.8	29.6	28.3	↓
Middle	32.8	30.1	28.2	↓
Old	31.3	28.9	28.5	—
% Protein				
Young	15.6	15.6	15.1	—
Middle	14.7	15.6	15.8	↑
Old	16.1	16.4	15.5	—

[1]LC = Longitudinal change, $P < 0.05$.

The men were divided into supplemented and unsupplemented age categories. About one-third of the men took supplements. Men taking supplements had higher PLP levels. Among unsupplemented men a significant decline in PLP with age was observed. Only 3% of men under 40 had PLP levels below 5 ng/ml, but 12% of those over 80 would be considered deficient. If 10 ng/ml is considered as the minimum acceptable level, then 28% of men under 40 and 83% of those over 80 were deficient. Reduced absorption or impaired formation of pyridoxal phophate or increased urinary excretion may be responsible for the decline with age in B_6 levels (Suter and Russell 1987).

Many researchers have reported declining overall intakes of food with aging. McGandy *et al.* (1966) examined the reasons for this decline by plotting differences with age in physical activity, basal energy expenditure and dietary intake. Along with 7-day diet records, 252 men aged 20–99 years completed detailed physical activity records and had basal oxygen consumption measured. Total calorie intake decreased from about 2700 kcal in men in their 20s to about 2100 kcal in men over 75 (Table 4.13). Basal metabolic rate declined from about 1600 to 1300 kcal, only about half of the reduction in intake. The rest of the difference is the result of the decline in expenditure from physical activity which fell from 44% of total intake

TABLE 4.11
LONGITUDINAL ANALYSIS BY AGE GROUPS

	1960	1970	1980	LC[1]
% Fat				
Young	42.1	41.9	36.7	↓
Middle	41.8	40.2	34.6	↓
Old	43.3	41.7	35.2	↓
% Carbohydrate				
Young	39.8	38.5	42.8	—
Middle	39.2	37.9	43.1	↑
Old	38.0	38.8	46.3	↑
% Ethanol				
Young	2.3	4.5	5.5	↑
Middle	4.2	6.2	6.4	—
Old	2.5	3.1	3.0	—
Cholesterol (mg)				
Young	627	480	415	↓
Middle	567	495	361	↓
Old	687	502	413	↓
P/S ratio				
Young	0.30	0.47	0.53	↑
Middle	0.33	0.43	0.54	↑
Old	0.34	0.50	0.62	↑
Fiber intake				
Young	4.4	4.6	4.9	—
Middle	4.2	4.3	5.6	↑
Old	4.6	4.5	6.7	↑

[1]LC = Longitudinal change, $P < 0.05$.

calories for men in their 20s to 31% for men over 75 years. Much more elaborate techniques are available for measures of energy expenditure than when this paper was published in 1966, but its conclusions have been repeatedly confirmed (Forbes and Reina 1973; Munro 1982). Much of the reduction in intake as people age can be attributed to a decrease physical activity.

One of the most potentially important aspects of the long-term collection of data from the BLSA is that now previous diet intake can be related to physical conditions and diseases or risk factors for them which appear much later in life. Herschcopf *et al.* (1982) examined changes in serum cholesterol, a well-known risk factor for cardiovascular disease, in relation to dietary variables. Serum levels were determined in 783 men from 1963 to 1977. Each of these men provided at least two blood samples over the 14-year span and were taking no drug or had no disease known to affect serum cholesterol. Over this period a significant drop in serum cholesterol was noted. Cholesterol level increased to age 60 and then declined; but for each age group the level was lower in the 1970s than in the 1960s, indicating both secular and aging differences. Changes in diet which occurred over this time that were not

TABLE 4.12
EFFECT OF AGE AND B_6 SUPPLEMENTATION
ON PLASMA PYRIDOXAL PHOSPHATE LEVELS

Age	n	No Supplement	%	Supplement	%
18–29	35	14.6	74	25.4	26
30–39	58	14.8	74	19.6	26
40–49	111	13.2	74	20.3	26
50–59	153	11.6	75	24.6	25
60–69	111	12.2	53	20.8	47
70–79	117	11.8	56	18.0	44
80–90	32	7.7	75	13.3	25
	617	12.3	67	20.5	33

Source: Rose *et al.* (1976).

related to changes in cholesterol were an increase in polyunsaturated fatty acids and decreases in saturated fatty acids and cholesterol. These changes would all be expected to lower cholesterol. A number of nutrient variables were analyzed with respect to these changes. Changes in cholesterol were correlated with changes in weight, BMI, and kilocalories which would suggest that weight loss is the most important change one could make to lower blood cholesterol. Different fractions of cholesterol and many more dietary variables now are being measured to more fully understand the relationship between diet and serum cholesterol.

Serum cholesterol and a number of other risk factors for cardiovascular disease were examined in relation to fiber intake (Hallfrisch *et al.* 1988c). Longitudinal changes in fiber intake of 380 men showed an increase with age in all age groups (Fig. 4.1). After adjusting for age and obesity, effects of fiber intake on serum cholesterol, triglycerides, fasting and 2-h glucose, and systolic and diastolic blood pressure were determined. Men were divided into quintiles of fiber intake. For each variable, men taking drugs or with conditions which would affect that variable were removed from the analysis. Serum cholesterol data from 557 men were used. Men

TABLE 4.13
ENERGY INTAKE AND EXPENDITURE FROM PHYSICAL ACTIVITY
OF MEN OF DIFFERENT AGES

Age	n	Intake	Expenditure	%
20–34	13	2688	1175	44
35–44	32	2639	1166	44
45–54	41	2454	982	40
55–64	34	2332	950	41
65–74	36	2297	928	40
75–99	13	2093	640	31

Source: McGandy *et al.* (1966).

consuming the most fiber had the lowest cholesterol levels, though the effect was not statistically significant. For serum triglycerides, data were transformed to logarithms due to nonhomogeneity of variance. Men who consumed the most fiber had significantly lower plasma triglycerides than men consuming the least fiber ($P < 0.05$). For fasting and 2-h glucose levels, similar patterns were seen. For fasting glucose the inverse relationship between fiber and glucose intake was statistically significant ($P < 0.002$). Both systolic and diastolic blood pressure were analyzed in relation to fiber intake ($n = 739$). All data were adjusted for age and BMI. Fiber intake again was inversely related to both systolic ($P < 0.005$) and diastolic blood pressure ($P < 0.05$). Thus, for all six risk factors for cardiovascular disease, higher fiber intake was associated with lower risk.

Since the longitudinal study has been in progress for almost 30 years, it is now possible to begin relating previous dietary intake to development of various diseases. A number of projects are in initial analysis or planning stages. Preliminary results of a case-control study examining the effects of diet on the development of colon polyps indicate a number of differences between the diets of 36 cases compared with controls matched for age, date of visit and occupation (Cheskin *et al.* 1987). Subjects consumed less fiber, complex carbohydrate and more alcohol than controls. A similar prospective case-control study examined diet and cardiovascular death (Hallfrisch *et al.* 1985). Men who died of cardiovascular disease were matched for age, BMI and smoking class. Diets of controls were compared to diets of men who died of cardiovascular disease. Men over 75 who died consumed less fiber and had a lower P/S ratio than survivors. They actually consumed less total kcal and kcal/kg

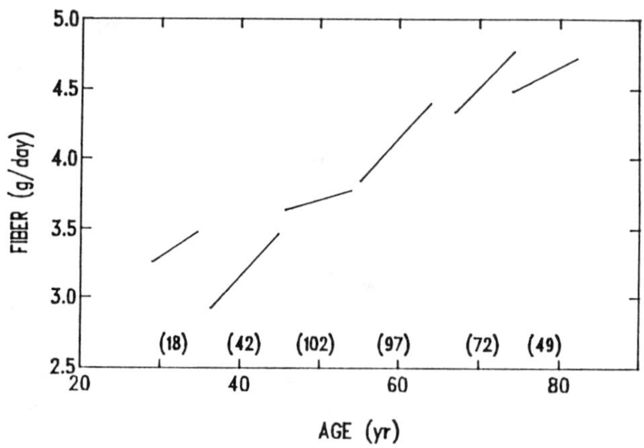

From Hallfrisch et al. (1988c)

FIG. 4.1. LONGITUDINAL ANALYSIS OF CRUDE FIBER INTAKE (ADJUSTED FOR TOTAL CALORIES) VERSUS AGE IN 380 MEN OF THE BALTIMORE LONGITUDINAL STUDY OF AGING and less total fat than controls. This observation may be related to differences in physical activity. Mortality from stroke is being examined in relation to diet and sodium and potassium excretion.

According to the free-radical theory of aging, aging occurs as a result of the cell's inability to remove damaging superoxide and peroxide radicals (Harmon 1981). Superoxide dismutase, an enzyme that detoxifies these compounds has been measured in about 400 subjects aged 17–93 (Hallfrisch *et al.* 1986). Levels declined with age in women. These results will be evaluated in relation to both intake and plasma levels of antioxidant vitamins. Retinol, β-carotene, and α-tocopherol levels were measured in the entire BLSA population (Hallfrisch *et al.* 1988a). About 40% of the women and 30% of the men were taking a supplement containing one of these vitamins. In people taking no supplements, retinol was higher in men than women and tended to increase with age. β-Carotene levels were higher in women than men. People taking vitamin A supplements had higher levels of β-carotene than those who did not, but retinol levels were not affected by vitamin A supplementation. α-Tocopherol levels did not differ between the sexes, but were significantly higher in people taking supplements. These results will also be used to examine the relationships of these vitamins to pulmonary function and to macular degeneration.

There is no doubt that diet plays a role in maintenance of health into later years. Thus, the detailed longitudinal nutrition intake information combined with biochemical parameters of nutritional status and medical, physiological and psychological data collected in the Baltimore Study provides an impressive bank of information that can be used to examine nutrition and aging in the years to come.

REFERENCES

BEISEL, W. R. 1982. Single nutrients and immunity. Am. J. Clin. Nutri. *35* (Suppl.), 417–468.

CHANDRA, R. K. and PURI, S. 1985. Nutritional support improves antibody response to influenza virus vaccine in the elderly. Brit. Med. J. *291*, 705–706.

CHESKIN, L. J., GITTINGS, N. and HALLFRISCH, J. 1987. Dietary history and the risk of colorectal polyps in the Baltimore Longitudinal Study population, 1961–75. Gastroenterology *92*, 1343. (Abstr.)

DELUCA, L., MAESTRI, N., BONANNI, F. and NELSON, D. 1972. Maintenance of epithelial cell differentiation: The mode of action of vitamin A. Cancer *30*, 1326–1331.

ELAHI, V. K. *et al.* 1983. A longitudinal study of nutritional intake in men. J. Gerontol. *38*, 162–180.

FORBES, G. B. and REINA, J. C. 1973. Adult lean body declines with age some longitudinal observation. Metabolism *19*, 653–663.

HALLFRISCH, J. *et al.* 1985. Diet and cardiovascular death in men of the Baltimore Longitudinal Study on Aging. *In* Proceeding of the XIII International Congress of Nutrition, T. G. Taylor and M. K. Jenkins (eds.). John Libby, London.

HALLFRISCH, J., ANDRES, R. and MULLER, D. 1986. Erythrocyte superoxide dismutase in the Baltimore Longitudinal Study on Aging. Fed. Proc. *45*, 828 (Abstr.)

HALLFRISCH, J., MULLER, D., ANDRES, R. and SINGH, V. N. 1988a. Plasma levels and supplement use of fat soluble antioxidant vitamins in the Baltimore Study. Gerontologist *28*, 230A.

HALLFRISCH, J. *et al.* 1988b. Diet trends: The Baltimore Longitudinal Study (1961–1986). FASEB J. *2*, A1423.

HALLFRISCH, J., TOBIN, J. D., MULLER, D. C., ANDRES, R. 1988C. Fiber intake, age, and other coronary risk factors in men of the Baltimore Longitudinal Study (1959–1975). J. Gerontol. Medical Sci. *43*, M64–M68.

HARMON, D. 1981. The aging process. Proc. Natl. Acad. Sci. *78*, 7124–7128.

HEBERT, J. R. and MILLER, D. R. 1988. Methodologic considerations for investigating the diet-cancer link. Am. J. Clin. Nutri. *47*, 1068–1077.

HERSCHCOPF, R. J. *et al.* 1982. Longitudinal changes in serum cholesterol in man: An epidemiologic search for an etiology. J. Chron. Dis. *35*, 101–114.

KEYS, A., TAYLOR , H. L. and GRANDE, F. 1973. Basal metabolism and age of adult men. Metabolism *22*, 579–587.

McCARRON, D. A., HENRY, H. J. and MORRIS, C. D. 1982. Human nutrition and blood pressure regulation: An integrated approach. Hypertension *4*(5), 2–13.

McGANDY, R. B. *et al.* 1966. Nutrient intakes and energy expenditure in men of different ages. J. Gerontol. *21*, 581–587.

MUNRO, H. N. 1982. Nutritional requirements in the elderly. Hosp. Pract. *17*, 143.

National Center for Health Statistics. 1986. Current Estimates from the National Health Interview Survey, United States, 1985. Vital and Health Statistics, Ser. 10, No. 160. DHHS Publ. 86–1588.

National Center for Health Statistics. 1988. Monthly Vital Stat. Rep. *37*, (1).

ROSE, C. S. *et al.* 1976. Age differences in vitamin B_6 status of 617 men. Am. J. Clin. Nutri. *29*, 847–853.

SONDIK, E. J., YOUNG, J. L., HORN, J. W. and RIES, L. A. 1987. Annual Cancer Statistics Review. NIH Publ. No. 87–2789. National Cancer Institute, Bethesda, MD.

Subcommittee of the 1984 Joint National Committee. 1985. Hypertension prevalence and the status of awareness, treatment and control in the United States. Final report. Hypertension *7*, 457–468.

SUTER, P. M. and RUSSELL, R. M. 1987. Vitamin requirements of the elderly. Am. J. Clin. Nutr. *45*, 501–512.

U.S.Dept. of Agriculture. 1988. Composition of Foods-raw, processed, prepared. Handbook No. 8. USDA, Washington, D.C.

U.S. DHHS. 1988. The Surgeon General's Report on Nutrition and Health. DHHS(PHS) Publ. No. 88-50210. U.S. Dept. of Health and Human Services, Washington, D.C.

WATT, B. K. and MERRILL, A. L. 1975. Composition of Foods. Agriculture Handbook No. 8. USDA, Washington, D.C.

CHAPTER 5

METABOLIC CHANGES IN AGING AS PREDICTORS OF DISEASE: THE SWEDISH EXPERIENCE

ALVAR SVANBORG, M.D., Ph.D.
Department of Geriatric Medicine
University of Gothenburg
Gothenburg, Sweden
and
Section of Geriatric Medicine
College of Medicine
University of Illinois at Chicago
Chicago, Illinois

and

STAFFAN EDEN, M.D., Ph.D. and DAN MELLSTROM, M.D., Ph.D.
Department of Geriatric Medicine
University of Gothenburg
Gothenburg, Sweden

The identification of changes in the metabolism at the cellular, organ, or organ system level primarily and directly caused by aging processes is obviously difficult. Changes in social roles, physical activity, eating habits with obvious metabolic consequences occur over the life span whether they are related to aging per se or not. In the global perspective, great variations of a cultural, socioeconomic, and demographic nature also limit possibilities to generalize about age-related metabolic changes. The differences between different species in life span, diet, body temperature, activity, etc., obviously also restrict the possibilities to generalize to the human from studies in experimental animals.

The metabolic consequences of aging can be expected to become most obvious when we are old, and the reserve capacities of organs are so limited that they influence, in general terms, "functional performance." At these ages morbidity, however, is common; and attempts have to be made to differentiate between physiology and pathology.

A prerequisite for studies of age-related metabolic changes in humans are, thus, broad and longitudinal population studies of biochemical, physiological, and morphological parameters in individuals whose state of health, lifestyle, and environment is known. In the epidemiologic perspective, it is also crucial to identify how representative a particular population studied is, i.e., to what extent samples studied allow generalizations to a whole population, or at least to a specified and identifiable part of a population.

The Swedish population has for several decades been the oldest in the world with a higher proportion reaching old age than in any other human population on earth. At the present time, about 18% are 65 years old or more (65+). Since 1971 a longitudinal study of 70 year olds has been performed in Gothenburg, which is the second largest city in Sweden with about 450,000 inhabitants in the downtown area and about 1 million in the metropolitan area. This population study (Rinder *et al.* 1975; Svanborg 1977; Svanborg *et al.* 1982; Svanborg 1988a) is different from most other longitudinal studies because the samples have been shown to be representative for the total population (Rinder *et al.* 1975; Berg 1980; Persson 1980; Nilsson-Ehle *et al.* 1988a, 1988b; Eriksson *et al.* 1987), the investigations are broad and cover areas of basic biology, clinical medicine, social and psychological perspectives. The longitudinal follow-ups have been performed without changes in the representativeness of the sample. The study includes also a comparison between 3 different age cohorts born within 5-year intervals (1901–02, 1906–07, 1911–12). At present (Table 5.1), the first age cohort has been followed from age 70 to age 85; the second, from age 70 to age 79; and to the third age cohort an intervention study has been added (Eriksson *et al.* 1987). The study thus allows a combination of longitudinal (retrospective and prospective) and cross-sectional comparisons (Svanborg 1988a).

This presentation is mainly based on results from this study of 70 year olds and will illustrate some observed age-associated morphological changes with obvious impact upon nutrition and metabolism, studies of the absorption of one nutrient (cobalamin) from the gastrointestinal tract, uptake of nutrients into muscle tissue and skeleton, and observations concerning age-associated changes in thyroid function. The analyses performed concern, e.g., diet and physical activity, height, body weight (BW) and body composition, a great number of blood components including blood glucose and free fatty acids (FFA), plasma cholesterol (CH), triglycerides (TG), total and individual phospholipids (PL), serum iron and cobalamin (B_{12}). Identical methods, or at least methods that allow comparison, have been used for some of these analyses in three epidemiological studies of younger adult age groups (Hallberg *et al.* 1966; Tibblin 1967; Bengtsson *et al.* 1973). This allows a combination of longitudinal, cross-sectional, and age cohort comparisons over a considerable

TABLE 5.1
THE PRESENT DESIGN OF THE LONGITUDINAL STUDY
OF 70 YEAR OLDS IN GOTEBORG, SWEDEN, SHOWING THE 3 AGE COHORTS

	Year		
Years of Investigation	*1901/02 H-70 (Age)*	*1906/07 H-70 (Age)*	*1911/12 IVEG[1] (Age)*
1971/72	70		
1976/77	75	70	
1980/81	79		
1981/82		75	70
1982/83	81		70
1983/84	82		72
1984/85	83		72
1985/86		79	
1986/87	85		
1987/88			76

[1]IVEG: Intervention programme (Inter-Vention Elderly in in Goteborg) added to the study of the third cohort.

part of the adult life span, as illustrated, e.g., by our previous studies of age-related changes in blood pressure (Landahl *et al.* 1986).

Analyses of dietary habits in this population sample have been reported from age 70 (Steen *et al.* 1977b; Steen 1987). Swedish dietary habits among elderly have also been reported from areas other than Gothenburg (Hansson *et al.* 1987; Steen *et al.* 1988; Nordstrom *et al.* 1988).

Earlier reports from numerous studies of age-related decline in body heights and body mass have generally been based on cross-sectional comparisons. They can, therefore, be misleading since ongoing age cohort differences in both heights and body weights in both males and females have influenced the conclusions.

In the Swedish population there is a slight decrease in height in the age interval 40–70, and there are reasons to believe that this decline is mainly due to an increased curvature of the spine, as well as in a few cases upon traumatic compression fractures of the vertebraes. During the same age period, BW increases (Larsson 1978).

Table 5.2 illustrates changes in height, BW, and body mass index [BMI = (body weight - height squared)] measured longitudinally between age 70 and 82 in the Gothenburg cohort born in 1901–02. Height declined at a similar rate in males and females, i.e., on an average with 0.21 cm/year in females and 0.2 cm/year in males. The average decline of BW was 0.6 kg (1% of BW) in females and 0.4 kg (0.5% of BW) in males.

Because of the differences in the age-related decline between height and BW, the BMI is thus higher at age 70 and above than at younger adult ages. Furthermore, we had expected to find a significant sex difference with a faster decline in height in females due to the well-known higher prevalence of osteoporosis in females than in males, but we found no obvious sex difference.

TABLE 5.2
LONGITUDINAL CHANGES IN HEIGHT, BODY WEIGHT AND BODY MASS INDEX (BMI) IN THE AGE INTERVAL OF 70–82 YEARS

	Females (N = 172)			*Males* (N = 110)		
Age	*Height (cm)*	*Weight (kg)*	*BMI*	*Height (cm)*	*Weight (kg)*	*BMI*
70	160.2±5.7	66.9±10.5	26.1±3.9	174.8±6.5	79.4±9.6	26.0±2.9
	$P < 0.001$	$P < 0.001$	$P < 0.05$	$P < 0.001$	$P < 0.001$	n.s.
75	159.3±5.6	65.4±10.3	25.8±4.0	173.4±6.5	77.5±10.0	25.8±3.1
	$P < 0.001$	$P < 0.001$	n.s.	$P < 0.001$	$P < 0.001$	$P < 0.05$
79	158.3±5.7	64.0±10.6	25.5±4.0	172.8±6.5	76.0±10.3	25.5±3.3
	$P < 0.01$	n.s.	n.s.	n.s.	$P < 0.001$	$P < 0.001$
81	158.0±5.9	63.7±11.0	25.5±4.4	172.8±6.4	74.6±10.3	25.0±3.3
	$P < 0.001$	$P < 0.001$	$P < 0.01$	$P < 0.001$	n.s.	n.s.
82	157.7±5.8	62.7±10.7	25.2±4.2	172.4±6.5	74.4±10.0	25.0±3.2

The marked individual differences in the rate of change in these morphological parameters are illustrated by the observation that at the same time as the BMI decreased, the standard deviation increased (Table 5.3). However, this increase in interindividual variation was observed only in the survivors and not in the total population. BMI decreased in the age interval 70–79 in 51% of the probands, was unchanged in 22%, but increased in 27%. It should be emphasized that this increase in BMI was not explained by disease factors, e.g., edema, and occurred generally in lean subjects (Svanborg 1988b).

On average, male smokers were found to have 4.5 kg lower BW than nonsmokers at age 70, and 7.0 kg lower BW at age 75, but their nutritional intake of energy and nutrients did not differ (Mellstrom *et al.* 1982). Smoking was not associated with any change in the mean concentration of free thyroxin (T4) in serum. The total T4 and the rT3 levels were marginally higher in smokers than in nonsmokers, but the thyrotropin (TSH) level was lower in smokers and ex-smokers than in nonsmokers (Eden *et al.* 1984). These results indicate that tobacco smoking, except for the well-known stimulation of certain enzymes, e.g., in the liver, may also cause long-term alterations in the thyroregulatory function. At the present time there seems to be no evidence that this effect of smoking should be characterized as an acceleration of the aging process within the thyroregulatory functions, although there is other evidence for a negative influence of tobacco smoking on aging (Mellstrom *et al.* 1982; Mellstrom and Svanborg 1987).

The body composition changes in the age interval 70–75 years implied for the total group studied that the proportion of cell mass of BW was generally unchanged but that the proportion of fat increased, and the proportion of extracellular water decreased (Steen *et al.* 1977a; Steen *et al.* 1980). The number of probands followed longitudinally from age 70 to 81 years was small (Steen *et al.* 1985) and the result, therefore, possibly inconclusive. The results indicate (Table 5.1) that BW loss in

TABLE 5.3
INCREASE IN INTERINDIVIDUAL VARIATION IN BODY MASS INDEX (BMI) WITH INCREASING AGE
Longitudinal survival (N = 137)

Age Group (Males)	*BMI*	*SD*
70	26.0	2.9
75	25.7	3.1
79	25.3	3.2
81	24.8	3.4

the eighth decade of life corresponded more to the loss of body cell mass in males and more to the loss of body fat in females. In both sexes, the most important cause of BW decline was a decrease of extracellular water, which might be related to some extent to the decreasing ability in urine concentration (Larsson *et al.* 1986).

In the Swedish population of elderly males, the prevalence of partially gastrectomized subjects (the Billroth operations) was found to be high. In the first age cohort of 70 year olds in Gothenburg, no less than 10% had been partially gastrectomized (Mellstrom and Rundgren 1982), and the prevalence in the 3 age cohorts averaged 7.5%. Thus, in these generations of elderly males, the proportion of males with partial gastrectomy was similar to the prevalence of diabetes. In comparison with the nonoperated group, the operated group showed a lower body weight of about 6 kg at the age of 70 and 11 kg at 75. The intake of energy and nutrients, e.g., calcium and iron, did not differ. The prevalence of anemia and the lifetime incidence of bone fracture at age 75 years was, however, higher in the gastrectomized group, and the density of the skeleton was lower. The prevalence of tobacco smokers was higher among operated subjects (26 versus 12%), as was the incidence of smoking-related cancer. When adjustments were made for smoking habits, the difference in cancer incidence disappeared, but the BII-operated group still had a lower density of the skeleton. The group of partially gastrectomized elderly, thus, represents a risk group from the perspective of nutrition and aging.

From the analyses of possible age-related changes in gastrointestinal function, this presentation will be restricted to the analyses of the resorption of cobalamin (B_{12}). There was no decrease in the reference value (10–38%) for B_{12} resorption from the food (Schilling Test) in healthy elderly subjects (Nilsson-Ehle *et al.* 1986, 1988a). Low values (< 130 pmol/L) appeared to be caused by definable disorders. The serum B_{12} values are examples of blood concentrations that do not show increasing interindividual differences at increasing ages, at least not in the age intervals we have studied.

Physical activity was found to have a significant stimulatory effect on not only muscle strength but also on muscle fiber activity (Aniansson and Gustavsson 1981), and this is the case still, at least, at the age of 82 years. Indirectly we can, therefore, conclude that more physical activity can be expected to increase the uptake of glucose and amino acids in the muscle still at the age of 82 years. Activity in combination

TABLE 5.4
PLASMA PROTEIN CONCENTRATION (g/L) FOLLOWED LONGITUDINALLY FROM AGE 70 TO 79 IN 302 FEMALES AND 198 MALES

	Females		*Males*	
Age	*M*	*SD*	*M*	*SD*
70	78.4	5.08	78.3	5.51
75	71.9	4.50	72.1	4.03
79	67.8	4.62	68.8	5.10

with adequate nutrition will thus direct the nutrients to one of the organ systems to be influenced positively and not to the adipose tissue.

Regarding the homeostasis of blood components during aging, no or only minor variations of most serum electrolytes, e.g., total calcium were found. As previously reported (Landahl *et al.* 1981), plasma protein was found to be one of the blood components analyzed normally distributed in probands without definable disease at age 70. Table 5.4 shows the plasma protein concentrations followed longitudinally from age 70 to age 79. The protein concentrations did not show any sex difference at age 70 and 75 but a higher value ($P > 0.02$) in males than in females at age 79. There was a significant age-related decline both in females ($P > 0.000$) and males ($P > 0.000$) in the age interval 70–79. A similar declining trend has been observed also between age 79, 81 and 82. Plasma albumin was analyzed longitudinally from age 79–81 and decreased in both sexes.

Plasma lipid changes with age have been extensively studied previously in many populations, as well as in Gothenburg, Sweden (Svanborg *et al.* 1977). Our present material (Eden *et al.* 1990) allows us to show age-related changes in plasma lipids from age 70–82 years in (1) the total population, in (2) survivors to age 82 years, and in (3) those who at these extensive examinations did not show any symptoms or signs of definable disorders and, therefore, were called "healthy."

Females had higher CH and PL concentration than males, but there were no significant concentration differences among the three groups. In survivors followed longitudinally from age 70 to 85, an age-related decline was observed in females after age 70 years, but in males only after age 79. Interindividual variations were similar in both sexes and did not change with age.

The TG concentration was higher in the total population than in survivors and "healthy" probands. It showed no significant age-related longitudinal decline in females, but a decline in the total group of males from age 70 years, and in male survivors from age 79 years. Within the PL fraction the proportion of lysolecithin (LL) was lower in females than in males, but the proportion of lecithin (L) was higher. The L/LL quotient is an indicator of the relationship between estrogenic and androgenic activity (for a review see Eden *et al.* 1987).

At these ages no positive relationship was observed between the CH level and mortality. A high TG level was, on the other hand, still at these ages positively correlated with ischemic heart disease in males and females, even after the exclusion of probands with diabetes which is accompanied by an increase in the TG level.

These studies of changes in plasma lipid concentrations indicate that a decline in plasma CH and PL occurs as a consequence of aging, but that age-related changes in the homeostasis of TG start later in males and even later, if ever, in females. The reason for these age-related changes are obviously multifactorial.

The differences observed from the comparison of our three representative cohort population samples indicate both positive and negative trends for the future (Svanborg *et al.* 1984; Svanborg 1988a, 1988b). One of the negative trends concerns the incidence of hip fractures which shows a very sharp increase (Zetterberg and Andersson 1982) in Gothenburg. Recent observations (Mannius *et al.* 1987) illustrate, however, marked regional differences in these negative trends, e.g., between rural and urban areas.

To what extent nutritional factors, such as the intake of calcium, in our industrialized countries serve as one of the causative roles for these age cohort differences has to be clarified. One of the positive trends observed at the cohort comparisons was a significant ongoing improvement in dental status, which obviously will have an impact on dietary habits. In the first cohort, 50% of the population were edentolus; in the second about 40%; and in the third 33%. The very fact that a global evaluation of the vitality and state of health of the elderly shows a positive trend will obviously, as long as this positive trend exists, imply better prerequisites for nutrition and activity in the future generations.

Although our population study in Gothenburg includes both retrospective and prospective information, the complicated interaction between nutrition, physical activity, age-related morphological, biochemical and circulatory changes in organ metabolism, hormone secretion and target effects, etc., obviously limit the possibilities to identify possible specific nutritional impacts upon the rate and functional consequences of aging.

CONCLUSION

Aging above age 70 is accompanied by changes in body mass and body composition which obviously must influence nutritional requirement and have an impact upon the metabolism at the cellular, organ, and organ system levels. It should, however, be emphasized that age-related morphological changes show great interindividual variations also in groups of individuals without such disorders that are known to influence nutrition and metabolism. Furthermore, smoking has a profound influence upon basic metabolic processes, more so than upon dietary habits, and elderly smokers have considerably lower body weight than non- and ex-smokers. Certain medical treatments that a patient may have experienced and may have been cured by earlier in life might constitute a risk for malnutrition in the longer perspective. Among those operated upon because of peptic gastric or duodenal ulcer with partial gastric resection, a high proportion represented a risk group in the perspective of nutrition and aging. Physical activity has obvious positive effects not only through the concomitant demand for increased intake of calories and nutrients, but also for the direction of nutrients to the muscle tissue and not to storage in the form of fat in the adipose tissue.

The homeostasis of certain metabolic components in the blood show age-related changes. Plasma protein concentration declined in the age interval 70–82. Before age 70 several blood lipid fractions show an age-related increase. Cholesterol and phospholipids are examples of blood components that increase up to age 70 but then decrease. Our studies indicate also that at ages above 70 a higher cholesterol level is no longer to the same extent as in younger adult ages a risk factor for mortality. The level of triglycerides in blood that shows a different age-related change than cholesterol at ages above 70 constitutes, however, still at these ages a significant positive relationship to cardiovascular disease and mortality.

Cohort comparisons at age 70 show both positive and negative age-related trends influencing or influenced by nutrition and age-related changes in metabolism.

REFERENCES

ANIANSSON, A. and GUSTAVSSON, O. 1981. Physical training in elderly men with special reference to quadriceps muscle strength and morphology. Clin. Physiol. *1*, 87–98.

BENGTSSON, C. *et al.* 1973. The study of women in Gothenburg 1968–69, a population study: general design, purpose and sampling result. Acta Med. Scand. *193*, 311–318.

BERG, S. 1980. Psychological functioning in 70- and 75-year-old people: A study in an industrialized city. Acta Psychiatr. Scand. *62* (Suppl.), 288.

EDEN, S *et al.* 1984. Thyroregulatory changes associated with smoking in 70-year-old men. Clin. Endocrinol. *21*, 605–610.

EDEN, S., OSCARSSON, J., JANSSON, J. -O. and SVANBORG, A. 1987. The influence of gonadal steroids and the pituitary on the levels and composition of plasma phospholipids in the rat. Metabolism *36*(6), 527–532.

EDEN, S., OSCARSSON, J. and SVANBORG, A. 1990. Plasma lipid changes in the age interval 70–82. (In preparation)

ERIKKSON, G. B., MELLSTROM, D. and SVANBORG, A. 1987. A medical-social intervention in a 70-year-old Swedish population. Compr. Gerontol. *1*, 49–56.

HALLBERG, L., HOGDAHL, A. -M., SVANBORG, A. and VIKROT, O. 1966. Plasma lipids in women. Acta Med. Scand. *180*, 697.

HANSSON, B. S., MAHISSON, J. and STEEN, B. 1987. Dietary intake and psychosocial factors in 68-year old men. A population study. Compr. Gerontol. B *1*, 62–67.

LANDAHL, S. *et al.* 1986. Age-related changes in blood pressure. Hypertension *8*(11) 1044–1049.

LANDAHL, S., JAGENBURG, R. and SVANBORG, A. 1981. Blood components in a 70-year old population. Clin. Chim. Acta *112*, 301–304.

LARSSON, B. 1978. Obesity. A population study of men, with special reference to development and consequences for the health. Thesis. Gothenburg.

LARSSON, M., JAGENBURG, R. and LANDAHL, S. 1986. Renal function in an elderly population. Scand. J. Clin. Lab. Invest. *46*, 593–598.

LINDSTEDT, G. *et al.* 1983. Factors influencing serum free T in 70-year-old men. Implications for reference intervals in the elderly. Scand. J. Clin. Lab. Invest. *43*, 401–413.

LUNDGREN, B. K., STEEN, B. and ISAKSSON, B. 1987. Dietary habits in 70- and 75-year-old males and females. Longitudinal and cohort data from a population study. Naringsforskning *31*, 53–56.

MANNIUS, S. *et al.* 1987. Incidence of hip fracture in Western Sweden 1974–1985. Acta. Orthoped. Scand. *58*, 38–42.

MELLSTROM, D. *et al.* 1982. Tobacco smoking, ageing and health among the elderly. A longitudinal population study of 70-year-olds and an age cohort comparison. Age Ageing *11*, 45–58.

MELLSTROM, D. and SVANBORG, A. 1987. Tobacco smoking—a major cause of sex differences in health. Compr. Gerontol. A *1*, 34–39.

NILSSON-EHLE, H. *et al.* 1986. Cyanocobalamin absorption in the elderly: results for healthy subjects and for subjects with low serum cobalamin concentration. Clin. Chem. *32*, 1368–1371.

NILSSON-EHLE, H. *et al.* 1988a. Haematological abnormalities and reference intervals in the elderly. A cross-sectional comparative study of three urban Swedish population samples aged 70, 75 and 81 years. Acta Med. Scand. *224*, 505–604.

NILSSON-EHLE, H. *et al.* 1988b. Decline of blood haemoglobin in the aged. A longitudinal study of an urban Swedish population sample from age 70 to 81. Brit. J. Haematol. *71*(3), 437–442.

NORDSTROM, G. *et al.* 1988. Dietary habits in the 8th decade of life. Compr. Gerontol. A *2*, 29–39.

PERSSON, G. 1980. Prevalence of mental disorders in a 70-year-old urban population. Acta Psychiatr. Scand. *62*, 119–139.

RINDER, L., ROUPE, S., STEEN, B. and SVANBORG, A. 1975. Seventy-year-old-people in Gothenburg. A population study in an industrialized Swedish city. General design of the study. Acta Med. Scand. *198*, 397–407.

STEEN, B. 1987. Body Composition and Aging. Nutrition and Aging Seminar. Symposium held at Marabou, Sundbyberg, Sweden, June 12–14.

STEEN, B. *et al.* 1977a. Body composition in 70-year-old males and females in Gothenburg, Sweden. A population study. Acta Med. Scand. *611* (Suppl.), 87–112.

STEEN, B., ISAKSSON, B. and SVANBORG, A. 1977b. Intake of energy and nutrients and meal habits in 70-year-old males and females in Gothenburg, Sweden. A population study. Acta Med. Scand. *611*, (Suppl.), 39–86.

STEEN, B., ISAKSSON, B. and SVANBORG, A. 1980. Longitudinal studies of body composition in high age groups. Aktuelle Gerontol. *10*, 325.

STEEN, B., LUNDGREN, B. K. and ISAKSSON, B. 1985. Body composition at Age 70, 75, 79, and 81 years: A longitudinal population study. *In* Nutrition, Immunity, and Illness in the Elderly, R. K. Chandra (ed.). Pergamon Press. New York.

STEEN, B., NILSSON, K., ROBERTSSON, E. and OSTBERG, H. 1988. Age retirement in women. II. Dietary habits and body composition. Compr. Gerontol. A *2*, 78–82.

SVANBORG, A. 1977. Seventy-year-old people in Gothenburg. A population study in an industrialized Swedish city. General presentation of social and medical conditions. Acta Med. Scand. *611* (Suppl.), 5–37.

SVANBORG, A. *et al.* 1977. Plasma lipid changes in the female in aging and the menopause.

Results from three population studies. Clin. Chim. Acta *79*, 299–307.

SVANBORG, A. 1988a. The health of the elderly population: Results from longitudinal studies with age-cohort comparisons. *In* Research and the Ageing Population. Wiley, Chichester (Ciba Foundation Symposium 134).

SVANBORG, A. 1988b. Cohort differences in the Goteborg studies of Swedish 70-year-olds. *In* Epidemiology and Aging, J. A. Brody and G. L. Maddox (eds.). Springer, New York.

SVANBORG, A., BERG, S., NILSSON, L. and PERSSON, G. 1984. A cohort comparison of functional ability and mental disorders in two representative samples of 70-year-olds. *In* Senile Dementia: Outlook for the Future. Modern Aging Research, Vol. 5. J. Wertheimer and M. Marois (eds.). A. R. Liss, New York.

SVANBORG, A., LANDAHL, S. and MELLSTROM, D. 1982. Basic issues of health care. *In* New Perspectives on Old Age, H. Thomas and G. Maddox (eds.). Springer, New York.

TIBBLIN, G. 1967. High blood pressure in men aged 50: A population study of men born in 1913. Acta Med. Scand. *470* (Suppl.), 1–84.

ZETTERBERG, C. and ANDERSSON, G. 1982. Fractures of the proximal end of the femur in Goteborg, Sweden, 1940–1979. Acta Orthop. Scand. *53*, 419–426.

CHAPTER 6

AGING AND NUTRITION: A JAPANESE PERSPECTIVE

SHUICHI HATANO, M.D.
Faculty of Social Welfare, Shukutoku University, Chiba
and
Department of Epidemiology, The Institute of Public Health
Tokyo, Japan
and
KAZUE YAMAOKA, Ph.D.
Faculty of Jurisprudence, Teikyo University, Tokyo
and
Department of Epidemiology
The Institute of Public Health
Tokyo, Japan

INTRODUCTION

Aging is expressed in variety of ways and can be measured at different levels, e.g., intracellular micromolecules, cell components, organ systems, individuals and also in populations, from different aspects of physicochemical, physiological, mental or social functions. All of these are interrelated and stem from the common basis of aging, but specific factors operate at different levels. What is essential at the cellular level may play a less significant role at the individual level and what was valid in one person may not be applicable to another. A causative role of nutrition in age-related diseases has been the subject of considerable study. The analysis of the relationship of diet to the processes of aging as distinguished from geriatric diseases has been a difficult challenge to epidemiology because of the complexity and diversity of aging. Among the various manifestations of aging processes, the most finite expression would be the terminating point of individuals summarily expressed as the death rate in populations. Finding the causes of premature death that occurred earlier than the average life expectancy might give us insights for intervention into the processes of aging. Aging processes are influenced by the long-term effects of environment, which has been changing rapidly in industrialized nations, especially in Japan. We, therefore, present the secular trends of mortality and nutrition and the results of some related epidemiological studies in Japan.

TRENDS IN MORTALITY

Japan has become the top-ranking country in life expectancy. Decreased mortality is observed not only in infancy but also in older people of both sexes (Fig. 6.1) (Kosei Tokei Kyokai, Annual). To understand the reasons for decreased mortality, trends of major causes of death are shown (Fig. 6.2) (Kosei Tokei Kyokai, Annual). Communicable diseases, such as pneumonia and tuberculosis, dropped sharply soon after the end of World War II. Cerebrovascular disease increased initially but has

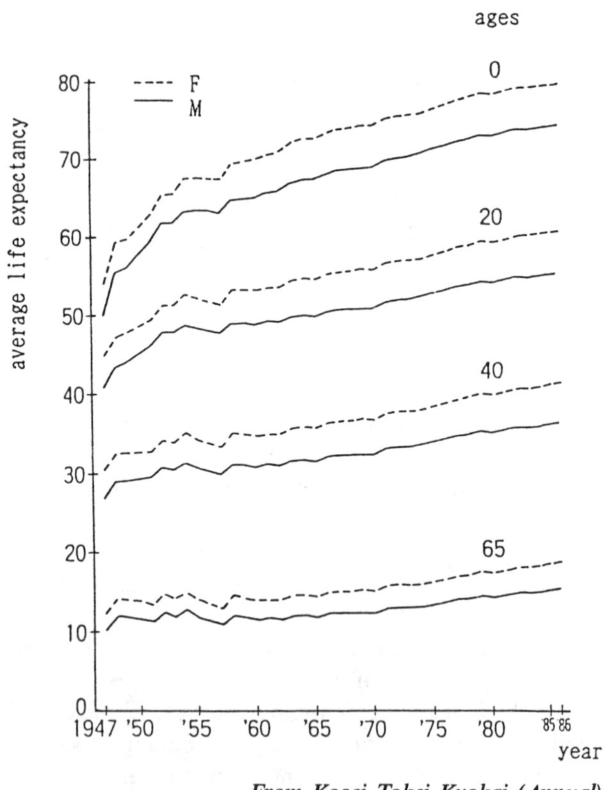

From Kosei Tokei Kyokai (Annual)
FIG. 6.1. SECULAR TRENDS OF LIFE EXPECTANCY FOR 4 AGE GROUPS OF MEN AND WOMEN

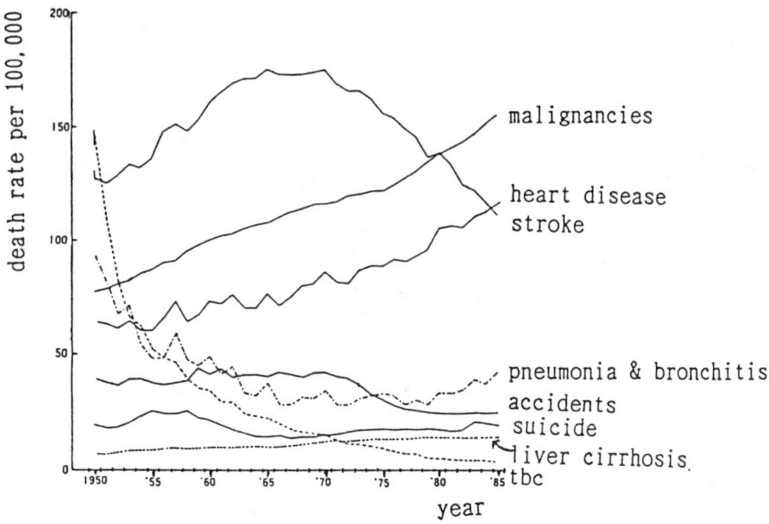

From Kosei Tokei Kyokai (Annual)

FIG. 6.2. SECULAR TRENDS OF CRUDE MORTALITY RATE FROM 8 MAJOR CAUSES OF DEATH IN JAPAN

been falling rapidly since 1970. Cancer and heart disease also decreased when age was adjusted (Fig. 6.3) (Ministry of Health and Welfare 1988; Hatano 1989). Most people die before their full life potential has been reached because of chronic diseases. The practical recourse for attaining a long life is to prevent cancer, heart disease and stroke, the major causes of premature death. Pneumonia has recently shown a small increase, presumably due to an increased incidence among the very old.

Geographical differences in mortality were seen between urban and rural populations in Japan (Fig. 6.3) (Bureau of Statistics and Information 1988). Age-adjusted mortality from stroke was higher in populations from rural areas. Conversely, mortality from cancer was higher in urban areas. Mortality due to heart disease was about half the stroke rate and does not show urban-rural differences since the late 1960s when higher rates were observed in rural areas. Whereas mortality due to stroke decreased rapidly, that from heart disease decreased slowly. Cancer mortality had been decreasing in women but was almost stable or increasing slightly in men. The urban-rural gap in stroke mortality has diminished over time. The initial higher mortality of heart disease in rural areas may possibly be caused by a greater incidence of hypertensive heart disease that went undiagnosed.

Why has mortality from so many diseases declined? This must be related to dramatic environmental and lifestyle changes after World War II. Among the various changes, industrial development and the subsequent improvement in living standards, including diet, are obvious. In addition, technological progress reduced strenuous physical labor for rural as well as urban workers. These changes may have contributed to reductions in high blood pressure due to stress, although the tendency toward over-

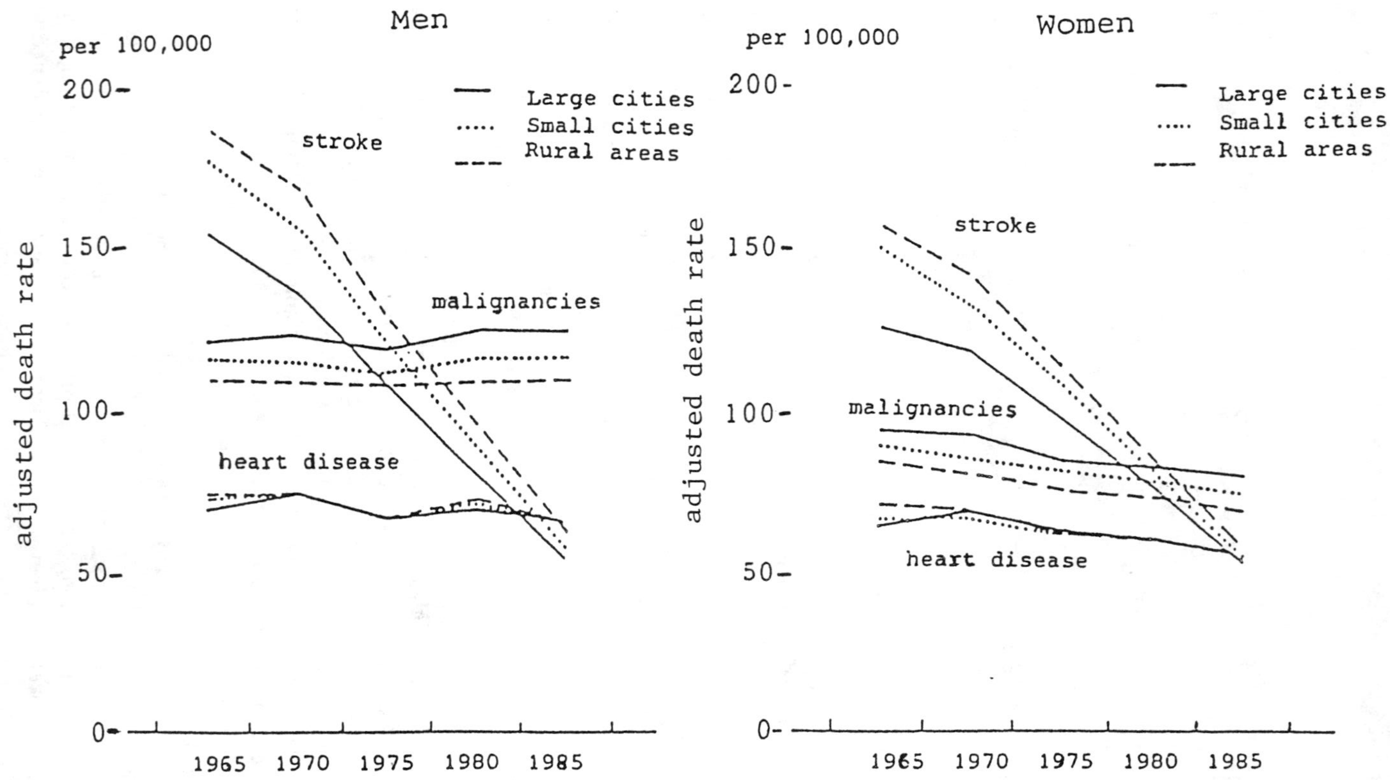

From Bureau of Statistics and Information (1988)

FIG. 6.3. SECULAR TRENDS OF AGE-ADJUSTED MORTALITY RATE FOR 3 MAJOR CAUSES OF DEATH IN URBAN AND RURAL AREAS OF JAPAN weight by reduced energy consumption at work may have acted to the contrary. Dietary changes are regarded as one of the most important variables with regard to the improved health of populations.

JAPANESE DIET: PAST AND PRESENT

The Japanese Ministry of Health and Welfare conducts an annual national nutrition survey (Ministry of Health and Welfare, Annual). The national and district average diet and nutritional intake per person have been estimated by actual weighings of food consumed at each meal in a random household sample over 3 successive days. The average diet was composed mainly of carbohydrate (81%) with a very small proportion of fat (7%) and protein (12%) just after the World War II (Fig. 6.4). Subsequently, fat intake increased and carbohydrate decreased every year. By 1985, energy intake from fat reached about a quarter of the total, whereas that from carbohydrate was only 60%, with the remainder from protein. Over this period, total energy intake had been rather stable. Consumption of animal foods increased

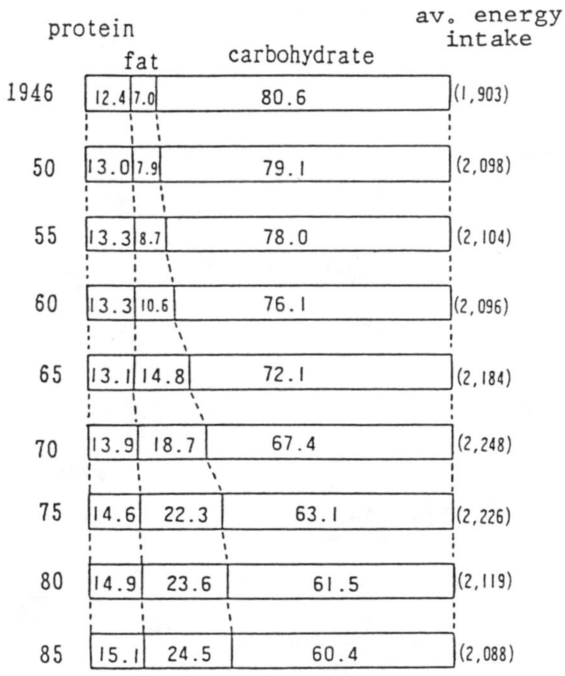

From Ministry of Health and Welfare (Annual) and Oda (1987)
FIG. 6.4. SECULAR TRENDS OF TOTAL AND PROPORTIONAL ENERGY INTAKE

every year. The intake of fat, particularly animal fat and animal protein increased dramatically by 4–5 times (Fig. 6.5) (Kosei Tokei Kyokai, Annual; Ministry of Health and Welfare, Annual; Oda *et al.* 1987). This trend, however, had practically ceased after 1970, which was a few years prior to the first oil crisis. Thus, the consumption was unrelated to economic pressures. The exact reasons are unknown but may reflect, at least in part, traditional habits and the results of public education. Although the

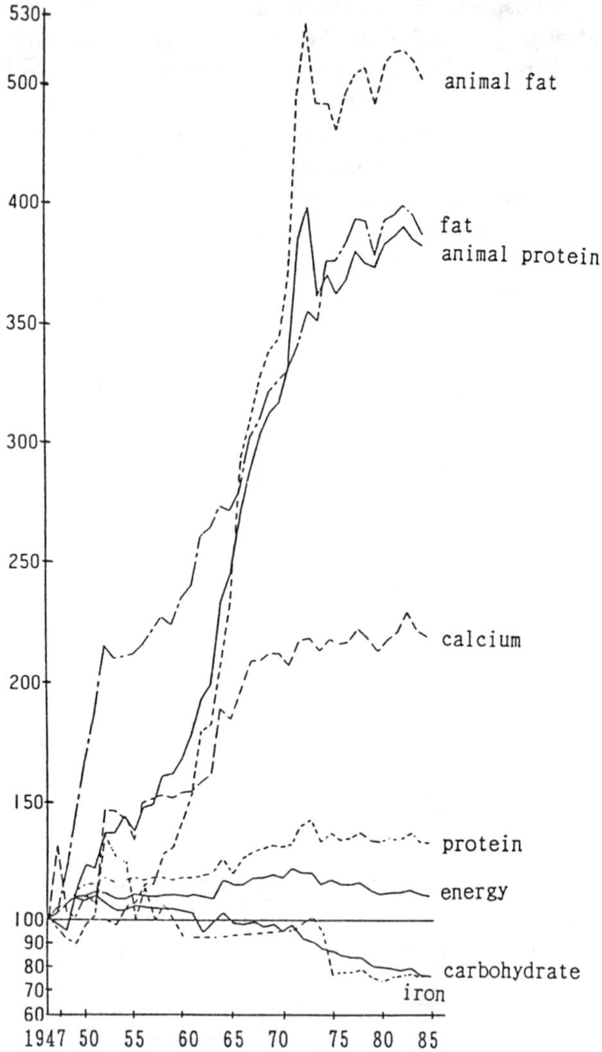

FIG. 6.5. SECULAR TRENDS OF PROPORTIONAL CHANGES OF AVERAGE NUTRITIONAL INTAKE OF THE JAPANESE (1946 = 100)

increases appear extraordinary as a percentage, it must be remembered that the initial values were very low. Fat consumption, particularly animal fat consumption, in Japan is such an example. The average amount of fat consumption was only 15 g per day in 1946 and increased to 57 g in 1985; however, this level is still lower than that recommended for U.S. citizens. The average daily protein intake was small (less than 80 g) in 1946, but changed dramatically with increasing consumption of animal proteins (Fig. 6.5). Calcium intake is, however, still low (91% of the recommended level) despite having risen to more than double the 1946 level (Ministry of Health and Welfare, Annual; Oda *et al.* 1987).

As to the kinds of animal protein consumed in Japan, fish was the primary protein source during late 1940s and early 1950s, but has since decreased, possibly due to the availability of other foods and partly due to rising fish prices. Consumption of milk and dairy products has increased almost linearly since 1946. Meat and egg consumption increased at a slower rate through 1970 and then leveled off, especially for eggs. In 1985, the average daily consumption of meat had reached 60 g, a very modest and safe level of consumption by U.S. standards.

In the East Asian tradition, the Japanese diet used rice as a main staple food, along with a few other additional side dishes. Rice had been a major energy and protein source. In addition, salt was used as a major ingredient to add taste in situations when very small amounts of food from animal sources were consumed. Soy sauce, made from soybean and wheat, was also added to almost every dish, even to salted pickles. Soup, another traditional staple, was usually made with the salted and

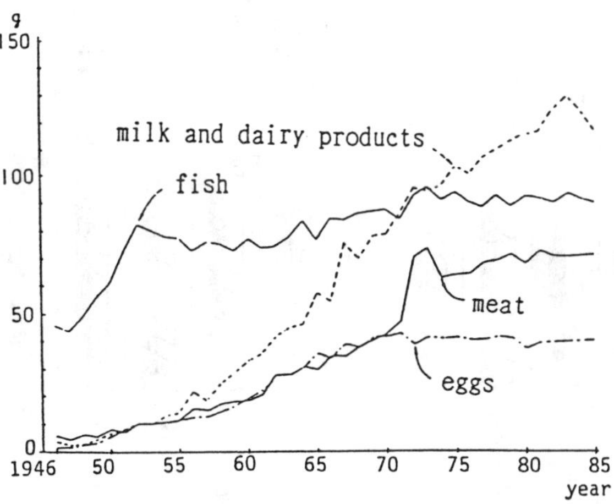

From Kosei Tokei Kyokai (Annual), Ministry of Health and Welfare (Annual) and Oda (1987)

FIG. 6.6. SECULAR TRENDS OF AVERAGE DAILY INTAKE OF MAJOR FOODS OF ANIMAL ORIGIN fermented bean paste "miso" and at times with soy sauce. The drinking of multiple cups of miso soup at each meal was usual, particularly in rural areas. The commonest side dishes were miso soup, salted vegetable pickles and sometimes salted and dried fish. These foods still comprise the standard basic meal for many Japanese families. Soy sauce and miso have been the major source of salt intake in the traditional Japanese diet.

The Japanese farmer's traditional diet was mostly dependent on local agricultural products. The use of a variety of foods was possible only in large cities before mass delivery systems were developed. Such urban-rural differences in foods could be a factor for the urban-rural difference in stroke and heart disease mortality in the past (Fig.6.3). The reasons for a higher death rate for cancer in urban areas are not yet known, but higher intake of saturated fat is a possibility (Kesteloot 1988). Less dependence on rice is associated with appreciation of many other types of tastes and seasonings and less use of salt (Akabane 1981). The Ministry of Health and Welfare recommends the diet consist of more than 30 kinds of food items every day as a practical approach to improve quality of diet and to prevent cardiovascular diseases and cancer.

The average daily salt intake was 15 g or higher, varying between individuals and geographic areas. The average salt consumption in recent 3 sequential time periods are illustrated by 3 connected bars for 12 districts in Japan (Fig. 6.7). (Ministry of Health and Welfare, Annual; Oda 1987). Districts from the northeast to the southwest are arranged from the left to the right in the graph. The district

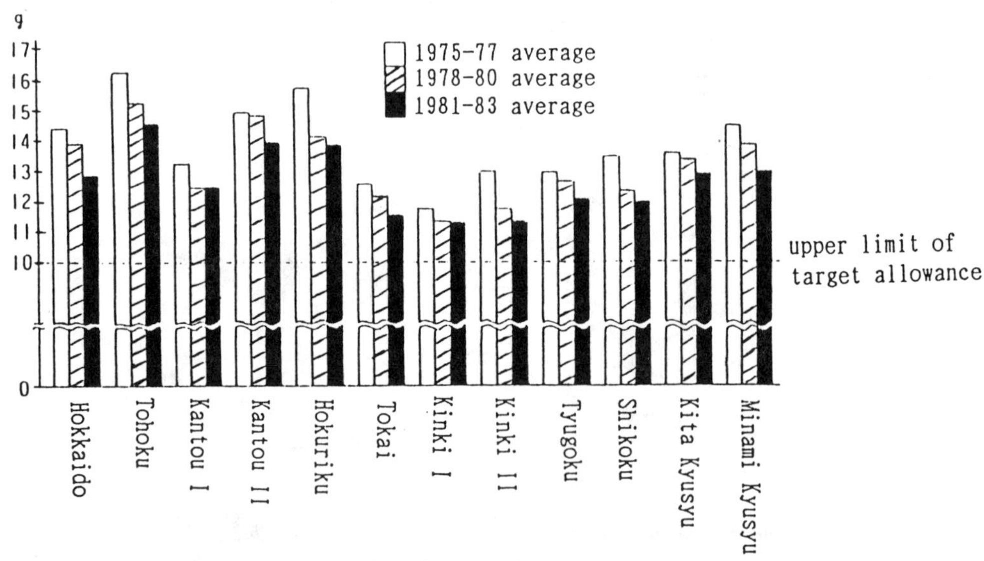

From Kosei Tokei Kyokai (Annual) and Ministry of Health and Welfare (Annual)

FIG. 6.7. SECULAR TRENDS OF AVERAGE DAILY SALT INTAKE IN 12 DISTRICTS OF JAPAN rank order remained, but a clear decreasing trend has been observed nationwide. The highest average daily consumption was 16.2 g per day in Tohoku followed by Hokuriku and northern Kanto II. The lowest were Kinki I and II districts with 11 g, followed by Tokai district. This geographic distribution was parallel to the geographical difference in stroke mortality. The Ministry of Health and Welfare of Japan set 10 g as a target allowance for daily salt consumption, but this has not been achieved in any district yet.

RISK FACTORS

Body Build

With an increase in the amount of energy and protein, height and weight of the Japanese have been increasing. Younger generations have grown faster and larger (Fig. 6.8) (Kosei Tokei Kyokai, Annual, Ministry of Health and Welfare, Annual). The only exception was young girls whose average weight was nearly constant, perhaps reflecting a conscious effort for esthetic considerations.

According to a large scale Life Insurance Study (Tsukamoto 1986a), mortality rate revealed a U-shape curve on DAW (percent Departure from Average Weight), because not only obese but also too slim people showed a higher mortality, and the lowest mortality was distributed around the average DAW.

DAW (%) = (observed weight − average weight* / average weight*

Death rates from heart disease, stroke, and liver diseases were all higher on the obese side, regardless of sex. However, death rates from all causes combined in women, including malignancies and respiratory diseases, were lower on the obese side than the average (Tsukamoto 1986b). The suicide mortality curve was flatter but still showed a gentle U-shape. Hospitalization rates also showed the same trend. Although not significant, our observations of mortality in old people's homes (Haga 1981) and in Koganei City, Tokyo (Hatano *et al.* 1984), were consistent with this finding, since the upper tertile of height, weight and obesity had the least mortality during a 5-year follow-up.

Hypertension

Despite a tendency for the Japanese to be more obese, hypertension has been decreasing (Table 6.1). The prevalence rate in four separate years was taken from the national nutrition surveys (Ministry of Health and Welfare, Annual). Age and sex difference were obvious. A declining trend in the prevalence of hypertension has been observed in all sex and age subgroups. The degree of reduction was larger in older populations. These declines, at least partly, could be attributed to intensive annual health screening addressed to citizens aged 40 and over and obligatory health

*average weight was calculated for each sex, age and height classes and so was DAW.

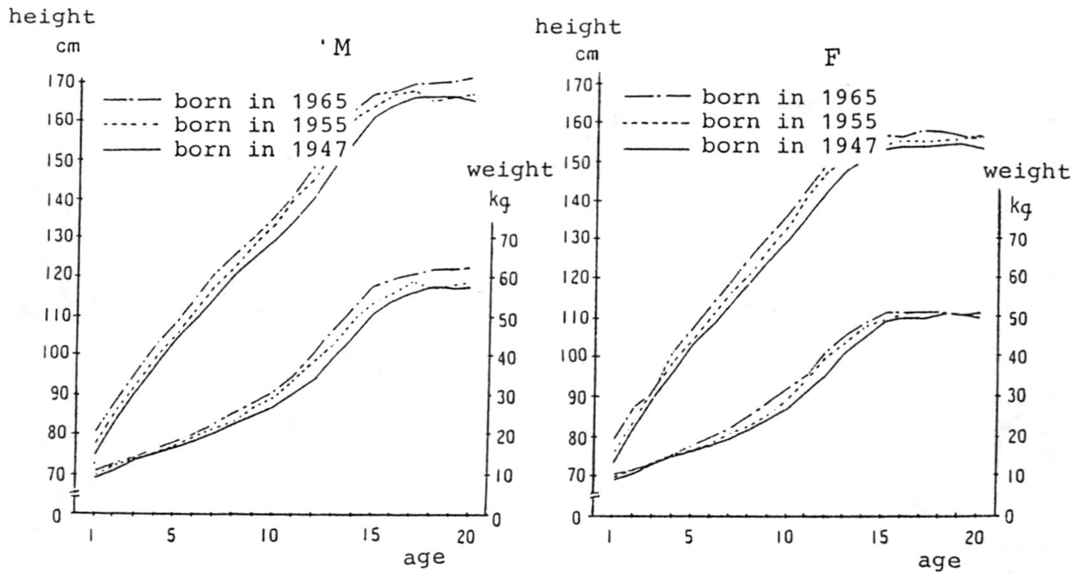

From Kosei Tokei Kyokai (Annual) and Ministry of Health and Welfare (Annual)

FIG. 6.8. SECULAR TRENDS OF AVERAGE HEIGHT AND WEIGHT IN 3 BIRTH COHORTS

TABLE 6.1
SECULAR TRENDS OF AGE- AND SEX-SPECIFIC PREVALENCE RATE OF HYPERTENSION (%)

	15-19	20-29	30-39	40-49	50-59	60-69	70+
Men							
1975	1.9	3.3	9.8	18.3	29.0	36.7	51.2
1980	0.8	3.8	9.2	19.3	28.7	35.9	44.0
1983	0.7	5.5	7.5	18.0	26.1	34.5	40.9
1985	0.8	2.6	8.0	16.5	24.8	29.0	35.2
Women							
1975	0.6	1.0	3.7	13.2	27.7	35.7	47.9
1980	0.2	0.7	2.9	12.0	21.1	30.3	41.9
1983	—	0.6	3.1	11.0	22.3	33.0	43.1
1985	0.2	—	2.8	9.9	18.9	28.3	39.1

Source: Ministry of Health and Welfare (Annual).

checks for all employees at firms since 1967. Pharmaceutical therapy of hypertension has been supported by nearly complete coverage of health insurance. Older populations had a higher participation rate and better compliance with treatment (Hatano *et al.* 1984). The major reason for the decrease in hypertension seems to be better treatment of hypertension. The potential effects of dietary changes, such as reduced energy and salt intake and an increased alcohol consumption (Omoto 1985), should also be taken into account.

Serum Cholesterol

Total serum cholesterol was measured in a nationwide cardiovascular survey (Ministry of Health and Welfare 1983) in 1980. The average was 186.4 mg/dL in men and 191.1 mg/dL in women aged 30 and over, reflecting the low fat consumption by the Japanese (Table 6.2). The average exceeded 200 mg/dL only in women aged 50 and over. Only 2.0% of men and 3.4% of women had serum cholesterol of 260 mg/dL or over.

EPIDEMIOLOGICAL STUDIES

In the longitudinal study of Komachi *et al.* (Komachi 1987), fat intake, serum cholesterol and the incidence rate of cardiovascular diseases in men aged 40–59 were compared between population groups. The results are a typical example of Japanese populations at different times. The average daily fat intake based on 24-h memory recall was 38 g, 35 g, 46 g and 48 g in rural areas, suburban areas, urban blue collar workers and urban white collar workers, respectively, in 1973–76. Fat intake increased to 42 g, 47 g, 52 g and 59 g, respectively, in 1980–82. The average total serum cholesterol in rural areas, urban blue collar workers and urban white collar

TABLE 6.2
SERUM TOTAL CHOLESTEROL IN THE JAPANESE POPULATION

Sex	Age	All Japan	Urban Tokyo
Males	30–39	186.7	194.1 mg/dL
	40–49	188.4	194.2
	50–59	188.6	199.5
	60–69	185.1	195.6
	70+	177.8	190.2
	30+	186.4	—
Females	30–39	176.9	182.1
	40–49	185.7	186.3
	50–59	202.7	210.4
	60–69	203.1	209.1
	70+	199.8	213.8
	30+	191.1	—

Source: Ministry of Health and Welfare (Annual).

workers was 175.7, 185.8 and 200.8 mg/dL in early 1970s and 179.4, 194.9 and 197.8 in early 1980s, respectively.

Incidence rates of stroke and acute myocardial infarction (AMI) were reported for the above three population groups (Inada *et al.* 1987). The high incidence rate of stroke decreased from about 10 to 6, 1.5 to 1.0 and 1.4 to 0.6 per thousand in rural populations, urban blue collar workers and white collar workers, and low incidence rate of AMI showed a trend of nonsignificant increase, i.e., from almost 0 to 0.2, 0.2 to 0.5 and 0.3 to 1.0, respectively, from the late 1960s to the early 1980s. Recent increases in fat consumption and the rise in the average serum cholesterol up to 200 mg/dL were not associated with a noticeable increase in incidence of myocardial infarction. However, those urban populations which had higher serum cholesterol since the 1940s have been observed to have a rising trend of ischemic heart disease occurrence recently. The higher incidence of stroke was associated with lower cholesterol levels, and the reverse was true with AMI.

The negative association between stroke and serum cholesterol was confirmed within populations as well (Bureau of Research Coordination 1979; Tanaka *et al.* 1982). Negative coefficients were stronger with cerebral hemorrhage in rural areas and weaker in cerebral infarction in urban populations.

Similar results on the negative association of stroke with other nutritional indicators, e.g., serum albumin/globulin ratio (Kimura *et al.* 1987) of fish containing sulfur-containing amino acids (Yamori *et al.* 1979) were reported in many other epidemiological cohort studies (Tanaka *et al.* 1982; Kimura *et al.* 1987; Yamori *et al.* 1979; Isomura and Sei 1987; Kagan *et al.* 1980) in Japan. No contradictory studies of this association have been reported to date. The higher incidence rate of stroke, particularly for cerebral hemorrhage, was associated with lower serum cholesterol. It is also noteworthy that such a negative association became weaker or nonexistent in recent epidemiological studies (Konishi *et al.* 1987; Shimamoto *et al.* 1985). Total serum cholesterol was a sensitive marker of better nutrition at a time when the quality of general nutrition was poor. The role of serum cholesterol as a marker diminished when the quality of the diet improved.

The elderly in an old people's home also showed an association of serum cholesterol with life expectancy according to Shinohara (1983). The elderly with total serum cholesterol between 195 and 214 mg/dL at entry had the best potential for survival, and three quarters of them survived for 5 years. The next best survival was experienced by a group with the highest level of over 214 mg/dL. The lower the initial cholesterol, the worse the survival. The lowest cholesterol group with the levels below 160 mg/dL showed the worst prognosis, about half died in 5 years. In other groups with the levels in between showed survival rates in between.

Few longitudinal studies have been undertaken on community-residing old people. The results of a small-scale population study of residents aged 70 ± 1 at entry in Koganei City, Tokyo (Hatano *et al.* 1988), are referred to here. A diet survey was carried out as a part of a comprehensive study asking weekly frequency of eating several common food items. In a 10 year follow-up, a significant difference in survival was manifested with some food items (Suyama *et al.* 1985). Daily milk drinking and alcohol drinking reduced total mortality in men. Other food items such as frequency of rice, noodles, bread, meat, eggs and fish consumption did not separate those who died and those who were alive until age 80. Milk and fat may be a marker of dietary styles for a variety of food items, i.e., those rich in protein and fat. Similarly, alcohol consumption may be an indicator of social activity (another protective factor, see below), and the possibility of their causal link cannot be dismissed.

In the Koganei Study, serum albumin and hemoglobin were negatively associated with mortality rate, but serum cholesterol was not (Hatano *et al.* 1988). The average serum albumin decreased from 4.41 to 4.14 g/dL in men and 4.47 to 4.22 in women from 70 to 75 years, and those who died by 75 had low average values (4.18 in men and 4.33 in women) at the age of 70. Serum albumin, however, was not related to a higher intake of protein rich diet; nor did a higher intake of protein in the elderly guarantee the augmentation of serum albumin. Serum albumin was thus understood as an indicator of biological age rather than a direct indicator of protein nutrition in this urban elderly population.

Since dietary factors may be only a part of the contributing factors, a multiple logistic regression analysis was carried out in the Koganei Study (Shibata 1988). Indeed, the levels of serum albumin, the memory score for a short visual memory retention test (Benton) and the composite social activity score were shown to be significant protective factors from premature death during a 10-year follow-up (Table 6.3). Maintaining an active lifestyle, nutritionally, intellectually and socially, thus seems to be associated with longevity. Although it can be a consequence and not a cause of biological age, to act accordingly would be more advisable than acting contrarily after summarizing all the changes and epidemiological data in Japan.

TABLE 6.3
MULTIPLE LOGISTIC REGRESSION COEFFICIENT
OF FOUR MAJOR RISK FACTORS FOR MORTALITY OF THE ELDERLY MEN AND WOMEN AGED 70 IN KOGANEI CITY, TOKYO

	Males (N = 194)	Females (N = 214)
Albumin	−0.172[1]	−0.072
Grasping power	0.014	−0.062
Benton score	−0.182[2]	−0.208[2]
Social activity score	−0.062[2]	−0.047
Constant	8.253	4.691

Source: Shibata (1988).
[1]$P < 0.01$.
[2]$P < 0.05$.

COMMENT

The Japanese people experienced rapid environmental changes after the end of the World War II: physical growth, improved diet, i.e., consuming a variety of foods rich in protein and fat and reduction of salt intake, reduced physical labor, introduction of effective heating systems to housing, community based hypertension control and a widespread campaign against cardiovascular risk factors. These changes developed in parallel, and it is difficult to separate the individual contribution of each factor now. A well-designed intervention study on modifying nutrition or hypertension control has not been undertaken in Japan, and evaluating separate effects of various factors is difficult. A long-term prospective study monitoring aging of individuals is still necessary to elucidate relationship between nutrition and aging. Such a study requires a large sample size and a long period of follow-up, and its feasibility is questionable. It would be practical and worthwhile, under these circumstances, to monitor secular trends of nutrition on the one hand, and those parameters of aging on the other, and to analyze their relationship carefully. The role of risk factors changes rather quickly, thus epidemiological studies on aging and nutrition must be continued for timely advice and intervention.

SUMMARY AND CONCLUSIONS

(1) The Japanese population offers a good opportunity to observe relationship between nutrition and longevity, since the Japanese are experiencing a rapid transition of diet and disease structure, leading to the longest life expectancy in the world.
(2) Secular trends, geographical variations, and urban and rural differences suggest shortcomings of the past traditional Japanese diet and the greater adequacy

of the present Japanese diet, which is close to dietary goals recommended in many countries (with the exception of a persistently high salt intake and a low intake of calcium).

(3) According to many epidemiological studies in Japan, serum cholesterol of around 200 mg/dL and higher serum albumin were associated with lower stroke mortality. These were indicators of good nutrition or biological age.

(4) In the preceding epidemiological studies of the elderly during the 1960s and 1970s, frequent intake of milk, alcohol and fat, higher serum albumin and cholesterol and more obese than the average were related to lower mortality.

(5) These studies suggest that improvement in quality of nutrition has helped the longevity of Japanese populations.

(6) No intervention study, however, has been conducted to prove causality.

ACKNOWLEDGMENT

We should like to express our great appreciation to the Health and Welfare Statistics Association and their contributors for generous permission to use their graphs and tables. We are grateful to colleagues in Tokyo Metropolitan Institute of Gerontology (H. Shibata, principal investigator) who kindly supplied data from the Koganei Study to this review article.

REFERENCES

AKABANE, M. 1981. Salt in diet and life. *In* A Handbook of Reducing Salt in Diet and Life—for Prevention of Hypertension, Stroke and Heart Disease. S. Hatano and M. Ohtaka (eds.). Shakaihoken Shuppan, Tokyo. (in Japanese)

Bureau of Research Coordination (The Office of Science and Technology). 1979. Prevention of hypertension and stroke. Office of Printing, Ministry of Finance, Tokyo. (in Japanese)

HAGA, H. *et al.* 1981. Prognosis for survival of the elderly in old people's homes in relation to the results of annual health examinations. (in Japanese)

HATANO, S. 1989. Changing coronary heart disease mortality and causes in Japan during 1955–1985. Int. J. Epidemiol. *18* (Suppl. 1), 149–158.

HATANO, S., FUJITA, T., TAKEUCHI, K. and TSUKAMOTO, M. 1984a. Current status of hypertension control and problems in Japan. Koketuatu (Hypertension) 7, 70. (in Japanese)

HATANO, S. *et al.* 1984b. Selection of variables related to early death of the elderly, The Koganei Study. Presented at the International Epidemiological Association, 10th Scientific Meeting, Aug. 19–25, Vancouver, Canada.

HATANO, S., *et al.* 1988. A prospective study of Japanese 70–year–olds: The Koganei Study. *In* Epidemiology and Aging. An International Perspective, J. A. Brody and G. L. Maddox (eds.). Springer Publishing Co., New York.

INADA, K. *et al.* 1987. Secular trends of incidence of stroke and ischemic heart disease and risk factors for stroke. *In* Changing Pattern of Cardiovascular Diseases: Correlation

Between Nutrition of Japanese and Their Living Environment, Y. Komachi *et al.* (eds.). Hokendojinsha, Tokyo. (in Japanese)

ISOMURA, K. and SEI, M. 1987. Changes in living environment and cardiovascular disease. *In* Changing Pattern of Cardiovascular Diseases: Correlation Between Nutrition of Japanese and Their Living Environment, Y. Komachi *et al.* (eds.). Hokendojinsha, Tokyo. (in Japanese)

KAGAN, A. *et al.* 1980. Factors related to stroke incidence in Hawaii—Japanese men. (The Honolulu Heart Study) Stroke *11*, 14.

KESTELOOT, H., YUAN, X.-Y. and JOOSSENS, J. V. 1988. Changing mortality patterns in men. Acta Cardiol. *XLIII*, 133–139.

KOMACHI, Y. 1987. A collaborative study on relationship between environmental factors, particularly nutritional factors, and stroke and ischemic heart disease, focusing at results of a study group in the Office of Science and Technology and Ministry of Health and Welfare 1975–1983. *In* Changing Pattern of Cardiovascular Diseases: Correlation Between Nutrition of Japanese and Their Living Environment, Y. Komachi *et al.* (eds.). Hokendojinsha, Tokyo. (in Japanese)

KONISHI, M., *et al.* 1987. The trend of coronary heart disease and its risk factors based on epidemiological investigations. Jpn. Circ. J. *51*, 319–324.

Kosei Tokei Kyokai (Health and Welfare Statistics Association). Annual. Kokumin eisei no doko (Trends of national health). Kosei no shihyo (Indic. Health Stat.) *35* (Suppl.), (9).

Ministry of Health and Welfare (Bureau of Statistics and Information). 1988. Age-adjusted mortality rate for major causes of death 1985. A special statistical report of population dynamics. Ministry of Health and Welfare, Tokyo. (in Japanese)

Ministry of Health and Welfare (Div. of Promotion of Health and Nutrition). Annual. Kokumin Eiyo no Genjyo (Current status of national nutrition). Daiichi Shuppan, Tokyo. (in Japanese)

Ministry of Health and Welfare (Div. of Tuberculosis and Adult Diseases). 1983. A Basic National Survey on Cardiovascular Diseases 1980. Japan Heart Foundation. Tokyo. (in Japanese with an English summary)

NAGAI, H. *et al.* 1984. Relationship between changes with aging in serum albumin in community residents and prognosis for survival. Jpn. J. Gerontol. Soc. *21*, 588–592. (in Japanese with English summary)

ODA, S., NAKAHARA, S. and INOUE, K. 1987. A 40-year history of the national nutrition survey. Kosei no Shihyo *34*, 4–60. (in Japanese)

OMOTO, M. 1985. Epidemiology of alcohol. Rinsho Eiyo (Clin. Nutr.) *67*, 653–665. (in Japanese)

SHIBATA, H. 1988. Predictive factors for death of the elderly. *In* Tokyo Metropol. Inst. Gerontol. : A comprehensive health survey of the elderly aged 70 in Koganei City—the 2nd report. A followup study during 10 years—. A report of a project research "Social and medical background of aging" (1982–1986).

SHIMAMOTO, T. *et al.* 1985. Changes of risk factors of stoke and ischemic heart disease accompanied with recent trends of lifestyles. Kosei no Shihyo *32* (14), 11–16. (in Japanese)

SHINOHARA, T. 1983. Middle-aged and old people and nutrition. *In* New Textbook of Nutrition, N. Hosoya (ed.). Karada no Kagaku. Suppl. 1. Nippon Hyoron sha, Tokyo. (in Japanese)

SUYAMA, Y. *et al.* 1985. Food intake of the elders in a community and prognosis for life. Jpn. J. Public Health *323* (10) (Suppl.), 385. A special issue for the 44th Annual Meeting of the Jpn. Public Health Assoc. (in Japanese)

TANAKA, H. *et al.* 1982. Risk factors for cerebral hemorrhage and cerebral infarction in a Japanese rural community. Stroke *13*, 62–73.

TSUKAMOTO, H. 1986a. An attempt for a new indicator of bodybuild. The Meiji Life Insurance Company Standard Weight Table. Rinsho Eiyo (Clin. Nutr.) *69*, 653–659. (in Japanese)

TSUKAMOTO, H. 1986b. Bodybuild of Japanese assessed from mortality rate. The Meiji Life Insurance Company Standard Weight Table. Kosei no Shihyo *33* (2), 3–14. (in Japanese)

UESHIMA, H., TATARA, K. and ASAKURA, S. 1987. Declining mortality from ischemic heart disease and changes in coronary risk factors in Japan, 1956–1980. Am. J. Epidemiol. *125*, 62–72.

YAMORI, Y. *et al.* 1979. Prophylactic effect of dietary protein on stroke and its mechanisms. *In* Prophylactic Approach to Hypertensive Diseases, Y. Yamori, W. Lovenberg and E. D. Freis (eds.). Raven Press, New York.

SECTION III

Effects of Caloric Restriction on Aging Phenomena

CHAPTER 7

RETARDATION OF AGING BY CALORIC RESTRICTION IN MICE

RICHARD WEINDRUCH, Ph.D.[1]
Biomedical Research and Clinical Medicine Program
National Institute on Aging
Bethesda, Maryland

INTRODUCTION

Dietary restriction (DR) of energy intake retards aging and disease processes in experimental animals. Most work has been conducted with mice or rats. Initiated by the studies of McCay *et al.* (1935) showing that rats on DR lived surprisingly long lives, reports published from 1940 to the mid-1970s emphasized DR's inhibitory effects on tumor growth (Tannenbaum 1947; Ross 1976) and marked the start of inquiry on DR's actions on the aging immune system (Gerbase-DeLima *et al.* 1975). In the mid-1970s the number of gerontologic studies on DR began to steadily increase, and their scope broadened.

It is now clear that mice and rats subjected to long-term, nonmalnutritional DR regimens show numerous desirable biological outcomes (see Holehan and Merry 1986; Masoro 1988; Walford *et al.* 1987; Weindruch and Walford 1988). Caloric restrictions of 30–70% of *ad libitum* intakes reduce incidences and delay onsets of many late-life diseases in rodents and increase average and maximum longevity. The rates of change for almost all of the age-sensitive biologic parameters tested to date are slowed by DR (Weindruch and Walford 1988). These effects of DR on rodents are unmatched by rival methods. As a result, rodents on DR are widely viewed as the best models available to study the biology of decelerated aging in homeothermic vertebrates.

Most of the DR investigations in rodents have tested DR started early in life (usually at 3–6 weeks) which retarded growth rates and delayed puberty onsets. Though less

[1]Present address: Department of Medicine, University of Wisconsin, Madison, Wisconsin.

studied, adult-onset DR is far more relevant from the perspective of potential human use. Also germane to humans is the lack of data on the effects of DR on aging in primate species.

The present comments briefly summarize parts of an extensive collaborative examination (Weindruch and Walford 1988) of DR's retardation of aging and disease processes. Although the subject of this essay is aging in mice subjected to DR, it is important to appreciate that DR increases average and maximum longevity in various nonrodent species (e.g., *Tokophyra* [a protozoan], *Daphnia* [the water flea], the bowl and doily spider [family *Linyphiidae*], *Lebistes* [the guppy]).

CALORIC RESTRICTION STARTED EARLY IN LIFE

A survey of the literature (Weindruch and Walford 1988) identified 21 studies where longevity was measured in mice on DR started in early life (usually 3–6 weeks). In rats, 26 such studies were found. Survival curves from these populations show that DR slows the actuarial aging rate and/or decreases the population's initial vulnerability to mortality. The very longest 10th decile life spans ($\sim$53 months) occurred for mice fed diets enriched in essential nutrients but in severely restricted amounts, with caloric intakes and peak body weights of DR animals being only about 40% as high as for unrestricted mice.

How good is the general health of DR rodents? Early studies reported high mortality in early life which may have been due to essential nutrient deficiency rather than simple caloric restriction. Modern studies are not reporting high infant mortality. Our experience in studies conducted at UCLA was that less than 2% of a large group of weanling mice died prior to 6 months of age and that this figure was the same for DR and control groups. As indicated in Table 7.1, our DR mice were fed diets enriched in content of proteins, vitamins and minerals relative to the diets fed to controls. These DR mice appeared quite healthy and were very active. The coats and appearances of DR rodents have long been found to be better maintained to older ages than for controls (McCay *et al.* 1935; Berg and Simms 1960), which accords with our observations for mice restricted either early or in mid life. Also, 31–35 month mice from our colony on early-onset DR outperformed age-matched controls in an age-sensitive maze test of learning capacities (Ingram *et al.* 1987).

Studies on Long-lived Mouse Strains

The use of an animal model which is a healthy and long-lived representative of its species is critically important in conducting interventive aging research. Long-lived models help to diminish the serious problems of separating aging-related phenomena from disease-related ones. An intervention which increases maximum life span in a long-lived model would likely be acting on basic aging processes. In contrast, another intervention which increases life span only in short-lived strains would probably be affecting diseases primarily.

TABLE 7.1
COMPOSITION OF DIETS

Ingredient	Diet 1[1] g/kg of Diet	Diet 1[1] g/Mouse per Week	Diet 2[2] g/kg of Diet	Diet 2[2] g/Mouse per Week
Casein	200.0	4.3	350.0	4.3
Cornstarch	260.8	5.7	157.6	2.0
Sucrose	260.8	5.7	157.6	2.0
Corn oil	135.0	2.9	135.0	1.7
Mineral mix, USP XIV	60.0	1.3	110.0	1.4
Fiber	56.4	1.2	40.0	0.5
Vitamin mixture	23.0	0.50	42.2	0.52
Brewer's yeast	4.0	0.09	7.4	0.09
Zinc oxide	0.05	1.1×10^{-3}	0.1	1.2×10^{-3}

Source: Adapted From Weindruch *et al.* (1986).

[1]Diet 1: Diet fed to control mice as seven 3.0–3.2 g feedings per week providing ~85 kcal/week. Composition is given as g ingredient/kg diet. The per week intake of each ingredient for each mouse is also given.

[2]Diet 2: Diet fed to restricted mice. This diet was enriched in casein, mineral and vitamin mixtures, brewer's yeast and zinc oxide. Fed as four 2.4–3.2 g feedings per week providing ~40–50 kcal/week to the various DR groups.

Growth curves for female mice of the long-lived $C3B10RF_1$ hybrid strain studied by our UCLA group are shown in Fig. 7.1. The heaviest mice were given free access to Purina Lab Chow™. The other diet groups were fed nutritionally adequate purified diets at 85, 50 or 40 kcal/week. Mice fed 85 kcal/week of Diet 1 served as controls but were themselves restricted by about 25% when compared to mice freely fed the Lab Chow™. As Fig. 7.2 illustrates, the longevity of $C3B10RF_1$ mice increased with the severity of DR.

Harrison *et al.* (1984) studied genetically obese (ob/ob) and normal female C57BL/6J (abbreviated B6) mice. Longevity was augmented by DR in both strains and strikingly so in ob/ob mice. Restricted ob/ob were still fatter (48% body fat) than +/+ mice fed normal (22% body fat) or restricted (13% body fat) diets, but had less body fat than ob/ob mice fed the control diet (67% body fat). DR may particularly benefit metabolically thrifty, fat-prone individuals. Increased longevity for genetically obese mice subjected to DR was also described by Goodrick *et al.* (1983).

Harrison and Archer (1987) next observed that DR prolonged life in both genetically obese (ob/ob) B6 male mice and normal weight male $B6CBAF_1$ mice but not in genetically normal B6 male mice. This lack of effect of DR in B6 mice contrasts with their initial results (Harrison *et al.* 1984) and our findings at UCLA (Gerbase-DeLima *et al.* 1975; Cheney *et al.* 1980; Weindruch and Walford 1982). The study of Harrison and Archer (1987) produced the longest-lived mouse, described in a peer-reviewed publication. This mouse was switched from DR to *ad libitum* feeding at 51 months of age and died at 57 months.

Apparently, meal-timing does not affect longevity in mice subjected to DR (Nelson and Halberg 1986). In this study, food was presented either as a single meal during

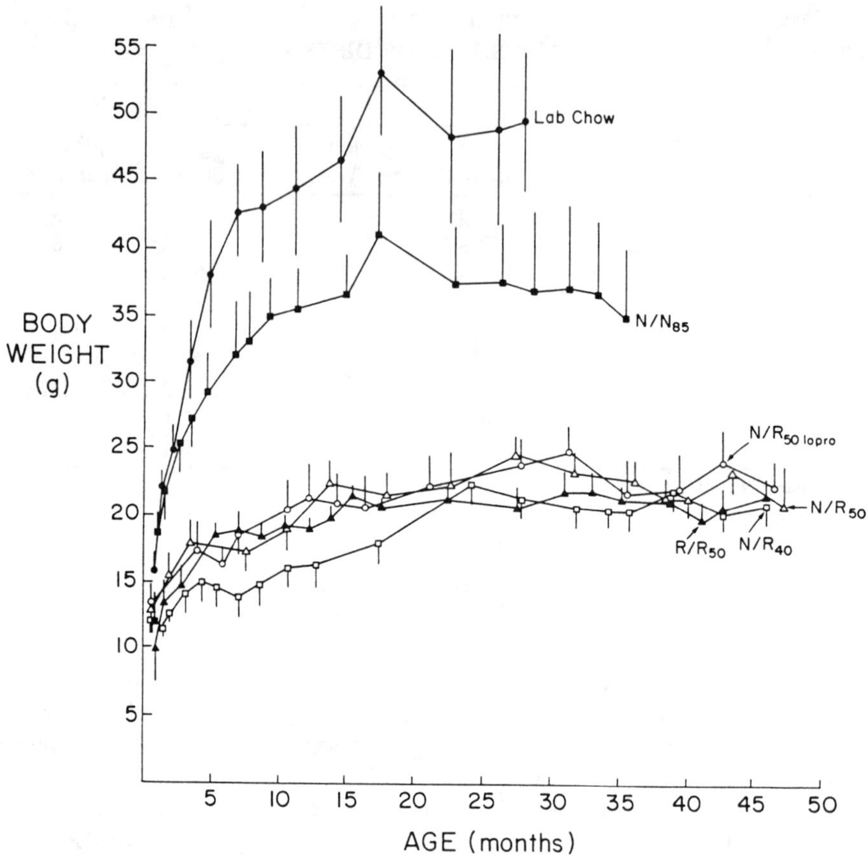

From Weindruch et al. (1986)

FIG. 7.1. INFLUENCES OF DIET ON BODY WEIGHT OF FEMALE C3B10RF$_1$ MICE Values represent mean ± SD. Diet groups: Lab Chow, Purina Lab Chow™ *ad libitum*; N/N$_{85}$, fed normally before and after weaning, postweaning diet fed at 85 kcal/week (25% less than *ad libitum*); N/R$_{50}$, fed normally before weaning, restricted postweaning to 50 kcal/week; R/R$_{50lopro}$, restricted after weaning to 50 kcal/week with a decrease with age in the protein content of the diet; N/R$_{40}$, restricted after weaning to 40 kcal/week.

early lightness, early darkness, or as 6 very small meals at 2-hour intervals. All DR groups showed maximum decile life spans of 41–43 months versus 35 months for controls.

Studies in Short-lived Mouse Strains

Longevity is also increased by early-onset DR in short-lived, disease-prone strains of mice. This work was pioneered by Robert Good's group which has found that DR inhibits diseases in four short-lived mouse strains: NZB (which develop autoim-

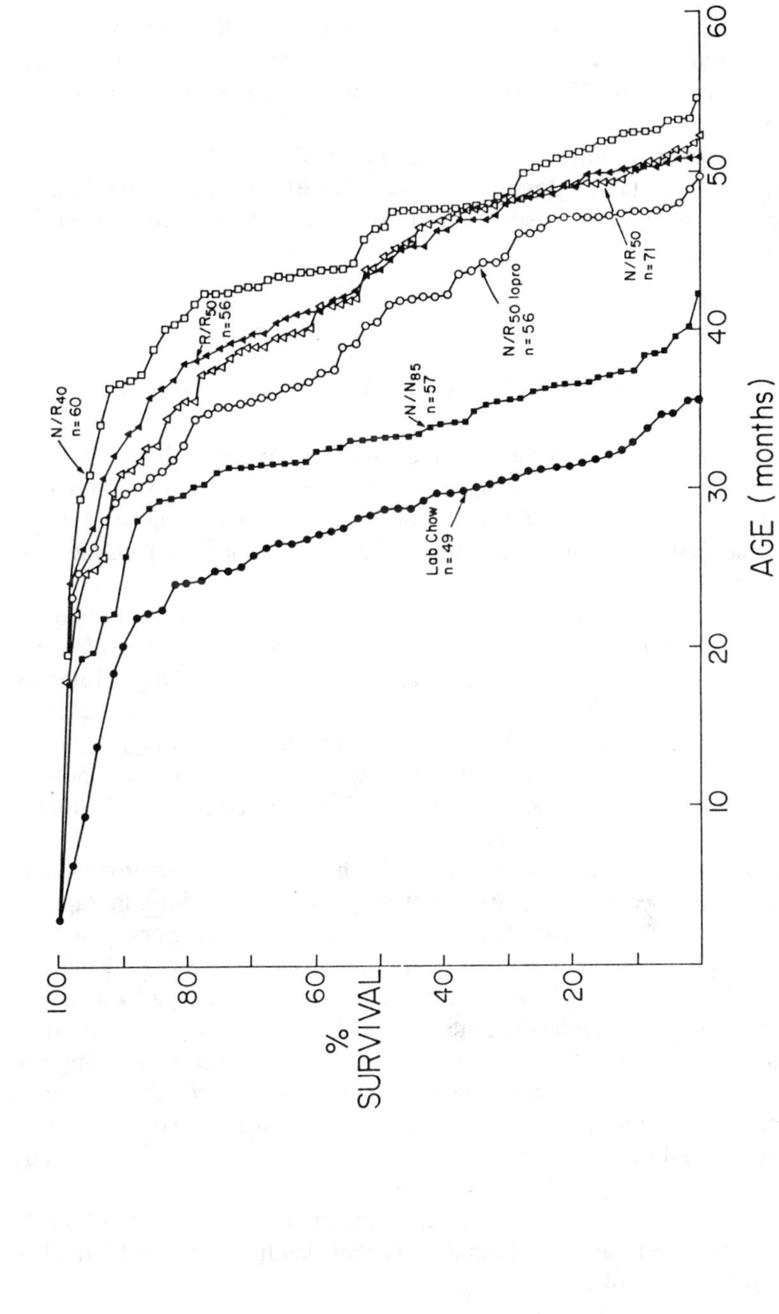

From Weindruch et al. (1986)

FIG. 7.2. INFLUENCES OF EARLY-ONSET DR ON SURVIVAL OF C3B10RF$_1$ FEMALE MICE
Each symbol represents an individual mouse. See Fig. 7.1 for diet groups.

mune hemolytic anemia during the first year of life), C3H/Umc females (which develop fatal mammary adenocarcinomas), B/WF_1 (a lupus model), and kd/kd (afflicted by renal disease). Good and Gajjar (1986) review these studies.

Recently, Good's group varied the fat and protein contents of the diets fed to energy-restricted B/WF_1 female mice. Kubo *et al.* (1987) found that life spans were most strikingly prolonged by DR when moderate fat intakes (38% of energy as fat) and not very high fat intakes (69% of energy as fat) were used. Variation of protein level in DR mice did not alter longevity (Gajjar *et al.* 1987).

DR need not be severe to improve longevity in short-lived mouse strains. Tucker (1979) and Rehm *et al.* (1985) found that mild DR (80% of *ad libitum* diet) led to 20–30% gains in average and maximum life spans over those of *ad libitum* fed, heavy weight (50 g) controls.

CALORIC RESTRICTION STARTED IN MIDADULTHOOD

For DR started at or beyond 3 months, the survey by Weindruch and Walford (1988) located 5 reports where longevity was measured in mice and 12 studies involving rats. As Fig. 7.3 illustrates for mice from a medium- and a long-lived strain, caloric restriction first started in midadulthood (12 months) increased average and maximum longevity by 10–20%.

The size of the increase in longevity brought on by adult-onset DR can approach that which follows early-onset DR (Table 7.2). Only three studies measured the longevity of populations subjected to early-onset DR, adult-onset DR and normal feeding. As shown in Table 7.2, in all three studies adult-onset DR resulted in average and maximum life spans which were 89–95% as great as those following early-onset DR. This consistency is interesting in view of the short age gap (4.5 months) separating early and later onset DR in the study of Yu *et al.* (1985) and the longer period (11–13 months) in the other studies.

Adult-onset DR has also been observed to benefit short-lived, disease-prone mouse strains with ongoing disease (i.e., to exert not only a preventive but a therapeutic effect). Friend *et al.* (1978) restricted B/WF_1 mice at either weaning or 4–5 months (at which time their lupus-like syndrome was clinically manifest). At about 9 months, mice on early or later onset DR showed far less autoimmune nephropathy than controls (longevity was not determined). Later studies in MRL/lpr mice (afflicted by an autoimmune lymphoproliferative condition early in life) revealed a strong impact of adult-onset DR on this syndrome and on life span. Mark *et al.* (1984) reported that 5–6 month mice, previously fed *ad libitum*, and then restricted, showed a much improved appearance 4–6 weeks thereafter. The mice were more active than fully fed controls and greatly outlived them (all controls were dead by 11 months of age versus 40% of the the DR group still alive at 13 months). Kubo *et al.* (1984) subjected MRL/lpr mice to DR at about 3 months. The median life span was 15 months, versus 7 months for controls.

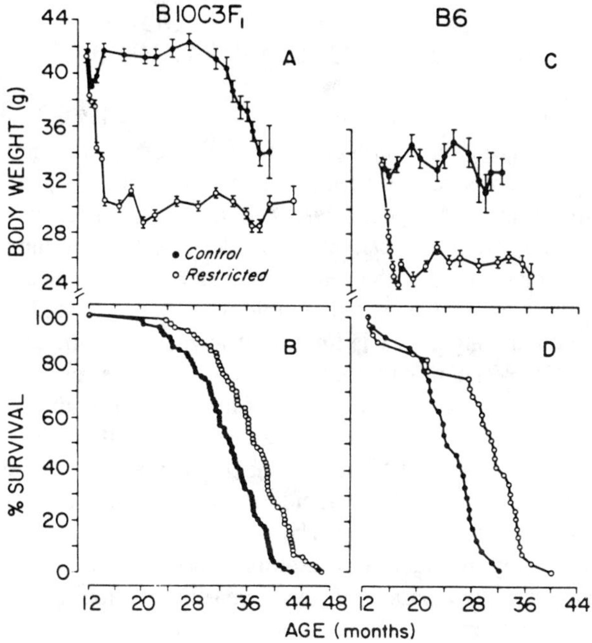

From Weindruch and Walford (1982)

FIG. 7.3. BODY WEIGHTS AND SURVIVAL CURVES OF B10C3F$_1$ MICE (A AND B) AND B6 MICE (C AND D) FED CONTROL OR ADULT-ONSET CALORICALLY RESTRICTED DIETS

The adult-onset DR started at 12 months. Each point in the survival curves represents one male mouse.

Knowledge about age-sensitive biological measures in animals started on DR at or beyond midadulthood is largely limited to indexes of immune system aging and most of these stay "younger longer" with underfeeding.

TABLE 7.2
THREE LONGEVITY STUDIES TESTING BOTH EARLY- AND ADULT-ONSET DR

Study[1], Animal	Onsets[2]	Avg. Life Span[3] C	EDR[2]	ADR[2]	A:E	Max. Life Span[4] C	EDR[2]	ADR[2]	A:E
(1) B10C3F$_1$ mice	1, 14	36	43	39	0.91	41	50	45	0.90
(2) F344 rats	1.5, 6	23	35	31	0.89	27	41	39	0.95
(3) Wistar rats	1, 12	31	38	35	0.92	39	46	41	0.89

[1](1) Cheney *et al.* (1983); (2) Yu *et al.* (1985); (3) Beauchene *et al.* (1986).
[2]The onsets (in months) for early-onset DR (EDR) and adult-onset DR (ADR) groups.
[3]Values are the average life spans in months. "C" gives values for controls. A:E gives the ratio for the life spans of the ADR:EDR groups.
[4]The value given is the average life span (in months) for each group's longest-lived 10%. Adapted from Weindruch and Walford (1988).

MECHANISMS: HOW DOES CALORIC RESTRICTION RETARD AGING?

Two main facts should be kept in mind when considering DR's mode(s) of action. One is the apparent *phylogenetic independence* of the effect. It is not simply a "rodent phenomenon"! Life span is extended by DR in nearly all species so far tested (the few exceptions seem to be special cases). A second main fact is that *only energy restriction retards aging in mammals.* Without calorie restriction, maximum life span has not been prolonged beyond that which is usual for the species.

Although nearly all of the age-sensitive biologic parameters studied to date in DR rodents stay "younger longer," it is important to recognize the existence of some age-sensitive but DR-resistant parameters (Table 7.3). The few DR-resistant ones may have little to do with basic aging (even if they change with age), or they may be responsible for DR animals not living even longer (Walford *et al.* 1987). Thus, for the DR paradigm, so-called "negative data" may be important data.

Future work carrying the goal of elucidating mechanisms behind DR's actions cannot succeed if it merely demonstrates by ever more sophisticated means that DR animals are functionally younger. For example, there is a tendency to reason that because a given age-sensitive parameter (e.g., gene expression) is sometimes greater (= functionally "younger") in DR animals, the mechanism of DR's action is to increase gene expression; but such an increase may merely mean that the animal has been kept functionally "younger" by some other nongene expression mechanism.

To elucidate how DR retards aging and extends life span is very difficult, especially in view of the present level of understanding on the etiology of aging. However, with this caveat in mind, comments on four classes of leading nonmutually exclusive possibilities follow which have been discussed and referenced more extensively elsewhere (Weindruch and Walford 1988).

TABLE 7.3
AGE-SENSITIVE BUT DR-RESISTANT PARAMETERS[1]

Parameter	Age Change	Ref.[2]
Circulating TSH (thyrotropin)	↓	1
Insulin secretion (islets *in vitro*)	↓	2
Insulin secretion (per volume of islet)	↓	3
Antilipolytic effect of insulin	↓	4
Oxidative damage products in urine	↑	5
Blood pressure	↑	6
Forskolin-stimulating adenylate cyclase activity	↓	7
Protein synthetic activity in brain	↓	8
β-oxidation in liver	↓	9

[1]Certain of these findings require repetition using DR regimens proven to extend maximum life span.
[2]Complete references are in Weindruch and Walford (1988): (1) Sarkar *et al.* (1982); (2) Reaven and Reaven (1981b); (3) Reaven *et al.* (1983a); (4) DiGirolamo *et al.* (1984); (5) Saul *et al.* (1987); (6) Yu *et al.* (1985); (7) Scarpace and Yu (1987); (8) Sparks *et al.* (1983); (9) Rumsey *et al.* (1987).

Energy Metabolism

All DR regimens extending maximum life span restrict energy intake. Thus, major energy-producing and energy-using operations, as well as processes which detoxify noxious byproducts of energy metabolism, merit serious attention in considering DR's basic actions. Four nonmutually exclusive, energy-based possibilities are that DR acts by: (1) lowering the metabolic rate at some critical but unappreciated level (e.g., per whole animal or per total mass of internal organs) or locale (e.g., per brain or per physiologic "sensing center"); (2) increasing metabolic efficiency; (3) decreasing heat and free radical production, with less damage to mitochondria and/or other sites; and (4) increasing detoxification of metabolically generated active oxygen.

Possibility 1: Metabolic Rate Reduction. The finding by McCarter *et al.* (1985) that O_2 consumption per lean body weight of rat is unaltered by DR seems to be an insufficient basis on which to abandon metabolic rate reduction as contributing to DR's effects. How closely does O_2 consumption by the intact animal gauge actual rates of oxidative metabolism? What percentage of the total O_2 consumed is used for mitochondrial energy metabolism versus O_2 used otherwise (e.g., mixed function oxidases, oxygenases)? Clearly, O_2 consumption is much lower (30% per whole DR animal. Also, O_2 use needs to be considered on a tissue-by-tissue basis because DR strongly reduces the weight of most tissues (e.g., lymphoid tissues, muscle, fat) but not others (e.g., brain).

Possibility 2: Increased Metabolic Efficiency. Metabolic efficiency can be viewed from two standpoints. The efficiency of energy generation represents the fraction of the energy ingested and absorbed which is recaptured in a biologically usable form. The efficiency of energy usage can be thought of as the percentage of the trapped energy used for essential physiologic functions, versus that wasted as heat generation, or in maintaining the tissues of an obese animal, or in other nonessential ways. Perhaps DR increases these efficiencies.

Possibility 3: Reduced Free Radical Production. The hypothesis that DR lowers free radical production by either or both of two metabolic effects (↓ rate, ↑ efficiency) is supported by indirect evidence showing that long-term DR lowers tissue levels of lipid peroxides and lipofuscin, but is not supported by direct proof. This hypothesis requires testing using assays which precisely detect free radicals and oxygen radical inflicted damage.

Possibility 4: Increased Detoxification. The prospect that DR increases the capacity to detoxify metabolically generated active oxygen is also supported by recent data. In a collaborative study (Koizumi *et al.* 1987), we compared livers of 12 and 24 month mice fed control (C, 95 kcal/week) and restricted (R, 55 kcal/week) diets since 3 weeks of age (Table 7.4). Many enzyme activities were measured including several xenobiotic metabolizers, radical scavengers (catalase, superoxide dismutase,

TABLE 7.4
EFFECTS OF DIETARY RESTRICTION AND AGE ON ACTIVITIES OF SUPEROXIDE DISMUTASE, CATALASE AND β-OXIDATION, AND ON LIPID PEROXIDATION IN MICE[1]

Diet	Age	SOD	Catalase	β-oxidation	Lipid Peroxidation
C	12	43 ± 14^{A}	210 ± 29^{C}	2.2 ± 0.8^{A}	27 ± 4^{AB}
R	12	43 ± 8^{A}	298 ± 31^{B}	1.7 ± 0.5^{A}	19 ± 2^{C}
C→R	12	41 ± 3^{A}	198 ± 31^{C}	ND	24 ± 3^{B}
C	24	39 ± 4^{A}	212 ± 15^{C}	ND	31 ± 6^{A}
R	24	39 ± 7^{A}	347 ± 64^{A}	ND	27 ± 5^{AB}

Source: Adapted from Koizumi *et al.* (1987).

[1]Ages are in months, other values are means ± SD. Abbreviations: SOD, superoxide dismutase; ND, not determined; pro, protein; C, control; R, restricted; C→R, C diet until 1 week before assay when switched to R. Five to ten mice were studied within each diet-age group. The values for SOD (units/mg pro), catalase (μmol/[mg pro·min]), and β-oxidation (palmitoyl CoA oxidation in nmol/[mg pro·min]) are enzyme or pathway activities. Lipid peroxidation (pmol/mg pro·h]) gives the amount of malondialdehyde formed in the TBA test. Means in each column not sharing a common superscript letter were significantly different ($P < 0.05$).

glutathione peroxidase), and superoxide sources (xanthine oxidase, peroxisomal β-oxidation). Lipid peroxidation was also measured. The strongest dietary effect was an increased catalase activity for DR mice (group R: 42% higher at 12 months, 64% at 24 months). The increase in catalase activity was not associated with peroxisomal proliferation. Lipid peroxidation was clearly lower in group R at 12 months (a 30% decrease) and somewhat lower (13%) at 24 months than in controls. These data suggest that if free radical damage is involved in aging, it may be damage that is partly prevented by a selective increase in catalase activity.

Protein Synthesis, DNA, Chromatin, Gene Expression, DNA Repair

These subjects are interrelated in terms both of aging theories and experimental evidence for age- and DR-related changes. A large gerontologic literature exists for each of these areas; however, relatively few DR studies on these phenomena have been reported (Holehan and Merry 1986; Richardson 1988; Weindruch and Walford 1988). There is emerging evidence that DR increases rates of protein synthesis and turnover in certain tissues, gene expression, and UV-induced DNA repair. More intensive study of DR in relation to these areas is needed.

Neuroendocrine and Immunologic Explanations

These interpretations imply that in highly organized animals cellular function and survival and perhaps aging depend largely on the extracellular homeostatic and integrative mechanisms. This approach is different from being preoccupied with molecular events in individual organ systems. The attractive possibility that DR acts via the neuroendocrine system is discussed by Meites (1988); however, ". . .the available information, while tantalizing, is insufficient and too disconnected to allow a clear formulation of possibilities" (Weindruch and Walford 1988).

The Basal/Induced Activity Hypothesis

Caloric restriction may act by slowing the basal turnover rate of proliferative or potentially proliferative cell populations, at the same time enhancing the proliferative as well perhaps as other responses to an inductive stimulus (Walford *et al.* 1987). This situation would retard programmatic or deteriorative aging while increasing environmental adaptability and would accord with the observation that DR animals are both long-lived and have increased resistance to disease. Our prior studies on natural killer cells support such a concept (Weindruch *et al.* 1983). Diminished natural killer cell activity was observed in unstimulated DR mice, but increased activity after stimulation, compared to controls.

SUMMARY

Dietary restriction (DR) of caloric intake increases life span in diverse species. In mice and rats, the most impressive results occur by feeding diets enriched in essential nutrients but in restricted amounts such that the caloric intakes and peak body weights of DR animals are only 30–60% those of controls. In mice, both DR started in early life and in midadulthood can increase longevity, and the results of the adult-onset regimens closely approach those of early-onset DR. Rodents on DR display retarded rates of change for most but not all age-sensitive biologic parameters tested to date. The age-sensitive but DR-insensitive factors may explain why DR rodents do not live even longer. The mechanisms whereby DR retards aging processes in rodents are unclear but the fact that dietary energy restriction is required may signal the importance of effects on energy metabolism. Future DR studies seeking to elucidate underlying mechanisms are doomed to fail if the investigations continue to show by ever more advanced methods that DR animals are functionally younger.

REFERENCES

BEAUCHENE, R. E. *et al.* 1986. Effect of age of initiation of feed restriction on growth, body composition, and longevity of rats. J. Gerontol. *41*, 13–19.

BERG, B. N. and SIMMS, H. S. 1960. Nutrition and longevity in the rat II. Longevity and onset of disease. J. Nutr. *71*, 255–263.

CHENEY, K. E. *et al.* 1980. Survival and disease patterns in C57BL/6J mice subjected to undernutrition. Exp. Gerontol. *15*, 237–258.

CHENEY, K. E. *et al.* 1983. The effect of dietary restriction of varying duration on survival, tumor patterns, immune function, and body temperature in $B10C3F_1$ mice. J. Gerontol. *38*, 420–430.

FRIEND, P. S. *et al.* 1978. Dietary restrictions early and late: effects on the nephropathy of the NZB x NZW mouse. Lab. Invest. *38*, 629–632.

GERBASE-DELIMA, M. *et al.* 1975. Immune function and survival in a long-lived mouse strain subjected to undernutrition. Gerontologia *21*, 184–202.

GAJJAR, A., KUBO, C., JOHNSON, B. C. and GOOD, R. A. 1987. Influence of extremes of protein and energy intake on survival of B/W mice. J. Nutr. *117*, 1136–1140.

GOOD, R. A. and GAJJAR, A. J. 1986. Diet, immunity, and longevity. *In* Nutrition and Aging, M. L. Hutchinson and H. N. Munro (eds.). Academic Press, New York.

GOODRICK, C. L. *et al.* 1983. Differential effects of dietary restriction on growth and lifespan in genetically obese mice. Age *6*, 145 (Abstr.).

HARRISON, D. E. and ARCHER, J. R. 1987. Genetic differences in effects of food restriction on aging in mice. J. Nutr. *117*, 376–382.

HARRISON, D. E., ARCHER, J. R. and ASTLE, C. M. 1984. Effects of food restriction on aging: Separation of food intake and adiposity. Proc. Natl. Acad. Sci. USA *81*, 1835–1838.

HOLEHAN, A. M. and MERRY, B. J. 1986. The experimental manipulation of ageing by diet. Biol. Rev. *61*, 329–368.

INGRAM, D. K. *et al.* 1987. Dietary restriction benefits learning and motor performance of aged mice. J. Gerontol. *42*, 78–81.

KOIZUMI, A., WEINDRUCH, R. and WALFORD, R. L. 1987. Influences of dietary restriction and age on liver enzyme activities and lipid peroxidation in mice. J. Nutr., *117*, 361–367.

KUBO, C., DAY, N. K. and GOOD, R. A. 1984. Influence of early or late dietary restriction on life span and immunological parameters in MRL/Mp-lpr/lpr mice. Proc. Natl. Acad. Sci. USA *81*, 5831–5835.

KUBO, C., JOHNSON, B. C., GAJJAR, A. and GOOD, R. A. 1987. Crucial dietary factors in maximizing life span and longevity in autoimmune-prone mice. J. Nutr. *117*, 1129–1135.

MARK, D. A. *et al.* 1984. Effects of nutrition on disease and life span. I. Immune responses, cardiovascular pathology, and life span in MRL mice. Am. J. Pathol. *117*, 110–124.

MASORO, E. J. 1988. Food restriction in rodents: An evaluation of its role in the study of aging. J. Gerontol. *43*, B59–B64.

MCCARTER, R., MASORO, E. J. and YU, B. P. 1985. Does food restriction retard aging by reducing the metabolic rate? Am. J. Physiol. *248*, E488–490.

MCCAY, C. M., CROWELL, M. F. and MAYNARD, L. A. 1935. The effect of retarded growth upon the length of the life span and upon the ultimate body size. J. Nutr. *10*, 63–79.

MEITES, J. 1988. Evidence that underfeeding acts via the neuroendocrine system to influence aging processes. *In* Dietary Restriction and Aging, D. Snyder (ed.). Alan R. Liss, New York.

NELSON, W. and HALBERG, F. 1986. Meal-timing, circadian rhythms and life span of mice. J. Nutr. *116*, 2244–2253.

REHM, S., RAPP, K. G. and DEERBERG, F. 1985. Influence of food restriction and body fat on life span and tumour incidence in female outbred Han:NMRI mice and two sublines. Z. Versuchtierkd. *27*, 249–283.

RICHARDSON, A. 1988. Effect of age and dietary restriction on the expression of $\alpha 2_u$-globulin. *In* Dietary Restriction and Aging, D. Snyder (ed.). Alan R. Liss, New York.

ROSS, M. H. 1976. Nutrition and longevity in experimental animals. *In* Nutrition and Aging, M. Winick (ed.). John Wiley & Sons, New York.

TANNENBAUM, A. 1947. Effects of varying caloric intake upon tumor incidence and tumor growth. Ann. N. Y. Acad. Sci. *49*, 5–18.

TUCKER, M. J. 1979. The effect of long-term food restriction on tumors in rodents. Int. J. Cancer *23*, 803–807.

WALFORD, R. L., HARRIS, S. and WEINDRUCH, R. 1987. Dietary restriction and aging: historical phases, mechanisms, current directions. J. Nutr. *117*, 1650–1654.

WEINDRUCH, R. and WALFORD, R. L. 1982. Dietary restriction in mice beginning at one year of age: Effects on lifespan and spontaneous cancer incidence. Science *215*, 1415–1418.

WEINDRUCH, R. and WALFORD, R. L. 1988. The Retardation of Aging and Disease by Dietary Restriction. Charles C. Thomas, Springfield, IL.

WEINDRUCH, R., DEVENS, B. H., RAFF, H. V. and WALFORD, R. L. 1983. Influence of dietary restriction and aging on natural killer cell activity in mice. J. Immunol. *130*, 993–996.

WEINDRUCH, R., WALFORD, R. L., FLIGIEL, S. and GUTHRIE, D. 1986. The retardation of aging by dietary restriction: longevity, cancer, immunity and lifetime energy intake. J. Nutr. *116*, 641–654.

YU, B. P., MASORO, E. J. and McMAHAN, C. A. 1985. Nutritional influences on aging of Fischer 344 rats: I. Physical, metabolic and longevity characteristics. J. Gerontol. *40*, 657–670.

CHAPTER 8

CALORIC RESTRICTION AND AGING IN RATS

EDWARD J. MASORO, Ph. D.
Department of Physiology
The University of Texas
Health Science Center at San Antonio
San Antonio, Texas

INTRODUCTION

This discussion focuses on the research on food restriction and related manipulations that our laboratory has carried out with rats. Our basic premise is that there are primary aging processes which are similar in all mammalian species. The rat was chosen for the investigation of these putative primary aging processes for 2 reasons: the short life span (less than 5 years) and the size (large enough to enable ready execution of physiological measurements and to provide goodly amounts of biological materials but small enough to be economical to maintain).

An approach long and successfully used in the study of basic physiological processes is to perturb the process and then describe the responses to and determine the mechanisms of action of the perturbation. It is our belief that aging processes can also be fruitfully investigated in this way. To do so, however, it is necessary to find manipulations that perturb the aging processes, and this has proven to be difficult to accomplish. At this point in time only food restriction has been shown to do so for a mammalian species; indeed the requisite evidence has only been obtained for rodent species.

PERTURBATION OF AGING PROCESSES BY FOOD RESTRICTION

The claim that food restriction perturbs the aging processes rests on the following evidence: increased longevity; retardation of age-associated changes in physiological processes; delay or prevention of age-associated diseases.

Longevity

The influence of food restriction on longevity is shown by the survival curves (Fig. 8.1) obtained in our laboratory (Yu *et al.* 1982) for male Fischer 344 fats fed *ad libitum* or 60% of the mean *ad libitum* food intake. Although life expectancy (mean length of life from birth) was clearly increased, this does not necessarily mean that the aging processes have been influenced. Increase in life expectancy can be due to prevention of premature deaths (e.g., the prevention of early human deaths due to infectious disease that occurred in the United States during the first half of this century). However, in addition to increasing life expectancy, food restriction also markedly increases life span (the length of life of the longest lived members of the population). For the study represented by the survival curves in Fig. 8.1, when the last of the 115 *ad libitum* fed rats died, approximately 70% of the 115 food-restricted rats were alive. According to concepts developed by Sacher (1977), such an increase in life span provides strong evidence that the aging processes have been retarded.

Age-associated Changes in Physiological Processes

Most age changes in physiological processes are delayed or partially prevented by food restriction (Masoro 1988). During our studies with the male Fisher 344 rat the following were found: blunting of age-related increases in serum lipids (Liepa

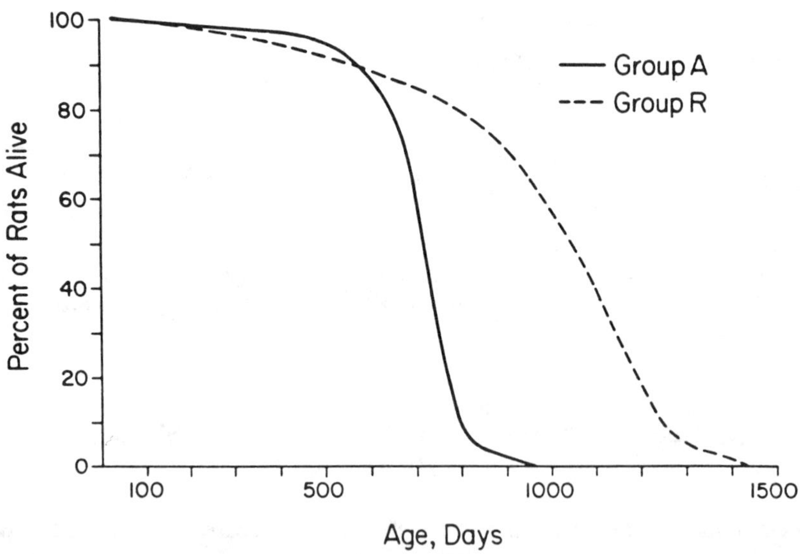

Courtesy of Yu et al. (1982)

FIG. 8.1 SURVIVAL CURVES FOR *AD LIBITUM* FED (GROUP A) AND RATS RESTRICTED TO 60% OF *AD LIBITUM* INTAKE (GROUP R)

et al. 1980; Masoro *et al.* 1983); blunting of age-related increases in serum parathyroid hormone and calcitonin concentrations (Kalu *et al.* 1988, 1983); modulation of the age-related loss in the responses of adipocytes to hormones (Bertrand *et al.* 1987; Yu *et al.* 1980; Voss *et al.* 1982); slowing of age-related changes in skeletal muscle structure and function (McCarter *et al.* 1982); prevention of age-related loss in tension development by vascular smooth muscle (Herlihy and Yu 1980); prevention of age-related decrease in spontaneous locomotor activity (Yu *et al.* 1985). The broad scope of action observed in our laboratory and in the laboratories of others with other rat strains and with mice provides strong evidence that the primary aging processes are being influenced by food restriction.

Age-associated Diseases

Food restriction retards most age-associated disease processes. In male Fischer 344 rats, the major ones are neoplastic disease, cardiomyopathy and chronic nephropathy. Food restriction was found to delay, but not prevent, the occurrence of neoplastic disease (Maeda *et al.* 1985). In contrast, it prevented the occurrence of severe cardiomyopathy and the progression of nephropathy to the point of renal failure (Maeda *et al.* 1985).

KIDNEY DISEASE: A CONFOUNDING ISSUE

Aging in rats, particularly in male Fischer 344 rats, is accompanied by a progressive nephropathy resulting in kidney failure in many rats by the time of their spontaneous death (Maeda *et al.* 1985). The question arises, therefore, as to whether the effects of food restriction on the aging processes in rats are due to the retardation of kidney disease rather than a direct action on the primary aging processes. To address this issue, extensive studies were carried out in our laboratory on the development of chronic nephropathy and its modulation by diet.

Grading of Lesions

The system used to grade the severity of the lesions of chronic nephropathy has been published (Yu *et al.* 1982) and is summarized in Table 8.1. The initial lesions involve the glomerular basement membrane and the mesangial matrix. The lesions progress to the tubules with thickening of the tubular basement membrane, obstruction of the tubular lumen with hyaline casts and interstitial lymphocyte infiltration. Eventually there is fibrosis of the glomeruli, tubules and interstitial tissue. Serum creatinine and BUN levels were used to evaluate the functional consequences of these lesions (Maeda *et al.* 1985). Rats with Grade 0 lesions (no lesions) and those with increasing severity lesions from Grade 1 (minimal lesions) through Grade 3 (moderate severity lesions) had similar serum creatinine and BUN levels. Rats with Grade 4

TABLE 8.1
SUMMARY OF THE SYSTEM FOR GRADING SEVERITY OF LESIONS OF CHRONIC NEPHROPATHY

Grade	Severity
0	No lesions
1	Thickening of mesangial matrix and glomerular basement membrane
2	Same as Grade 1 but more severe plus hyaline casts
3	Same as Grade 2 but more severe plus thickening of Bowman's capsule, lymphocyte infiltration and mild interstitial fibrosis
4	Same as Grade 3 but more severe plus glomerular sclerosis and frequent adhesions of glomerular tufts to Bowman's capsule
5	Same as Grade 4 but the glomerular sclerosis is widespread, as is interstitial fibrosis and calcification

lesions (very severe lesions) had small but significantly elevated serum creatinine and BUN levels. Rats with Grade E lesions (the most severe lesions) had markedly elevated serum creatinine and BUN levels along with parathyroid hyperplasia, osteodystrophy and metastatic calcification. Thus, rats with Grade E lesions appear to be in renal failure.

Food Restriction and Chronic Nephropathy

Male Fischer 344 rats fed our standard semisynthetic diet (containing 21% casein) showed a marked progression with age in the severity of chronic nephropathy, but rats restricted to 60% of the *ad libitum* fed intake did not. This is reflected in the difference between those two groups in regard to renal disease to the time of their spontaneous death (Table 8.2). Grade 4 or E lesions were found in 68% of the *ad libitum* fed rats compared to only 1% of the food restricted rats while 78% of the food restricted rats had Grade 0 or 1 lesions compared to 4% of the *ad libitum* fed rats. These findings are even more striking in light of the fact that food-restricted rats were much older at the time of death than *ad libitum* fed animals.

Protein Restriction and Chronic Nephropathy

Brenner *et al.* (1982) have proposed dietary protein causes the age-associated progression of chronic nephropathy. If so, food restriction may be retarding chronic nephropathy by reducing protein intake. To explore this further, dietary protein (casein) was restricted without restricting calories or other nutrients. Data on renal lesions at the time of spontaneous death are shown in Table 8.3. Although restricting dietary protein without restricting calories retarded the progression of chronic nephropathy, it was not as effective as food restriction which included caloric restriction.

TABLE 8.2
SEVERITY OF CHRONIC NEPHROPATHY AT TIME OF SPONTANEOUS DEATH OF RATS *AD LIBITUM* FED THE STANDARD CASEIN-CONTAINING DIET OR RESTRICTED TO 60% OF THE *AD LIBITUM* INTAKE

Dietary Regimen	Number of Rats Examined	% of Rats with Lesions of Grade 0	1	2	3	4	E
Ad libitum	182	0	4	14	14	23	45
Food restricted	145	6	72	15	6	0	1

Source: Data in this table are derived from Maeda *et al.* (1985) and Masoro *et al.* (1989a).

Soy Protein and Chronic Nephropathy

In a further study it was found that not only did the quantity of dietary protein influence nephropathy, but the nature of the protein did, too. The study used casein and soy protein as sources of dietary protein. The caloric intakes of the rats eating the soy protein and casein diets were similar but the severity of nephropathy was much less marked for rats on the soy protein diet (lesions at the time of spontaneous death are summarized in Table 8.4).

Comparison of Influence of Protein and Calories on Nephropathy

The relative importance of dietary protein and calories in nephropathy was further explored by comparing rats on restricted protein and caloric intake to those restricted in caloric but not protein (casein) intake. Lesions at the time of spontaneous death are reported in Table 8.5. Caloric restriction in the absence of protein restriction was almost as effective as caloric restriction which includes protein restriction in retarding the progression of chronic nephropathy. It should be noted that the rats on the caloric restriction regimen in the absence of protein restriction had a casein intake per gram body weight 1.7 times that of the *ad libitum* fed rats and lived much longer than the *ad libitum* fed rats.

TABLE 8.3
SEVERITY OF CHRONIC NEPHROPATHY AT TIME OF SPONTANEOUS DEATH OF RATS *AD LIBITUM* FED THE STANDARD (21% CASEIN) DIET OR A 12.6% CASEIN DIET

Dietary Regimen	Number of Rats Examined	% of Rats with Lesions of Grade 0	1	2	3	4	E
Standard (21% casein)	182	0	4	14	14	23	45
Protein restricted (12.6% casein)	68	2	15	25	22	26	10

Source: Data in this table are derived from Maeda *et al.* (1985) and Masoro *et al.* (1989a).

TABLE 8.4
SEVERITY OF CHRONIC NEPHROPATHY AT TIME OF SPONTANEOUS DEATH OF RATS FED *AD LIBITUM* STANDARD CASEIN DIET OR SOY PROTEIN DIET

Dietary Regimen	Number of Rats Examined	% of Rats with Lesions of Grade					
		0	1	2	3	4	E
Standard casein diet	182	0	4	14	14	23	45
Soy protein diet	70	3	12	24	34	20	7

Source: Data in this table are derived from Iwasaki *et al.* (1988a), Maeda *et al.* (1985) and Masoro *et al.* (1989a).

Conclusions

On the basis of our studies on longevity (Yu *et al.* 1985; Iwasaki *et al.* 1988a), age changes in physiological processes (Kalu *et al.* 1988; Masoro *et al.* 1983; Masoro 1984) and pathologic lesions other than nephropathy (Maeda *et al.* 1985; Masoro *et al.* 1989a) it is concluded that the action of food restriction on most aging processes is not secondary to its effect on renal disease. However, some actions were found to be secondary to renal disease, e.g., the increase with age in male Fischer 344 rats of plasma parathyroid hormone concentration (Kalu *et al.* 1988). This emphasizes the need to be fully aware of coexisting pathology when interpreting functional changes that occur with advancing age.

These studies also have provided new insights in regard to age-associated renal disease resulting in the following conclusions:

(1) Restriction of dietary protein intake is not the major reason for the retardation of chronic nephropathy by food restriction.
(2) The findings point to caloric restriction as the major reason for the retardation of chronic nephropathy by food restriction.
(3) The current emphasis on protein restriction (Mitch 1984) in the treatment of humans with chronic renal failure should be reassessed.

TABLE 8.5
COMPARISON OF INFLUENCE OF DIETARY CALORIES AND DIETARY PROTEIN ON CHRONIC NEPHROPATHY

Dietary Regimen	Number of Rats Examined	% of Rats with Lesions of Grade					
		0	1	2	3	4	E
Standard diet *ad libitum*	182	0	4	14	14	23	45
Restricted in both caloric and protein intake	145	6	72	15	6	0	1
Restricted in caloric but not protein intake	63	2	41	33	16	2	6

Source: Data in this table are derived from Maeda *et al.* (1985) and Masoro *et al.* (1989a).

RESTRICTION OF INDIVIDUAL DIETARY COMPONENTS

Protein

A 40% reduction in protein intake with no reduction in caloric intake increased the median length of life and the life span of male Fischer 344 rats, but these increases were much less marked than those occurring when food intake is reduced by 40% (Yu *et al.* 1985). Exploration of the effects of these dietary manipulations on age changes in physiological and disease processes led to the conclusion that the effect of protein restriction on longevity was secondary to its action on renal disease and that food restriction did not extend life span primarily through its effect on renal disease, but rather extended it by influencing the primary aging processes. This view is further supported by our research comparing caloric restriction in the presence and absence of protein restriction (Masoro *et al.* 1989a). Under these circumstances, in which renal disease is not a major problem for either group, restricting protein intake did not increase longevity but rather marginally decreased it.

Fat

Restricting dietary fat intake to the same extent as in the food restriction regimen but with out reducing caloric intake did not influence longevity of male Fischer 344 rats (Iwasaki *et al.* 1988b). Parenthetically it should be noted that this finding does not necessarily disagree with the recommendation that people reduce fat intake: (1) the fat source in our standard diet is corn oil and not animal fat; (2) fat in our standard diet accounts for 20% of the calories rather than the 40% or so of the typical American diet.

Minerals

Restriction of dietary mineral intake to the same extent as in the food restriction regimen but without reducing caloric intake did not influence longevity of male Fischer 344 rats (Iwasaki *et al.* 1988b). This finding is counter to the often heard claim that rat diets contain excessive amounts of minerals.

Conclusions

The data from our studies (Yu *et al.* 1985; Maeda *et al.* 1985; Iwasaki *et al.* 1988b; Masoro *et al.* 1989a) directly rule out the reduction in intake of protein or fat or minerals or vitamins as major factors in the action of food restriction on the aging processes. Moreover, these data indirectly rule out carbohydrates as well. Our conclusion is that it is most likely the restriction of calories which is responsible for the retardation of the aging processes.

It has been suggested that the restriction of adventitious toxic substances in the diet is responsible for the effects of food restriction on aging. Our data plus the fact that the many studies demonstrating food restriction extended life span used a wide range of food sources (Weindruch 1985) make this suggestion unlikely.

MECHANISMS

The current research in our and other laboratories is focused on learning the mechanisms by which food restriction retards aging processes. A major reason for this focus is the belief that knowledge of these mechanisms will yield insights on the nature of the primary aging processes. Another reason is the likelihood that such knowledge will provide a basis for the development of interventions for use in human aging.

Growth and Development Hypothesis

Initial studies on food restriction (McCay 1935) were interpreted as indicating aging was retarded by the delaying of maturation and the slowing of growth. Recent work casts doubt on the validity of this hypothesis. Our research with male Fischer 344 rats (Yu *et al.* 1985; Maeda *et al.* 1985) has yielded strong evidence against this view. The data on life span from these studies are summarized in Table 8.6. Food restriction started soon after weaning but stopped at 6 months of age had only a small effect on life span and little effect on the age changes in the physiological systems and age-associated disease processes. In contrast, food restriction started either soon after weaning or in young adult life and continued until death were equally effective in markedly increasing life span, retarding age changes in the physiological systems and retarding age-associated disease processes. In spite of these findings the hypothesis that food restriction acts by retarding maturation still has some advocates. It appears to be particularly appealing to the evolutionary biologists.

Body Fat Hypothesis

Berg and Simms (1960) proposed that food restriction influences the aging processes by decreasing the body fat content. This has been a popular view because of the link between adiposity and longevity in humans. Food restricted male Fischer 344 rats are leaner than *ad libitum* fed rats (Bertrand *et al.* 1980), and presumably this is also true of other rat strains and mice. With the *ad libitum* fed male Fischer 344 rats no correlation was found between body fat content and the length of life and with the food-restricted animals there was a positive correlation. Bertrand *et al.* (1980) concluded that, although food restricted rats are leaner than *ad libitum* fed rats, this leanness is not causally related to the actions of food restriction on

TABLE 8.6
INFLUENCES OF DIETARY RESTRICTION APPLIED AT DIFFERENT STAGES OF LIFE ON THE LIFE SPAN

Dietary Program	Age of 10th Percentile Survivor Days	Maximum Length of Life Days
Ad libitum fed through life	822	941
Food restricted from 6 weeks of age	1226	1296
Food restricted from 6 weeks to 6 months of age	918	1040
Food restricted from 6 months of age	1177	1299

Source: Data in this table are derived from Yu *et al.* (1985).

the aging processes. Stuchlíková *et al.* (1975) came to a similar conclusion from their studies with male Wistar rats as did Harrison *et al.* (1984) from their studies with mice.

Metabolic Rate Hypothesis

The hypothesis which has had the greatest impact is that of Sacher (1977) in which he proposed food restriction retards the aging processes by lowering the metabolic rate. The reasons for such a great impact are two: First, the long history of the belief that aging is inversely related to metabolic rate (Masoro 1985) and second the linkage between metabolic rate and the generation of oxygen free radicals (Harman 1981). This hypothesis was directly tested in our laboratory (McCarter *et al.* 1985) in a study in which the metabolic rate in *ad libitum* fed and food restricted male Fischer 344 rats was measured under conditions similar to those of the usual living environment. The metabolic rate per 24 h per unit of lean body mass (or "metabolic mass") was found not to be decreased by food restriction. Many find these results difficult to accept because of the body of evidence showing a fall in metabolic rate in response to a reduction in food intake. McCarter and McGee (1988) have recently addressed this issue and have indeed found that there is a fall in metabolic rate in response to food restriction but the decrease is transient, lasting less than six weeks. Since in earlier work (Yu *et al.* 1985), it was found that it is prolonged rather than short-term food restriction that retards the aging processes it is not likely that the transient decrease in metabolic rate plays a major role. Thus on the basis of the work of our laboratory, it must be concluded that food restriction need not lower the metabolic rate per unit of "metabolic mass" to retard the aging processes.

GENERAL CONCLUSIONS AND FUTURE DIRECTIONS

During our assessment of the Sacher hypotheses, data were collected and analyzed on the influence of food restriction started at 6 weeks of age with male Fischer 344 rats on the intake of calories and other nutrients per gram of lean body mass (Masoro *et al.* 1982). Of course, at the start, food intake per gram lean body mass was less in food restricted than *ad libitum* fed rats, but this difference rapidly disappeared during the first six weeks. Thus, for most of the life span food restricted rats did not have a reduced intake of calories or any other nutrient per unit of lean body mass. Quite simply the lean body mass of the food restricted rats rapidly changed in such a fashion that caloric intake per unit of lean body mass was the same in food restricted rats as in *ad libitum* fed rats, a finding totally in agreement with our metabolic rate findings.

Therefore, it is the decreased nutrient intake per rat (animal) not per unit of lean body mass (or "metabolic" mass) that retards the aging processes. Since a reduced flux of calories (or other nutrient) per unit tissue mass cannot be the factor responsible for retarding aging, the challenge is to learn how the intake of calories per rat (animal) is coupled to the aging processes.

We propose the following working hypothesis: Food restriction is coupled to the aging processes through its action on the endocrine and/or neural regulatory systems. In this schema, the reduced food intake signals the neural and endocrine regulatory centers by either neural or humoral afferent pathways. The regulatory centers respond to this input by sending neural or humoral efferent messages to target sites which result in the occurrence of molecular events opposed to the aging processes.

A logical place to initiate research on this hypothesis would be studies aimed at identifying the afferent pathways including sensors or receptors. Unfortunately, no information is currently available to serve as guides for such an approach. For this reason, our initial studies are focused on identifying the neural and endocrine systems involved. Identification of these systems should provide a basis for designing research aimed at understanding the afferent pathways.

Two guidelines have been used in choosing the endocrine and neural systems to be studied. One is the evidence that the system may be involved in aging. The other is the likelihood that food restriction can influence the system.

Based on these criteria, the adrenal cortical glucocorticoid system is a good candidate for study. First, Dallman (1984) points out the large body of evidence which shows a strong interaction between food intake and plasma glucocorticoid levels. Second, Sapolsky *et al.* (1986) on the basis of their studies with rats have proposed the "Glucocorticoid Cascade Hypothesis of Aging." The essence of this theory is the loss with age in the regulatory control of glucocorticoid secretion which Sapolsky *et al.* showed occurs with rats. The resulting hyperadrenocorticism is viewed to further compromise this regulatory control and ultimately to promote aging processes in target tissues. Food restriction could, therefore, retard the aging processes by preventing the loss with age in this regulatory control of the glucocorticoid system. The initial results from our explorations of this possibility do not support such an action of food restriction. Measurement of the diurnal concentrations of plasma corticosterone over the age range of 3–13 months in a longitudinal study of our *ad libitum* fed and food-restricted male Fischer 344 rats showed that the food-restricted rats tended to have higher rather than lower plasma corticosterone levels. On the basis of the "Glucocorticoid Cascade Hypothesis of Aging" the opposite results would have been anticipated if the antiaging action of food restriction relates to a modulation of age changes in the regulatory control of the adrenal cortical glucocorticoid system. However, such an influence may only occur at more advanced ages. Therefore, any definitive conclusion must await completion of this longitudinal study.

Another likely candidate is the glucose-insulin system. Cerami (1985) proposed glucose to be a mediator of aging in what might be called the "Glycation Theory of Aging." This theory is based on the fact that glucose nonenzymatically glycosylates proteins and nucleic acids. With time reactions involving these glycosylated materials occur which result in the formation of advanced glycosylation end-products. The resulting alterations in protein and nucleic acid structure including cross-linking are proposed to cause functional change characterized as aging. The extent to which these end-products are formed directly relates to the concentration of glucose and the time of exposure of proteins and nucleic acids to the glucose concentration. Of course, it is likely that food restriction influences the glucose-insulin system making that system a good candidate for study. The initial results of our research on this possibility are promising. Food-restricted rats maintained plasma glucose levels below that of the *ad libitum* fed rats throughout the day (mean 24 h levels being 15 mg/dL below the *ad libitum* fed) and a glycosylated hemoglobin level significantly below that of the *ad libitum* fed (Masoro *et al.* 1989b). However, much more work is needed to establish that food restriction retards the aging processes by its influence on plasma glucose levels.

Similar arguments can be made for the thyroid gland and the sympathetic nervous system as candidates for the coupling of food restriction to the aging processes. Research on these candidates has also been initiated in our laboratory.

The influence of food restriction on molecular responses in target tissues to food restriction has been the focus of much study. On the basis of the findings, two general areas have emerged as promising avenues for future research.

One is based on the hypothesis of Cheung and Richardson (1982) that a fundamental change during aging is the reduction in the rate of protein turnover which comprises cellular homeostasis. Evidence has been obtained in our laboratory (Ward 1988a, 1988b) and by Richardson's group (Birchenall-Sparks *et al.* 1985; Ricketts *et al.* 1985) that a higher rate of protein turnover is maintained for most of the life span in food-restricted rats compared to *ad libitum* fed animals. Moreover, in a study using male Fischer 344 rats from our laboratory, Richardson *et al.* (1987) found that the transcription of α_{2u}-globulin gene by isolated liver nuclei is markedly decreased with increasing age and that food restriction retards this age-related decrease in α_{2u}-globulin expression. Further work is needed in this important area and much is under way.

The other area is based on the free-radical theory of aging (Harman 1981). Laganiere and Yu (1987) reported that food restriction inhibits the increase with age in malondialdehyde production by membranes isolated from the liver of male Fischer 344 rats and retards the age-related increase in the lipid peroxide content of these membranes. These findings are similar to those reported for mice (Chipalkatti *et al.* 1983; Koizumi *et al.* 1987). Laganiere and Yu suggest that these findings are in part due to the inhibition by food restriction of the age-related increase in the content of membrane 22:5 fatty acid, thereby reducing the peroxidizability of membrane lipids. In this view food restriction acts to retard the deterioration of membrane structure and function with advancing age. These findings and suggestions are provocative and this research area should be a high priority one.

How these changes in the target tissues are linked to neural and endocrine coupling systems has yet to be addressed. However, it is to be expected that as our knowledge of the involvement of the neural and endocrine systems and of the molecular events in the target tissues develops, the nature of this linkage will probably become evident.

ACKNOWLEDGMENTS

The research of the author has been supported by grant number AGO1188 from the National Institute on Aging of the National Institutes of Health.

REFERENCES

BERG, B. N. and SIMMS, H. S. 1960. Nutrition and longevity in the rat. II. Longevity and onset of disease with different levels of intake. J. Nutr. *71*, 255–263.

BERTRAND, H. A., ANDERSON, W. R., MASORO, E. J. and YU, B. P. 1987. Action of food restriction on age-related changes in adipocyte lipolysis. J. Gerontol. *42*, 666–673.

BERTRAND, H. A., LYND, F. T., MASORO, E. J. and YU, B. P. 1980. Changes in adipose mass and cellularity through the adult life of rats fed ad libitum or a life prolonging restricted diet. J. Gerontol. *35*, 827–835.

BIRCHENALL-SPARKS, M. G. *et al.* 1985. Effect of dietary restriction on liver protein synthesis in rats. J. Nutr. *115*, 944–950.

BRENNER, B. M., MEYER, T. W. and HOSTETTER, T. H. 1982. Dietary protein intake and the progressive nature of kidney disease. N. Engl. J. Med. *307*, 652–659.

CERAMI, A. 1985. Hypothesis: glucose as a mediator of aging. J. Am. Geriat. Soc. *33*, 626–634.

CHEUNG, H. T. and RICHARDSON, A. 1982. The relationship between age-related changes in gene expression, protein turnover and the responsiveness of an organism to stimuli. Life Sci. *31*, 605–613.

CHIPALKATTI, S., DE, A. K. and AIYAR, A. N. 1983. Effect of diet restriction on some biochemical parameters related to aging in mice. J. Nutr. *113*, 944–950.

DALLMAN, M. F. 1984. Viewing the ventromedial hypothalamus from the adrenal gland. Am. J. Physiol. *246*, R1–12.

HARMAN, D. 1981. The aging process. Proc. Natl. Acad. Sci. USA *78*, 7124–7128.

HARRISON, D. E., ARCHER, J. R. and ASTLE, C. M. 1984. Effects of food restriction on aging: separation of food intake and adiposity. Proc. Natl. Acad. Sci. USA *81*, 1835–1838.

HERLIHY, J. R. and YU, B. P. 1980. Dietary manipulation of age-related decline in vascular smooth muscle function. Am. J. Physiol. *238*, H652–655.

IWASAKI, K. *et al.* 1988a. The influence of dietary protein source on longevity and age-related disease processes of Fischer rats. J. Gerontol. Biol. Sci. *43*. B5–12.

IWASAKI, K. *et al.* 1988b. Influence of the restriction of individual dietary components on longevity and age-related disease of Fischer rats: the fat component and the mineral component. J. Gerontol. Biol. Sci. *43*, B13–21.

KALU, D. N., COCKERHAM, R., YU, B. P. and ROOS, B. A. 1983. Lifelong dietary modulation of calcitonin levels in rats. Endocrinology *113*, 2010–2016.

KALU, D. N. *et al.* 1988. Modulation of age-related hyperparathyroidism and senile bone loss in Fischer rats by soy protein and food restriction. Endocrinology *122*, 1847–1854.

KOIZUMI, A., WEINDRUCH, R. and WALFORD, R. L. 1987. Influences of dietary restriction and age on liver enzyme activities and lipid peroxidation in mice. J. Nutr. *117*, 361–367.

LAGANIERE, S. and YU, B. P. 1987. Anti-lipoperoxidation action of food restriction. Biochem. Biophys. Res. Comms. *145*, 1185–1197.

LIEPA, G. U., MASORO, E. J., BERTRAND, H. A. and YU, B. P. 1980. Food restriction as a modulator of age-related changes in serum lipids. Am. J. Physiol. *238*, E253–257.

MAEDA, H. *et al.* 1985. Nutritional influences on aging of Fischer 344 rats: II. Pathology. J. Gerontol. *40*, 671–688.

MASORO, E. J. 1984. Nutrition as a modulator of the aging processes. Physiologist *27*, 98–101.

MASORO, E. J. 1985. Metabolism. *In* Handbook of the Biology of Aging, 2nd Ed., C. Finch and E. L. Schneider (eds.). Van Nostrand Reinhold, New York.

MASORO, E. J. 1988. Food restriction in rodents: an evaluation of its role in the study of aging. J. Gerontol. Biol. Sci. *43*, B59–64.

MASORO, E. J., COMPTON, C., YU, B. P. and BERTRAND, H. 1983. Temporal and compositional dietary restrictions modulate age-related changes in serum lipids. J. Nutr. *113*, 880–892.

MASORO, E. J. *et al.* 1989a. Dietary modulation of the progression of nephropathy in aging rats: an exploration of the importance of protein. Am. J. Clin. Nutr. *49*, 1217–1227.

MASORO, E. J., KATZ, M. S. and McMAHAN, C. A. 1989b. Evidence for glycation hypothesis of aging from food-restricted rodent model. J. Gerontol. Biol. Sci. *44*, B20–22.

MASORO, E. J., YU, B. P. and BERTRAND, H. A. 1982. Action of food restriction in delaying the aging process. Proc. Natl. Acad. Sci. USA *79*, 4239–4241.

McCARTER, R. J. M., MASORO, E. J. and YU, B. P. 1982. Rat muscle structure and metabolism in relation to age and food intake. Am. J. Physiol. *242*, R89–93.

McCARTER, R. J. M., MASORO, E. J. and YU, B. P. 1985. Does food restriction retard aging by reducing metabolic rate? Am. J. Physiol. *248*, E488–490.

McCARTER, R. J. M. and McGEE, J. 1988. Food restriction and metabolic rate: different adaptive time courses of BMR and 24-hour metabolic rate. FASEB J. *2*, A1208.

McCAY, C., CROWELL, M. and MAYNARD, L. 1935. The effect of retarded growth upon the length of life and upon ultimate size. J. Nutr. *10*, 63–79.

MITCH, W. E. 1984. The influence of diet on the progression of renal insufficiency. Annu. Rev. Med. *35*, 249–264.

RICHARDSON, A. *et al.* 1987. Effect of age and dietary restriction on the expression of α_{2u}-globulin. J. Biol. Chem. *262*, 12821–12825.

RICKETTS, W. G., BIRCHENALL-SPARKS, M. C., HARDWICK, J. P. and RICHARD-

SON, A. 1985. Effect of age and dietary restriction on protein synthesis by isolated kidney cells. J. Cell. Physiol. *125*, 492–498.

SACHER, G. A. 1977. Life table modifications and life prolongation. *In* Handbook of the Biology of Aging, C. Finch and L. Hayflick (eds.). Van Nostrand Reinhold, New York.

SAPOLSKY, R. M., KREY, L. C. and McEWEN, B. S. 1986. The neuroendocrinology of stress and aging: the glucocorticoid cascade hypothesis. Endoc. Rev. *7*, 284–301.

STUCHLIKOVÁ, E., JURICOVA-HORAKOVÁ, M. and DEYL, Z. 1975. New aspects of dietary effect of life prolongation in rodents. What is the role of obesity in aging? Exp. Gerontol. *10*, 141–145.

VOSS, K. H., MASORO, E. J. and ANDERSON, W. 1982. Modulation of age-related loss of glucagon-promoted lipolysis by food restriction. Mech. Age. Dev. *18*, 135–149.

WARD, W. F. 1988a. Enhancement by food restriction of liver protein synthesis in aging Fischer 344 rats. J. Gerontol. Biol. Sci. *43*, B50–53.

WARD, W. F. 1988b. Food restriction enhances the proteolytic capacity of aging rat livers. J. Gerontol. Biol. Sci. *43*, B121–124.

WEINDRUCH, R. 1985. Aging in rodents fed restricted diets. J. Am. Geriat. Soc. *22*, 125–132.

YU, B. P., BERTRAND, H. A. and MASORO, E. J. 1980. Nutrition-aging influence of catecholamine-promoted lipolysis. Metabolism *29*, 438–444.

YU, B. P., MASORO, E. J. and McMAHAN, C. A. 1985. Nutritional influences on aging Fischer 344 rats: I. Physical, metabolic and longevity characteristics. J. Gerontol. *40*, 657–670.

YU, B. P. *et al.* 1982. Life span study of SPF Fischer 344 male rats fed *ad libitum* or restricted diets: longevity, growth, lean body mass and disease. J. Gerontol. *37*, 130–141.

CHAPTER 9

GENOTYPE MODULATES THE EFFECTS OF CALORIC RESTRICTION ON AGING PROCESSES IN RODENTS

DAVID E. HARRISON, Ph.D., and JONATHAN R. ARCHER
The Jackson Laboratory
Bar Harbor, Maine

INTRODUCTION

The only treatment that consistently retards aging in mammals is the nutritional manipulation, food restriction. It extends life spans of short-lived rodents if begun early in life (McCay *et al.* 1939; Ross 1976; Barrows and Kokkonen 1977; Young 1979; Yu *et al.* 1985; Weindruch *et al.* 1986). Knowledge of how food restriction retards aging processes might suggest clinically useful treatments.

Retarding age-associated depression of immune function, or reducing long-term metabolic rates, are two strongly supported hypotheses describing how food restriction may act. In collaborative experiments, we found that T-cell precursor frequencies remain near young levels in old, food-restricted B6CBAF$_1$ hybrids. On the other hand, genetically obese C57BL/6J female longevities are extended without improving their immune responses. Genetically obese mice are thus important because they seem to have reduced metabolic rates without improved immune responses, and thus separate the immune and metabolic hypotheses.

Aging in a variety of biological systems was retarded in food-restricted B6CBAF$_1$ males, consistent with their increased longevities. Results were similar in food-restricted C57BL/6J males, except for hair regrowth rates. This was the only system correctly predicting that the same food restriction treatment that benefited B6CBAF$_1$ and C57BL/6J obese males reduced longevity in C57BL/6J males. Using defined diets so that only carbohydrates and fats were reduced, C57BL/6J males were benefited by food restriction. These results suggest that food restriction (and probably all treatments to retard aging) may have beneficial effects by different mechanisms in different genotypes and that a treatment beneficial for some individuals may not be beneficial for all.

A proposed evolutionary mechanism that would produce this response to limited food supplies predicts that the extension of longevities should be more effective in species with shorter life spans. Nevertheless, food restriction is the best available model for treatments that retard aging rates in mammals, and knowledge of how it operates should be useful in man.

DEFINING THE MECHANISMS OF THE FOOD RESTRICTION EFFECT

Retarding Immune Dysfunction With Age

Food restriction preserves immune responses in normal aging mice (Walford *et al.* 1974; Weindruch and Suffin 1980; Weindruch *et al.* 1982) and retards immunopathological changes in autoimmunity-prone mice (Fernandes *et al.* 1978). T-cell precursor frequencies remain near young levels in old, food-restricted B6CBAF$_1$ hybrids (Miller and Harrison 1985). These data fit the idea that immune dysfunctions are important in causing aging and suggest that beneficial effects of food restriction result from retarding immune dysfunction with age. Higher levels of immune function obviously would contribute to extended longevity by increasing resistance to infectious agents and to certain tumors. In addition, autoimmunity may increase with age as normal immune responses decline, and autoimmune reactions may cause many of the deleterious effects of aging (Walford 1969).

However, other sets of data contradict the idea that immune dysfunctions are important in aging. Some immune responses are reduced in food-restricted mice (Christadoss *et al.* 1984), and life spans of genetically obese C57BL/6J (B6)-*ob/ob* female mice are extended without improving their immune responses (Harrison *et al.* 1984). B6-*ob/ob* mice have impaired cellular immunity (Mead and Sheena 1979) expressed when mutants are sensitized *in vivo* (Nichols *et al.* 1978). While there may be an immunosuppression caused by the elevated insulin and corticosteroid levels of *ob/ob* mice, levels of these hormones were elevated at young ages when the splenic immune responses were normal. The immune responses per spleen then showed accelerated rates of declines with age (Harrison *et al.* 1984) that food restriction failed to alter.

Reducing Long-term Metabolic Rates

Food restriction may also retard aging by reducing metabolic rates. Rubner (1908) calculated that domestic animals of a wide range of sizes use over their lifetimes a similar number of calories per gram of body mass. Pearl (1928) proposed the "rate of living'' hypothesis: the higher the metabolic rate per gram of body mass, the shorter the life span of a species. Thus, food restriction might extend longevity by retarding metabolic rates.

Why reducing metabolic rates may reduce aging rates is explained by current theories that aging is caused by free-radical damage (Harman 1981), mostly from toxic oxygen radicals, so the rate of O_2 utilization should affect rates of aging. This is supported by the finding of Sacher and Duffy (1979) that longevities in 26 mouse strains and F1 hybrids were negatively correlated with average O_2 consumption. Sacher's (1977) calculations using data published by Ross (1969) showed that rats fed different diets had a wide range of longevities, but all groups had similar lifetime calorie intakes per gram body weight. In precise studies of metabolic rates over 3–4 weeks, young Sprague-Dawley rats adapted to a restricted diet by reducing their O_2 consumption (Forsum *et al.* 1981), and the degree of reduction in metabolic rate of Wistar rats was proportional to the reduction in body weight (Hill *et al.* 1985). However, 3–4 weeks does not represent long-term food restriction.

In the only study that measured effects of food restriction over a long time, F344 rats consumed equal amounts of O_2/g lean body mass per day whether food was restricted or fed *ad libitum* (McCarter *et al.* 1985). This contradicts the metabolic hypothesis, and fits life-long food restriction studies, in which Masoro *et al.* (1982) and Weindruch *et al.* (1986) found that rats and mice limited to one half to two thirds of normal caloric consumption were much smaller and longer lived, and so consumed more calories per gram during their lives than did *ad libitum* fed controls.

These results do not necessarily contradict the idea that an important cause of aging is free-radical damage. Increased O_2 utilization might not be harmful if protective mechanisms against free radicals (such as antioxidants) were also increased proportionally. While it is vital to test protective measures, unfortunately there are too many antioxidants and enzymes with potential protective action to measure practically. The critical point is the rate of oxidative damage to the organism. Total lipid peroxidation reactions in tissue homogenates may be measured by methods that correlate with species maximum life span potentials (Cutler 1985). Direct measures of oxidative damage to long-lasting molecules such as DNA (Cathcart *et al.* 1984) should also be used to determine whether food restriction reduces such damage.

Obese Mouse Models

B6-*ob/ob* mice are important because they greatly increase weight gain and adiposity when fed the same amount as normal mice (Coleman 1985). Thus, they appear to have reduced metabolic rates. Food restriction extends longevities of *ob/ob* mice (Lane and Dickie 1958; Harrison *et al.* 1984; Harrison and Archer 1987), although in the 1984 study, they rapidly lost immune responses with age.

Assays for Aging

Objective measures of aging rates in different biological systems are vital for evaluating effects of antiaging treatments such as food restriction. We have defined a series of assays of "biomarkers," changes with age in a variety of biological systems that can all be measured in single mice without significantly affecting longevities (Harrison and Archer 1983, 1987, 1988b). For example, six biomarkers that changed with age in B6 and $B6CBAF_1$ males are: tail collagen denaturation rate, wound healing rate, hemoglobin and hematocrit levels, urine concentrating ability, hair regrowth rate, and neuromuscular function (tight wire).

Values for most of these assays were significantly more like than those of younger mice in food restricted than in *ad libitum* fed (C57BL/6J × CBA/HT6J) F_1 hybrid ($B6CBAF_1$) males, as expected from their increased longevities. In food restricted B6 +/+ males, biomarkers gave similar results except hair regrowth rates were faster in *ad libitum* fed mice. This was the only biomarker correctly predicting the surprising result that food restriction reduced longevity in B6 males (Harrison and Archer 1987). These results suggest that food restriction has beneficial effects on biomarkers by different mechanisms in different genotypes, and that these may not correlate with longevities.

METHODS AND MATERIALS

Since this chapter reviews many studies that have already been reported, the references will be given, but methods used from them will only be summarized. Methods will be detailed when they have not been published elsewhere.

Mice

All mice were raised and tested at The Jackson Laboratory, and were free from known pathogens when tested for 10 standard mouse viruses by Microbiological Associates. A description of the health monitoring procedures used in this colony has been published (Harrison and Archer 1983). Only mice appearing healthy to an experienced observer were used for tests of physiological systems. Health assessment was based on normal activity and responses to handling, normal external appearance including eyes and pelt, absence of palpable lumps, and absence of recent weight loss. Even more important, the tests did not harm the subjects, so subsequent longevities were determined after testing.

Food Restriction Protocols

Protocol I. In studies, mice were housed 4 per side of cage at 4 weeks of age. In the earlier food restriction protocol used for most of the data in this paper (Harrison *et al.* 1984; Miller and Harrison 1985; Harrison and Archer 1987), all mice were fed a grain-based, pelleted, pasteurized diet (96WA, Emory Morse, Guilford, CT), containing 22% protein, 7% fat, 50% nitrogen-free extract (mostly carbohydrates), and 357 Kcal/100 g. Restricted mice received their rations each day in a single feeding between 12:00 and 2:00 PM, 6 days a week, with double rations on the sixth, day, and none on the seventh. *Ad libitum* fed mice had access to food at all times. These feeding regimens were continued throughout life. Restricted mice were given two-thirds of the amount of food consumed by *ad libitum* fed mice, with one or more food pellets each when fed. There were no unusual losses from fighting among food restricted mice, and the variations in body weights of cage-mates were similar in fed and restricted groups, suggesting that the dominant mouse did not consume an unusually large share of food in the restricted cages.

Protocol II. In our new protocol, total amounts of all nutrients except carbohydrates and fats are the same among animals fed *ad libitum* and food restricted, and the fiber percentage is the same. The diet is semichemically defined, based on the AIN 76 diet, as described by Bieri *et al.* (1977), but altered as follows. We reduced protein, and changed starches from 50% sucrose plus 15% corn starch to 27.4% sucrose, 32.3% corn starch, and 5% dextrose. This increases amounts of complex starches, and the resulting powder can still be pelleted, if necessary. The vitamin and mineral mix supplements are those recommended by the AIN 76 committee (Bieri *et al.* 1977), but amounts are increased by a factor of 1.5 to insure against potential deficiencies developing with age. In addition, Vitamin K has been increased 10-fold in the vitamin mix. This diet, detailed in Table 9.1, is purchased from TEKLAB and was designed with the help of Dr. R. J. Rose.

TABLE 9.1
SEMICHEMICALLY DEFINED DIETS[1]

Percentage Weight Ingredient	Fed *Ad Libitum* Mouse	Restricted Mouse
Casein	18.0	25.56
DL-Methionine	0.27	0.382
Sucrose	27.42	23.21
Corn starch	32.26	27.49
Dextrose (monohydrate)	5.0	4.24
Fiber (cellulose-type)	5.0	5.0
Corn oil	5.0	4.14
AIN-76 mineral mix	5.25	7.43
AIN-76 vitamin mix	1.50	2.12
Choline bitartrate	0.30	0.424

[1]Details of the diets in food restriction protocol II. Food-restricted mice are given 72% the weight of diets eaten by *ad libitum* fed animals. Amounts of most nutrients are constant, but caloric intake is reduced to 68% by reducing the amount of carbohydrate and oil.

Measurements in Different Biological Systems

Food (given in food restriction experiments) is the amount eaten recorded as grams per day per mouse and measured for one week during the period when the physiological systems were being tested. Weight is body weight in grams measured when the other tests were performed. Tail length is measured in centimeters from the root of the tail where it joins the rectum to the tip of the tail.

Tail collagen aging is given as the denaturation rate, i.e., the number of minutes required for a single tendon fiber from the middle of the tail to be denatured in 7 M urea at 45 °C, so that it is broken by a 2 g weight (Harrison *et al.* 1978). Urine concentrating ability is measured as the osmolality in mOs/kg of urine from a mouse deprived of water for 48 h. Urine samples are held in capillary tubes to prevent evaporation, food remains present, and mice are injected with 1.0 mL saline intraperitoneally at time zero (Harrison and Archer 1983).

Thymus-dependent immune responses were measured using spleen cells, as detailed previously (Astle and Harrison 1984; Harrison *et al.* 1984). Formation of direct plaques in response to SRBC (sheep erythrocytes) was measured *in vivo* by a modified Jerne Plaque assay. Proliferation in response to the mitogen phytohemagglutinin (PHA) *in vitro* was measured by tritiated thymidine uptake. Since the spleen must be removed, these measures can only be done once and may affect subsequent longevity.

Limiting dilution assays were done using blood cells, as detailed previously (Miller 1984; Miller and Harrison 1985). Helper (pHTL) and killer (pCTL) cell frequencies were calculated from titration curves in which doses of 5, 10, 20, or 40 whole blood leukocyte responder cells were added to each microtiter well, which contained appropriate media, supplements, and filler cells. Each well was scored as positive, if its supernatant supported T lymphocyte proliferation (for helpers), or if its cells caused target cell lysis (for killers), at least three standard deviations above the control values for wells containing no responder cells.

Tight wire refers to a test measuring the time in seconds that a mouse can hold itself on a wire suspended above foam padding. Timing is begun after the mouse grips the wire with both front paws and one hind paw. There is no exit from the wire, but mice are removed and testing ends if they cling for 240 s in a single trial. Otherwise the maximum score of five trials is recorded (Campbell 1982). Correlations between tight-wire clinging times and body weights among mice of thc same age and genotype showed that only a small portion of the variance could be explained by increased weight causing decreased clinging times. For example, in B6 males at 500–614 days of age, correlation coefficients (r) between clinging times and body weights for *ad libitum* fed and food restricted +/+ mice and for food restricted *ob/ob* mice were −0.266, −0.159 and −0.409, explaining 7%, 3% and 17% respectively of the variances in clinging times (Harrison and Archer 1987).

Open field is a measure of the activity displayed during five minutes in a 80 cm square, well-lighted, open-topped box, measured as the number of 15 cm sided squares that the mouse crosses (Sprott and Eleftheriou 1974). Hair growth is a test measuring the fraction of a 2 cm square shaved area centered on the back near the tail into which hair has begun to regrow after 25 days. The subjective element in estimating the area is minimized by defining regrowth as the first appearance of hair, and dividing the shaved area to be scored into 8 equal portions with a transparent screen. Excellent repeatability was found when 22 mice were randomly recaged and retested an hour after the initial trial; 20 were scored exactly the same way both times, and scores of the other 2 varied by only one of the 8 screen divisions (Harrison and Archer 1987).

Wound healing is a test measuring the number of days required until the wound in the tail made in removing a portion of one of the dorsal tail tendon bundles for the tail collagen test feels smooth to the touch when running the index finger along the tail. Tails were checked 7 days after the wounds were made, and every 2–3 days thereafter. Since this test is subjective all animals in an experiment were scored by the same technician. In a blind test of repeatability, the correlation coefficient between successive runs was 0.88 with 16 mice. In the same experiment, one that was designed to evaluate the technician, wounds were made at different times over three weeks, but presented as if all had been made simultaneously. Expected healing times were 27.2, 34.5, 41.2 and 34.8 days for 4 groups of mice; reported times were 24.5, 36.5, 40.0 and 35.6 respectively, demonstrating good objectivity (Harrison and Archer 1987).

Hemoglobin is tested as the concentration of hemoglobin in blood, measured by taking blood from the retroorbital sinus in a 70 mL heparinized microhematocrit capillary tube (Fisher), mixing 10 mL blood with 2.50 mL Drabkin's reagent (1.0 g sodium bicarbonate, 0.05 g potassium cyanide, 0.20 g potassium ferricyanide dissolved in 1000 mL water) and measuring absorption 5–60 min later using a spectrophotometer (Helena Digispec) at a wave length of 540 nm.

Statistical significances of differences between groups were tested using the Student-Newman-Keuls multiple range test, or a multifactor Anova (using the Statview SE program by Abacus Concepts, Berkeley, CA), while correlation coefficients (r) were calculated for linear correlations using the same program.

RESULTS AND DISCUSSION

Food Restriction Effects on Obese and Normal B6 Females

Harrison *et al.* (1984) studied the effects of life-long food restriction beginning at 4 weeks of age in genetically obese (*ob/ob*) and normal B6 females (Table 9.2). Food restriction greatly reduced body mass in obese mice, but they retained very high percentages of body fat, nearly 50%. Kidney function, measured as urine concentration ability, was not impaired by obesity. Immune responses were normal in young obese mice (Table 9.2), but were less than 10% of normal in 500 day old obese mice. Food restriction failed to mitigate this rapid immunological aging (Table 9.2). Denaturation rates of tail collagen were accelerated in obese mice, but this accelerated aging process was greatly retarded by food restriction to exactly the same rate of collagen aging as found in food restricted normal mice (Table 9.2).

Food restriction extended longevities in the same pattern by which it retarded collagen aging: a great deal in obese mice, significantly in normal mice, and to a similar

TABLE 9.2
EFFECTS OF FOOD RESTRICTION AND OBESITY IN B6 FEMALES[1]

	B6-+/+ Females		B6-*ob/ob* Females	
Measure	Fed *Ad Libitum*	Restricted	Fed *Ad Libitum*	Restricted
Food	3.0	2.0	4.2	2.0
Weight	30 ± 1	20 ± 2	59 ± 5	28 ± 2
Fat as % weight	22 ± 6	13 ± 3	67 ± 5	48 ± 1
Tail collagen	46.5 ± 2.2	33.3 ± 0.8	77.0 ± 8.9	33.7 ± 0.9
Urine concentration	2600 ± 140	3000 ± 180	3400 ± 120	3400 ± 80
Immune Responses				
SRBC	6 ± 3	16 ± 8	2 ± 2	3 ± 2
PHA	124 ± 31	127 ± 28	33 ± 18	21 ± 15
Spleen weight	150 ± 8	78 ± 4	75 ± 17	36 ± 3

[1]Values are mean ± SEM, and units are: food, g/day; weight, g; tail length, cm; tail collagen, denaturation time in minutes; urine concentrating, mOsm, and the amount of fat is given as the % of body weight. Immune responses are given per spleen as number direct anti-SRBC plaques × 10^4 *in vivo*, and cpm tritiated Thymidine uptake × 10^5 *in vitro*, with spleen weights in mg. Mice in the first 3 lines were aged 180–360 days with ages matched in all groups, and 4–8 of each type tested. Tail collagen data are given for 488 day olds (4–6/group), urine concentrations for 329–364 day olds (13–17/group), and immune responses for groups averaging 550–560 days of age (8–14/group). *Ad libitum* fed 100 day old *ob/ob* controls had the following values for SRBC and PHA responses, and spleen weights with 21 mice: 31 ± 5 and 201 ± 41, and 105 ± 8. Values for 21 *ad libitum* fed 100 day old +/+ controls were: 27 ± 5 and 254 ± 18, and 112 ± 3. Most of these data were presented in Harrison *et al.* (1984), and food restriction was done using protocol I.

extent in obese and normal mice (Fig. 9.1). These results suggest that reduced food consumption and reduced collagen aging, but not reduced adiposity or improved immune functions, are essential in extended longevity of *ob/ob* mice. These data do not support the suggestions that food restriction extends longevity by reducing fat or improving immune responses, and suggest that food restriction acts by retarding collagen aging.

Food Restriction Effects on B6CBAF$_1$ Males and on Obese and Normal B6 Males

A similar food restriction experiment compared B6-*ob/ob* and +/+ males and B6CBAF$_1$ males (Harrison and Archer 1987). Food-restricted F$_1$ hybrid behaved as expected, having results significantly more like those of younger mice in most systems (tail collagen, urine concentration, hair regrowth, tight wire, and open field activity), but the opposite results in wound healing (Table 9.3). Longevities were extended from a mean of 974 days (already quite long lived) to 1180 days, and the longest life span was 1742 days, a new record for *Mus* (Fig. 9.2).

B6-*ob/ob* male mice greatly benefited from food restriction in all measures, as females had been (data not shown), and their longevities were greatly extended (Fig. 9.3). However, B6 +/+ males showed a dramatic difference in response to the same food restriction treatment, with longevities significantly reduced from a mean of 858 days to 593 days by food restriction (Fig. 9.3). Nevertheless, restricted B6 +/+

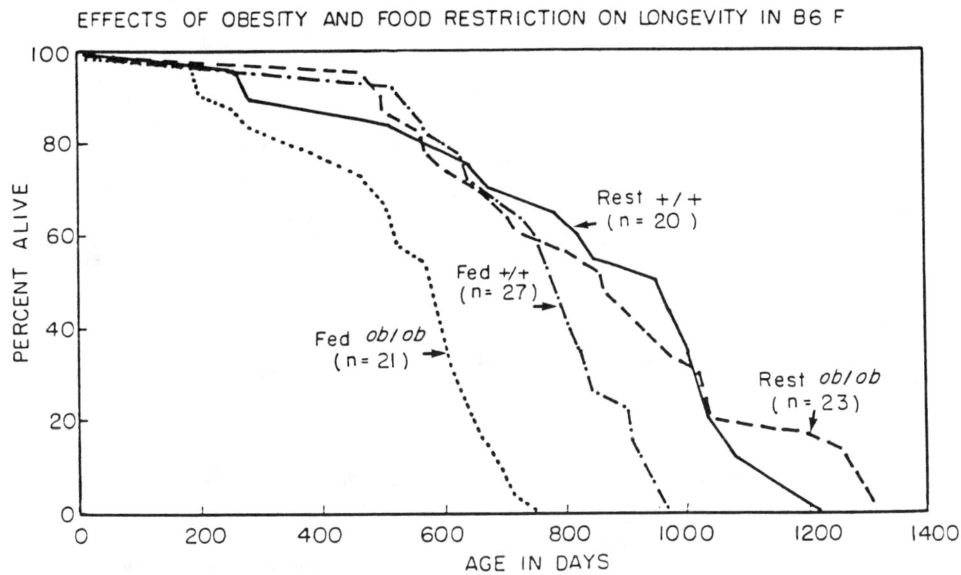

From Harrison and Archer (1984)

FIG. 9.1. FOOD RESTRICTION BY PROTOCOL I

Longevity plots as percentage remaining alive versus age in days for B6 females. Data for food restricted +/+ mice are plotted by the solid line, data for *ad libitum* fed *ob/ob* mice as the dotted line, data for food restricted *ob/ob* mice as the dashed line, and data for *ad libitum* fed +/+ mice as the dashed-dotted line. Data from the same mice, plus additional groups, are given in Table 9.5.

males had test results significantly more like those of younger mice than *ad libitum* fed B6 +/+ males in tail collagen, tight wire and open field activity. Hair regrowth, however, was much slower in the restricted B6 males, and was the only measure that predicted the reduction in longevity; wound healing was poorer, as it had been in F_1 males (Table 9.4).

Taken alone, the experiments with F_1 hybrids would have led to oversimplified conclusions. Longevities were extended by food restriction, and values were more like those of young animals in five physiological systems. If this had been the only group studied, it would have seemed reasonable to suggest that all five systems aged more slowly and could be used to evaluated antiaging treatments in any mouse genotype. However, food restriction reduced longevities in B6 +/+ males while maintaining three of the same five systems at levels characteristic of younger mice. Thus, the life-extending effects of a particular food restriction regimen may depend on the genotypes of the animals treated and the composition of the particular diets, and may not always correlate with effects in different biological systems. This illustrates how particular biological systems may age at different rates in different individuals.

TABLE 9.3
EFFECTS OF FOOD RESTRICTION ON B6CBAF$_1$ MALES[1]

	Food Restricted		*Ad Libitum* Fed	
Measure	Adult	Aged	Adult	Aged
Food	2.0	2.1	3.3	3.1
Weight	24.9 ± 0.3*	24.8 ± 0.5*	39.1 ± 0.7	40.0 ± 0.9
Tail length	10.4 ± 0.04*	10.9 ± 0.03	10.8 ± 0.04	11.0 ± 0.04
Tight wire	233 ± 4*	199 ± 10*	178 ± 11	77 ± 10
Open field	105 ± 7*	87 ± 4*	49 ± 4	58 ± 4
Tail collagen	33.5 ± 1.4*	95.9 ± 7.4*	40.6 ± 1.2	205 ± 7
Urine concentration	3929 ± 40*	3453 ± 98*	3156 ± 68	2831 ± 84
Hair growth	69.4 ± 6.3	67.2 ± 6.8*	53.3 ± 5.2	36.3 ± 6.9
Wound healing	19.4 ± 0.7	32.6 ± 3.6	16.2 ± 0.5*	20.0 ± 1.3*

Source: Harrison and Archer (1987).

[1]Values are mean ± SEM, with 30–36 mice per group; measures are defined in test. Adults were 294–389 days old, and aged mice 775–804 days old when tested, with ages matched in the two dietary groups. An asterisk (*) denotes values significantly different from others of the same age on the same line with $P < 0.05$ by the Student-Newman-Keuls multiple range test. Units are: food, g/day; weight, g; tail length, cm; tight wire-clinging time in seconds; open field, number of squares crossed; tail collagen, denaturation time in minutes; urine concentrating, mOsm; hair growth, percentage of shaved area regrowth in 25 days; wound healing number of days until healed. Food restriction was done using Protocol I.

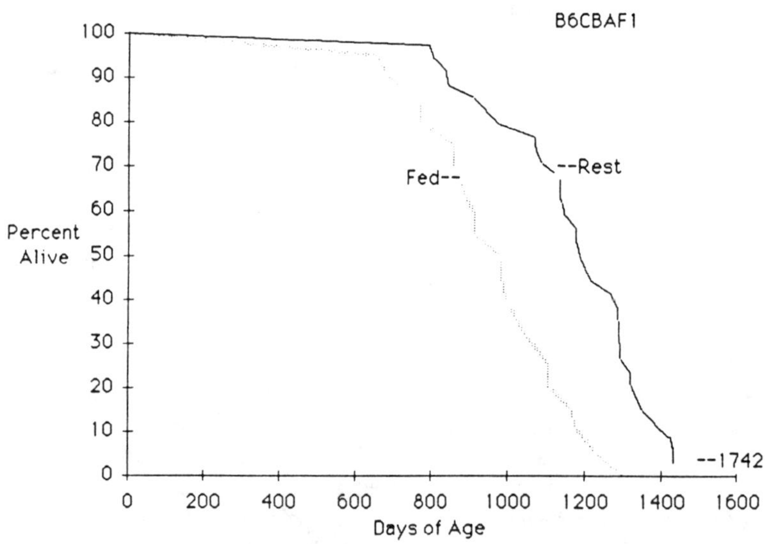

From Harrison and Archer (1987)

FIG. 9.2. FOOD RESTRICTION BY PROTOCOL I

Longevity plots as percentage remaining alive versus age in days for B6CBAF$_1$ males. Data for food-restricted mice are plotted by the sold line, while data for *ad libitum* fed mice are plotted as the dotted line. Data from the same mice are given in Table 9.5.

TABLE 9.4
EFFECTS OF FOOD RESTRICTION ON B6 MALES[1]

Measure	Food Restricted		*Ad Libitum* Fed	
	Adult	Aged	Adult	Aged
Food	1.8	2.1	3.0	2.8
Weight	22.5 ± 0.8*	24.0 ± 0.9*	33.3 ± 0.4	35.6 ± 0.6
Tail length	9.7 ± 0.06*	10.1 ± 0.04	10.0 ± 0.04	10.1 ± 0.06
Tight wire	149 ± 11.8*	60 ± 12.9*	77 ± 8.4	35 ± 6.2
Open field	116 ± 6.2	111 ± 10.3*	109 ± 5.2	83 ± 6.1
Tail collagen	25.6 ± 1.3	46.8 ± 4.3*	27.8 ± 1.3	60.3 ± 2.5
Hair growth	26.4 ± 3.8	18.3 ± 5.8	68.9 ± 3.7*	40.0 ± 6.6*
Wound healing	31.6 ± 2.8	42.7 ± 3.8	20.1 ± 0.7*	20.9 ± 0.9*

[1]Same as Table 9.3, except 44–53 mice per adult group and 17–24 per aged group. Adult mice were 260–373 days old and aged mice were 570–679 days old when tested, with ages matched in the two dietary groups. Urine concentration data were not affected by food restriction in B6 males, so were not included.

Why were B6 males damaged by exactly the same food restriction treatment that benefited females and obese mice of the same inbred strain, and $B6CBAF_1$ hybrids? The most likely possibility is that they required higher levels than the other groups of an essential nutrient that is not present in adequate amounts when they are restricted to about two-thirds of their normal food intake. Therefore B6 males were studied using food restriction protocol II with a defined diet (Table 9.1), so that amounts of protein and all micronutrients, and the percentage of fiber, are held constant in fed and restricted groups. When calories were restricted by reducing only carbohydrates and fats, B6 males were not harmed by food restriction, although they benefited only slightly (Fig. 9.4). There apparently was an unexpectedly specific requirement for some micronutrient in B6 males. This illustrates that an antiaging treatment that is successful in some individuals, may be harmful in other individuals, even if they are related.

Comparison of Longevity Patterns

Longevities of normal and obese B6 female mice food restricted using protocol I are shown in Fig. 9.1. Death rates increased more slowly with age in the food restricted groups than in the groups fed *ad libitum*. This caused maximum longevities in restricted +/+ mice to be about 30% greater than those of fed +/+ mice, although the former began dying at similar ages. This pattern of longevity curve suggests that food restriction did not benefit general health and reduce early mortality, but may have retarded some types of basic aging processes and increased maximum longevities. Food restricted obese mice began dying about 300 days later than fed obese mice, and maximum longevities were about increased even more, suggesting benefits on both general health and basic aging processes. The longevity summaries at the bottom of Table 9.5 show the same results for larger numbers of the same groups.

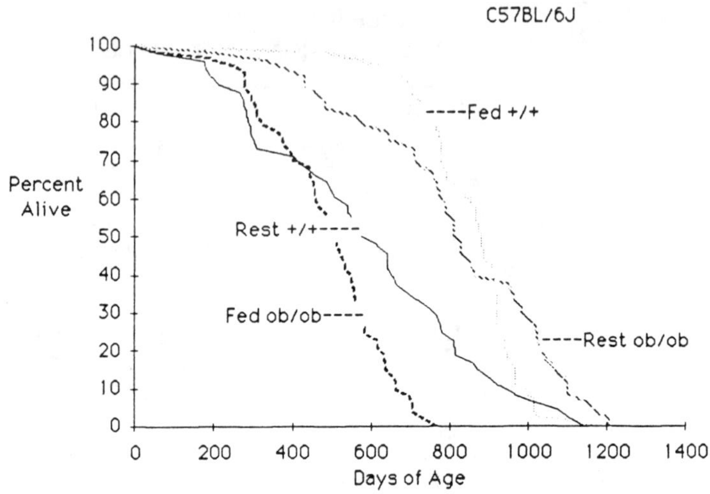

From Harrison and Archer (1987)

FIG. 9.3. FOOD RESTRICTION BY PROTOCOL I

Longevity plots as percentage remaining alive versus age in days for B6 males. Data for food restricted +/+ mice are plotted by the solid line, data for *ad libitum* fed +/+ mice as the dotted line, data for food restricted *ob/ob* mice as the dashed-dotted line, and data for *ad libitum* fed *ob/ob* mice as the dashed line. Data from the same mice are given in Table 9.5.

Fig. 9.2 compares longevities of F_1 hybrid mice food restricted using protocol I. Death rates increase with age in parallel, but the increase starts later in the food restricted group. Thus the median, mean and maximum longevities for restricted mice are about 200 days longer than those for fed groups, suggesting that some basic aging processes may have been retarded.

Longevities of normal and obese B6 male groups food restricted using protocol I are shown in Fig. 9.3. Death rates increased more slowly with age in the food-restricted groups than in the groups fed *ad libitum*. This caused maximum longevities in restricted +/+ mice to be almost as long as those of fed +/+ mice, although the former began dying at a much younger age. The decline in mean and median longevities as a result of food restriction in +/+ mice was over 260 days, while the decline in maximum longevity was only 27 days. This observation suggests that food restriction had most of its deleterious effects on health, reducing mean longevities, rather than on fundamental aging processes which would have reduced maximum longevities. Food-restricted obese mice began dying much later than fed obese mice with increases in mean and median longevities of about 300 days. Increases in maximum longevities were even greater, over 400 days, as expected if death rates increased with age more slowly in the restricted *ob/ob* group.

Figure 9.4 compares longevities of restricted and *ad libitum* fed B6 males given a defined diet so that calories were reduced two-thirds by reducing only carbohydrates

TABLE 9.5
EFFECTS OF FOOD RESTRICTION ON LONGEVITIES

Genotype	Gender	Treatment	Median	Mean	S E	N	Range Max. 10%
B6 +/+	M	*Ad Libitum* Fed[1]	855	817	40	20	1046–1105[2]
B6+/+	M	Restricted[1]	865	867	46	20	1126[2]–1129[2]
B6 +/+	M	*Ad Libitum* Fed	878	858	19	45	994–1172
B6 +/+	M	Restricted	591	593	40	48	967–1145
B6-*ob*/*ob*	M	*Ad Libitum* Fed	515	490	21	53	700–770
B6-*ob*/*ob*	M	Restricted	821	817	36	48	1102–1210
$B6CBAF_1$	M	*Ad Libitum* Fed	985	951	35	35	1188–1296
$B6CBAF_1$	M	Restricted	1191	1185	36	34	1432–1742[3]
B6 +/+	F	*Ad Libitum* Fed	799	771	28	32	954–976
B6 +/+	F	Restricted	850	810	48	38	1089–1287
B6-*ob*/*ob*	F	*Ad Libitum* Fed	552	526	36	29	776–893
B6-*ob*/*ob*	F	Restricted	814	823	46	39	1209–1307

[1]These mice were food restricted using protocol II. All other mice were food restricted using protocol I. In both cases, calories fed restricted groups were 66–70% of those fed *ad libitum*. All groups not separated by a space were studied over the same time period on the same diet, and are, from top to bottom, the same mice in Figs. 9.4, 9.2 + 9.3, and 9.1, respectively, with more mice added to those in Fig. 9.1.
[2]These mice were still alive 9/9/88, so the longevity data are minimums.
[3]The longest-lived mouse was fed *ad libitum* after 1541 days of age.

and fat. Death rates increase with age in parallel, but the increase may start later in the food restricted group. This is a preliminary experiment, and longevities may have been reduced because the mice around 800 days of age had to reside for several weeks in a new area with ventilated caging and 5–10°F lower temperatures than the normal area. During this period more than half the mice in the restricted group died; possibly the death rate was increased as a result of the changed environment. Nevertheless, food restriction clearly was not harmful to longevities.

Since the most accurate nutritional studies require the use of defined diets, such as AIN 76 on which our protocol II diets were based (Table 9.1), it is interesting to compare longevities of *ad libitum* fed B6 males given the defined diet (protocol II: Fig. 9.4 and line 1 of Table 9.5) with those given a Jackson Laboratory standard, grain-based diet (protocol I: Fig. 9.3 and line 3 of Table 9.5). Longevities appear similar, with medians of 855 and 878 days, respectively, suggesting that the defined diet does not cause important deleterious effects in this genotype.

Does Food Restriction Act by Retarding Collagen Aging?

The relationships between retarding collagen aging and extending longevities are not consistent. The tail tendon collagen test (Tcd) shows high correlation with chronological age, yet it does not correlate as expected with subsequent longevity of individuals or strain longevity (Harrison *et al.* 1978; Ingram *et al.* 1982), although collagen aging seemed slower in a long-lived mouse species (Harrison *et al.* 1978).

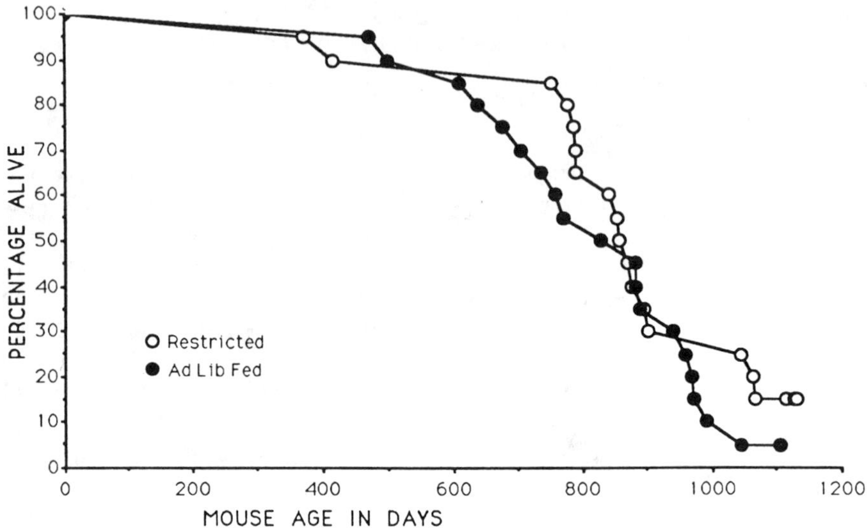

FIG. 9.4. FOOD RESTRICTION BY PROTOCOL II

Longevity plots as percentage remaining alive versus age in days for normal B6 males fed defined diets so that all nutrients were the same except carbohydrates and fats in both groups. Data for food-restricted mice are plotted by open circles, while data for *ad libitum* fed mice are plotted as the closed circles. Three restricted and one *ad libitum* fed mice remained alive when these data were collected (Sept. 1988). Data from the same mice are given in Table 9.5.

The agreement between reduced tail tendon collagen aging rates and increased longevities in restricted B6 female +/+ and *ob/ob* mice suggests that collagen aging is important to longevity in these animals (Table 9.2, Fig. 9.1). Collagen aging seems to be generally retarded by food restriction (Table 9.2–9.4) which generally extends longevities, yet collagen aging was also retarded in B6 +/+ males whose longevities were reduced by food restriction (Table 9.4, Fig. 9.3).

Does Food Restriction Act by Retarding Aging of Immune Responses?

Although food restriction extended longevities in female obese mice without retarding immune aging, it seemed to retard immune aging in the SRBC response of normal mice (Table 9.2). We also studied effects of food restriction on changes with age in frequencies of T helper and killer cell precursors using limiting dilution assays (Miller 1984; Miller and Harrison 1985). Even in extremely old (32–35 months) $B6CBAF_1$ mice that were restricted to 70% of the normal food intake, T-cell precursor frequencies in the circulation were almost at young levels (Table 9.6). This observation supports the idea that some of the benefits of food restriction result from retarding immune aging.

TABLE 9.6
EFFECTS OF FOOD RESTRICTION ON PRECURSOR T-CELL FREQUENCIES[1]

Age (Months)	Diet	Helpers	Killers
7–10	*Ad libitum*	105 ± 43(4)	55 ± 22(4)
32–35	*Ad libitum*	16 ± 7(6)	10 ± 4(6)
32–35	Restricted	56 ± 19(5)	45 ± 11(6)

Source: Miller and Harrison (1985).
[1]Frequencies are given as mean numbers of helper or killer precursor cells per 10^3 peripheral blood leukocytes determined by limiting dilution assays, ± standard deviation, with the number of individual mice tested given in parentheses. Mice were food restricted using protocol I.

Does Food Restriction Act by Retarding Metabolic Rates?

Food restricted B6-*ob/ob* females may have reduced metabolic rates, as they were fed identical amounts, but weighed 30% more and had 3–4 fold higher body fat percentages than restricted +/+ mice (Table 9.2). Thus, beneficial effects of food restriction on obese mice may be mediated through effects on metabolic rates. If metabolic rate is as greatly reduced by food restriction, as is implied by the weight and adiposity data, aging processes in which beneficial effects of food restriction result from retarding metabolic rate may be benefited more in restricted obese than in +/+ mice.

In the studies outlined in Tables 9.2, nutrient levels had been reduced to 70% of normal +/+ consumption during food restriction, perhaps causing deficiencies affecting spleen size or immune response, since food restricted mice were simply fed 70% of a standard 96WA diet. This problem can be corrected by feeding constant levels of nutrients to all mice using a defined diet, such as the one in Table 9.1. In the future, effects of the obese mutation on immune and metabolic function should be studied without confusion resulting from increased *ad libitum* food intake.

GENERAL IDEAS

Considerations in Designing Food Restriction Experiments

Although such experiments may be of great value in defining mechanisms of mammalian aging, they are even more difficult to do correctly than are conventional aging studies. All studies of mammalian aging require excellent environmental and genetic definition (Solleveld and Hollander 1984) including pathogen control and pathology, to get repeatable results and to distinguish aging from disease. However, the following considerations are also needed in food restriction studies:

(1) There should be controls to distinguish long-term benefits of food restriction from short-term benefits, since only the former could result from retarding aging processes. The latter might result from reversing aging processes, an

exciting possibility but one that must be carefully defined. Controls could be provided as follows: Six weeks before testing, an extra *ad libitum* group should be fed restricted amounts. Changes should be made gradually to avoid stress, while giving the equivalent of one month of full restriction.

(2) As mice are food restricted, it is vital to avoid malnutrition. Therefore, either the *ad libitum* fed animals must have an excess of all nutrients, or the restricted diet must be enriched by supplementation of each nutrient. In future studies, we will supplement the diet fed to restricted animals, to avoid confounding *ad libitum* feeding with feeding excessive nutrients. Our restricted mice have an enriched diet, but this should not cause problems because consumption of all nutrients except carbohydrates and fats will be the same among animals fed *ad libitum* and food restricted, and there will be adequate amounts of carbohydrates and essential fats.

(3) A potential source of error in food restriction studies is a different meal time for *ad libitum* fed and restricted groups, leading to different diurnal rhythms. To avoid this, in future experiments we will feed both *ad libitum* fed and restricted groups one meal per day, such that they will finish their rations in less than 4 h and retain similar diurnal rhythms. "*Ad libitum*" fed mice will be actually meal fed, receiving amounts with nearly the same caloric contents as those consumed by mice of the same genotype and age fed *ad libitum* with the conventional Jackson Laboratory 96WA diet. They finish their food in 4 h because they do not have food constantly present.

(4) To measure food intake and metabolic rates accurately, mice must be housed singly; however, this arrangement might be stressful and reduce longevities of the *ad libitum* controls, especially in males, perhaps due to decreased exercise. For example, even in colonies with excellent pathogen control, longevities of singly housed F344 male rats fed *ad libitum* (Bertrand *et al.* 1980) were 6 months less than those of the same strain housed in groups of 3 (Coleman *et al.* 1977). Multiply housed controls should be used to test if single-housed mice receiving the same diet differ in any changes with age or in longevity.

(5) Changes in efficiency of food use or in body composition as a result of food restriction should be tested. These require long-term metabolic measures and direct measures of body composition.

How the Response to Food Restriction May Have Evolved

We have suggested that the ability to retard aging in response to food restriction evolved due to the selective advantages for females whose reproductive life spans were extended by food restriction (Harrison and Archer 1988a). We should consider the enormous selective advantage of mice that could respond to a drought, or other long-term condition that severely reduced food supplies, by delaying reproductive senescence. This would be most important in females, as their reproductive senescence occurs at younger ages than that of males. After a drought outlasting the maximum female reproductive life span, a surviving female that is still able to reproduce could repopulate huge areas once weather conditions and food supplies became favorable. Survivors lacking the food restriction response would have reached female reproductive senescence before food supplies became adequate to raise offspring.

The hypothesis results in a unique and testable prediction: that the beneficial effects of food restriction will be greater in species with shorter female reproductive life spans. This would occur because selective pressure would be greater for mechanisms that prolong life in response to food restriction in species with shorter reproductive life spans. The shorter the reproductive life spans, the more likely are droughts that outlast maximum reproductive life spans.

Our hypothesis could be tested by comparing the two mouse species *Mus musculus* and *Peromyscus leucopus* because the latter live about twice as long as the former, despite their similar sizes and metabolic rates (Sacher and Hart 1978). We predict that food restriction will have significantly less benefit for *Peromyscus* mice because their female reproductive life spans are already twice as long as those of *Mus* mice.

This leads to a related hypothesis: that the same selective pressures favoring prolonged life spans in response to food restriction in *Mus*, also caused the extremely long life span potential in *Peromyscus*. Thus there are two ways for short-lived rodents to survive drought longer than the normal female reproductive period and retain the ability to reproduce and repopulate the area once food supplies improve. One is to increase maximum potential longevities in response to food restriction. The other, taken by *Peromyscus* mice, is to increase longevities in general, whether or not there is food restriction.

If the above hypotheses are correct, they lead to two important consequences: (1) Female reproductive senescence is regulated by at least some of the same mechanisms that control longevity, and thus is a good model for studies of aging. (2) The degree of genetic change required to extend longevity in response to food restriction is similar to that required to extend longevity in general, since at least one species, *Peromyscus*, adapted using the more general mechanism.

If the beneficial effects of food restriction are greater in species with shorter female reproductive life spans, the specific treatment of food restriction would have little beneficial effect on human longevity. However, studies of the underlying mechanisms by which food restriction retards aging in short-lived species would still be highly relevant to human health, since the same mechanisms might retard aging in man.

REFERENCES

ASTLE, C. M. and HARRISON, D. E. 1984. Effects of young and old marrow on immune responses: studies on the cellular level. J. Immunol. *132*, 673–677.

BARROWS, C. H. and KOKKONEN, C. G. 1977. Relationship between nutrition and aging. Adv. Nutr. Res. *1*, 253–298.

BERTRAND, H. A., FREDERICK, T. L., MASORO, E. J. and YU, B. P. 1980. Changes in adipose mass and cellularity through adult life of rats fed ad libitum or a life-prolonging restricted diet. J. Geront. *35*, 827–835.

BIERI, J. G. *et al.* 1977. Report of the American Institute of Nutrition ad hoc committee on standards for nutritional studies. J. Nutr. *107*, 1340–1348.

CAMPBELL, B. A. 1982. Behavioral markers of aging in the Fischer 344 rats. *In* Biological Markers of Aging, M. E. Reff and E. L. Schneider (eds.). NIH Pub. No. 82–2221.

CATHCART, R., SCHWIERS, E., SAUL, R. L. and AMES, B. N. 1984. Thymine glycol and thymidine glycol in humans and rat urine. Proc. Natl. Acad. Sci. *81*, 5633–5637.

CHRISTADOSS, P., TALAL, N., LINDSROM, J. and FERNANDEZ, G. 1984. Suppression of cellular and humoral immunity to T-dependent antigens by calorie restriction. Cell Immunol. *88*, 1–8.

COLEMAN, D. L. 1985. Increased metabolic efficiency in obese mutant mice. Int. J. Obesity *9*, 69–73.

COLEMAN, G. L. *et al.* 1977. Pathological changes during aging in barrier-reared Fischer 344 male rats. J. Gerontol. *32*, 258–278.

CUTLER, R. G. 1985. Peroxide-producing potential of tissues: inverse correlation with longevity of mammalian species. Proc. Natl. Acad. Sci. *82*, 4798–4802.

FERNANDES, G. P., FRIEND, P., YUNIS, E. J. and GOOD, R. A. 1978. Influence of dietary restriction on immunologic function and renal disease in (NZB / NZW)F_1 mice. Proc. Natl. Acad. Sci. *75*, 1500–1504.

FORSUM, E., HILLMAN, P. E. and ESHEIM, M. C. 1981. Effect of energy restriction on total heat production, basal metabolic rate, and specific dynamic action of food in rats. J. Nutr. *111*, 1691–1697.

HARMAN, D. 1981. The aging process. Proc. Natl. Acad. Sci. *78*, 7124–7128.

HARRISON, D. E. and ARCHER, J. R. 1983. Physiological assays for biological age in mice: relationship of collagen, renal function and longevity. Exp. Aging Res. *9*, 245–251.

HARRISON, D. E. and ARCHER, J. R. 1987. Genetic effects on responses to food restriction in aging mice. J. Nutr. *117*, 376–382.

HARRISON, D. E. and ARCHER, J. R. 1988a. Natural Selection for Extended Longevity for Food Restriction. Growth Dev. Aging *52*, 65.

HARRISON, D. E. and ARCHER, J. R. 1988b. Biomarkers of aging: Tissue markers. Future research needs, strategies, directions and priorities. Exp. Gerontol. *23*, 309–321.

HARRISON, D. E. ARCHER, J. R. and ASTLE, C. M. 1984. Effects of food restriction on aging: Separation of food intake and adiposity. Proc. Natl. Acad. Sci. *81*, 1835–1838.

HARRISON, D. E., ARCHER, J. R., SACHER, G. A. and BOYCE, F. M. 1978. Tail collagen aging in mice of thirteen different genotypes and two species: relationship to biological age. Exp. Gerontol. *13*, 63–73.

HILL, J. O., LATIFF, A. and DIGIROLAMO, M. 1985. Effects of variable caloric restriction on utilization of ingested energy in rats. Am. J. Physiol. *248*, R549–559.

INGRAM, D. K., ARCHER, J. R., HARRISON, D. E. and REYNOLDS, M. A. 1982. Physiological and behavioral correlates of life span in aged C57BL/6J mice. Exp. Gerontol. *17*, 295–303.

LANE, P. W. and DICKIE, M. M. 1958. The effect of restricted food intake on the life span of genetically obese mice. J. Nutr. *64*, 549–554.

MASORO, E. J., YU, B. P. and BERTRAND, H. A. 1982.Action of food restriction in delaying the aging process. Proc. Natl. Acad. Sci. *79*, 4239–4241.

McCARTER, R., MASORO, E. J. and YU, B. P. 1985. Does food restriction retard aging by reducing the metabolic rate? Am. J. Physiol. *248E*, 488–490.

McKAY, C. M., MAYNARD, L. A., SPERLING, G. and BARNES, L. L. 1939. Retarded growth, life span, ultimate body size and age changes in the albino rat after feeding diets restricted in calories. J. Nutr. *18*, 1–13.

MEAD, C. J. and SHEENA, J. 1979. Immunity in genetically obese rodents. 1979. *In* Animal Models of Obesity, M. F. W. Festing (ed.). Oxford University Press, New York.

MILLER, R. A. 1984. Age-associated decline in precursor frequency for different T-cell mediated reactions, with preservation of helper of cytotoxic effect per precursor cell. J. Immunol. *132*, 63–68.

MILLER, R. A. and HARRISON, D. E. 1985. Delayed reduction in cell precursor frequencies accompanies diet-induced life span extension. J. Immunol. *134*, 1426–1429.

NICHOLS, W. K., SPELLMAN, J. B. and DAYNES, R. A. 1978. Immune responses of diabetic animals. Diabetologia *14*, 343–349.

PEARL, R. 1928. The Rate of Living. Alfred Knopf, New York.

ROSS, M. H. 1969. Aging, nutrition and hepatic enzyme activity in the rat. J. Nutr. *97* (Suppl.) (11), 563–602.

ROSS, M. H. 1976. Nutrition and longevity in experimental animals. *In* Nutrition and Aging, M. Winick (ed.). John Wiley & Sons, New York.

RUBNER, M. 1908. Das Problem der Lebensdauer und seine Beziehungen zum Wachstum und Ernabrung. Oldenbourg, Munich.

SACHER, G. A. 1977. Life table modification and life prolongation. *In* Handbook of Biology of Aging, C. Finch and L. Hayflick (eds.). Van Nostrand Reinhold, New York.

SACHER, G. A. and DUFFY, P. H. 1979. Genetic relation of life span to metabolic rate for inbred mouse strains and their hybrids. Fed. Proc. *38*, 184–188.

SACHER, G. A. and HART, R. W. 1978. Longevity, aging and comparative cellular and molecular biology of the house mouse, *Mus musculus*, and the white-footed mouse, *Peromyscus leucopus*. Birth Defects: Orig. Article Ser. *14*, 71–96.

SOLLEVELD, H. A. and HOLLANDER, C. F. 1984. Animals in aging research: requirements, pitfalls and a challenge for the laboratory animal specialist. Vet. Q. *6*, 96–101.

SPROTT, R. L. and ELEFTHERIOU, B. E. 1974. Open-field behavior in aging inbred mice. Gerontology *20*, 155–162.

WALFORD, R. L. 1969. The Immunologic Theory of Aging. W. W. Norton and Co., New York.

WALFORD, R. L. *et al.* 1974. Long-term dietary restriction and immune function in mice: response to sheep red blood cells and to mitogenic agents. Mech. Age. Dev. *2*, 447–454.

WEINDRUCH, R., GOTTESMAN, S. R. S. and WALFORD, R. L. 1982. Modification of age-related immune decline in mice dietarily restricted from or after midadulthood. Proc. Natl. Acad. Sci. *79*, 898–902.

WEINDRUCH, R. H. and SUFFIN, S. C. 1980. Quantitative histologic effects on mouse thymus of controlled dietary restriction. J. Gerontol. *35*, 525–531.

WEINDRUCH, R, WALFORD, R. L., FLIGIEL, S. and GUTHRIE, D. 1986. The retardation of aging in mice by dietary restriction: Longevity, cancer, immunity and lifetime energy intake. J. Nutr. *116*, 641–654.

YOUNG, V. R. 1979. Diet as a modulator of aging and longevity. Fed. Proc. *38*, 1994–2000.

YU, B. P., MASORO, E. J. and McMAHAN, C. A. 1985. Nutritional influences on aging of Fischer 344 rats: physical, metabolic and longevity characteristics. J. Gerontol. *40*, 657–670.

CHAPTER 10

EFFECTS OF CALORIC RESTRICTION ON ENDOCRINE FUNCTION DURING AGING IN RATS

B. J. MERRY, Ph.D and ANNE M. HOLEHAN, Ph.D.
The Institute for Human Ageing
University of Liverpool
Liverpool, England

INTRODUCTION

Of the many attempts which have been made to develop experimental animal models of retarded aging, the most successful and reproducible have incorporated some form of dietary manipulation. The beneficial effect of restricted feeding on survival in populations of laboratory rodents is now well established, but elucidating the biochemical mechanism by which this is achieved is proving an extremely intractable scientific problem (Holehan and Merry 1986).

The early work of McCay had demonstrated that rats maintained for prolonged periods in a prepubertal state by severe underfeeding had extended lifespans (McCay *et al.* 1939). An inverse correlation was observed between the period of underfeeding, and the length of life remaining subsequent to accelerated growth and sexual maturation following the addition of carbohydrate and fat to the calorie–deficient diet. As the length of the sexually immature period and total lifespan increased, the period of life remaining after sexual maturation decreased. The observation of Mulinos and Pomerantz (1940) that severe prolonged undernutrition, particularly in adult animals, could induce a pseudo–hypophysectomized state led to the suggestion that restricted feeding operates through the neuroendocrine axis in a similar manner (Samuels 1946; Comfort 1979). This hypothesis received further support from the observations of Everitt (1976) that early postweaning hypophysectomy linked to selective hormone replacement therapy could mimic many of the aspects of the restricted feeding model. Everitt and Porter (1976) have further shown that food restriction, under certain conditions, will reduce the secretion of many anterior pituitary hormones, while Campbell *et al.* (1977) have demonstrated that very severe underfeeding in adult rats will decrease the synthesis of hypothalamic–releasing hormones. A colony of diet–restricted rats was established in 1975 to support an investigation into the endocrine hypothesis of enhanced survival in this model system.

THE DIET–RESTRICTED MODEL

Different experimental approaches have been adopted by a number of laboratories to induce chronic caloric restriction and extended survival in rodents. These have involved varying the composition of the diet or feeding the normal balanced diet on a limited basis, i.e., alternate day fasting and feeding or a fixed, reduced daily intake. The strategy adopted by this laboratory for all its studies is to feed a normal rat breeder diet, on a limited basis from weaning (21 days), to maintain the body weight of restricted rats at about 50% that of age–matched *ad libitum* fed control animals. Subsequent populations of diet–restricted animals have been matched to established growth curves, allowing for a simple, but highly reproducible animal model to be maintained. This procedure avoids repeated cycles of fasting and overeating induced by alternate day feeding. It also avoids the problem associated with the strategy of feeding a limited, but fixed amount of diet which results in a gradual increase in the severity of restriction during growth. The survival time of the last decile of the diet–restricted population compared with a population of fully fed rats is increased by 44%, and the median survival point and maximum lifespan are increased by 40% and 41%, respectively (Merry and Holehan 1981; Merry 1988). The time to double the rate of mortality increases from about 100 days in *ad libitum* fed animals to approximately 200 days for male rats maintained on a restricted diet during the postweaning period (Holehan and Merry 1986).

REPRODUCTIVE ENDOCRINOLOGY

Sexual Maturation

The hypothesis that the degree of restricted feeding necessary to significantly enhance survival also induced a "dietary hypophysectomy" and arrested sexual maturation was rejected on the basis of early work (Merry and Holehan 1979). Puberty was delayed but not inhibited in female CFY Sprague–Dawley rats (range of 63–189 days compared to 34–39 days in *ad libitum* fed controls) (Merry and Holehan 1979, 1985a). In contrast, puberty in male rats, as judged by fertility trials and the serum levels of testosterone, was delayed only 10–20 days (Fig. 10.1) (Merry and Holehan 1981).

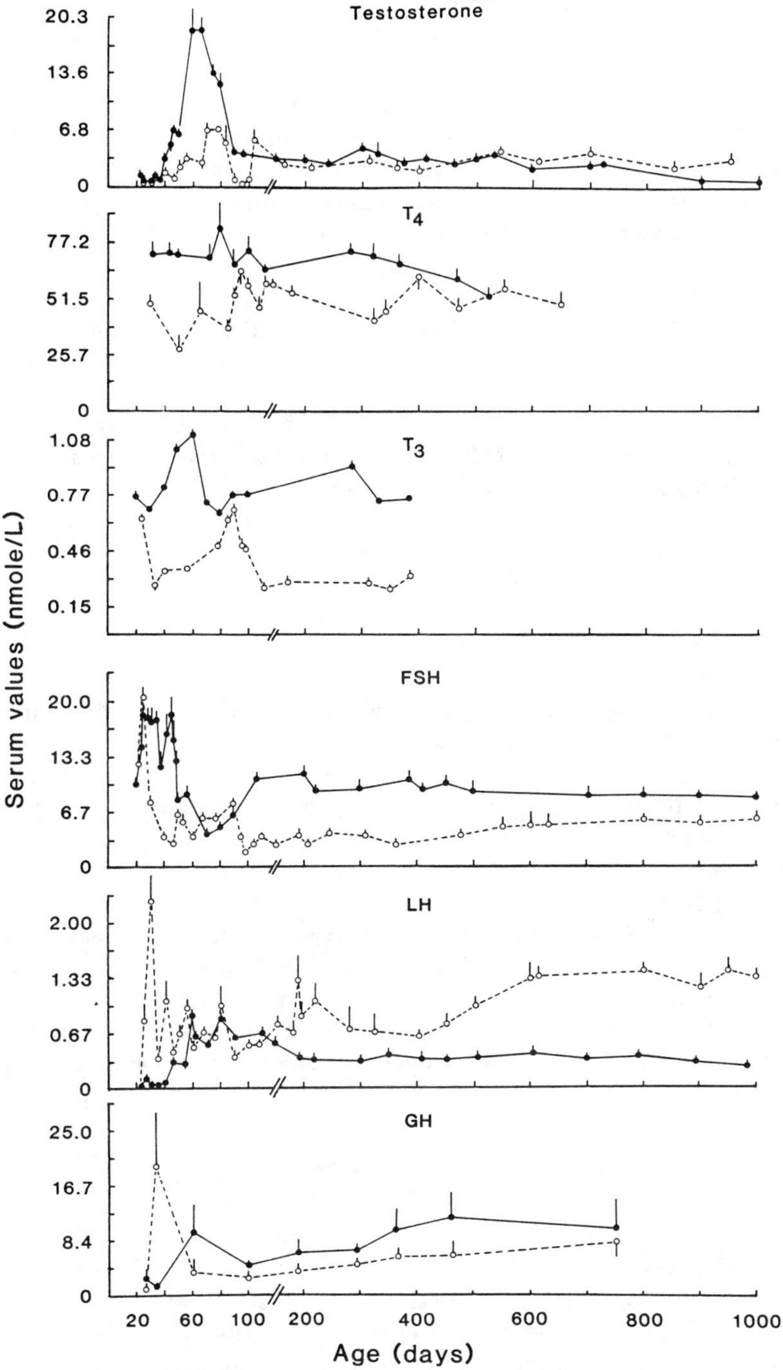

Reprinted with permission from Merry and Holehan (1985)

FIG. 10.1 AGE PROFILES FOR SERUM TESTOSTERONE, T_4, T_3, FSH, LH AND GH FOR MALE CFY *AD LIBITUM* (7) FED AND DIET-RESTRICTED (C) RATS

Each point represents the mean ± s.e.m for 10 animals.

Several factors have been suggested as the trigger for puberty. Frisch (1972) postulates a critical "pubertal" body weight or body composition (Frisch 1980) as the initiating cause. The finding that there was no significant difference at puberty in body weight between fully fed and diet-restricted females would support this idea.

The delay in puberty was associated with decreased serum levels of follicle stimulating hormone (FSH) in both sexes (Fig. 10.1) and with lowered serum progesterone and a 2–3 fold elevation of serum estradiol-17β in the female (Holehan and Merry 1985a). Due to the presence of estrogen-binding protein (α-fetoprotein), not all circulating estradiol-17β is biologically active. The biological activity of estradiol-17β increases prior to puberty as the fraction bound to α-fetoprotein falls. This increase in free estradiol-17β may act through negative feedback on the hypothalamic-pituitary axis to lower FSH release from the pituitary prior to puberty (Andrews and Ojeda 1977). The levels of α-fetoprotein in the diet-restricted rat have not been measured, and it is unclear whether the decreased serum levels of FSH result from enhanced negative feedback induced by elevated estradiol-17β or are a direct result of underfeeding on the hypothalamic control of pituitary FSH.

The decreased serum levels of progesterone which are observed in the prepubertal period result from insufficient ovarian stimulation by pituitary gonadotrophins and are not the result of a direct effect of chronic underfeeding on the ovary. This was demonstrated by the induction of superovulation in prepubertal fully fed and diet-restricted rats following the injection of 50 IU pregnant mare serum gonadotrophin (PMSG) and 25 IU human chorionic gonadotrophin. Circulating progesterone was elevated in both control and experimental animals at all ages tested and between 25–35 days, where a direct comparison between groups could be made, there was no significant difference in response. When the elevation in serum progesterone is expressed as a percentage increase over basal levels, maximum response occurred at 28 days in fully fed animals and 35 days in underfed females. After 35 days diet-restricted females showed a significant decline in the response to exogenous gonadotrophin stimulation (Fig. 10.2). In contrast to the increased synthesis and release of progesterone from superovulated diet-restricted animals, significantly fewer ova were recovered from the fallopian tubes than in superovulated fully fed animals (Merry and Holehan 1985a).

Estrus Cycles

Although the range for vaginal opening and first estrus is 63–189 days in diet-restricted animals, more than 90% demonstrated these criteria of puberty by 147 days. After vaginal opening and first estrus, more than 70% of control and diet-restricted animals exhibited normal 5-day estrous cycles (Holehan and Merry 1985a). In fully fed females at around 150 days, the first age-related changes in estrous cyclicity are seen with a significant increase in cycle length. Cycle length continues to increase with age to 5.8 ± 0.2 (s.e.m.) days at 400 days of age. No increase in estrous cycle length with age was observed in diet-restricted females, even though normal cycles were maintained to a greater age (Merry and Holehan 1979). With

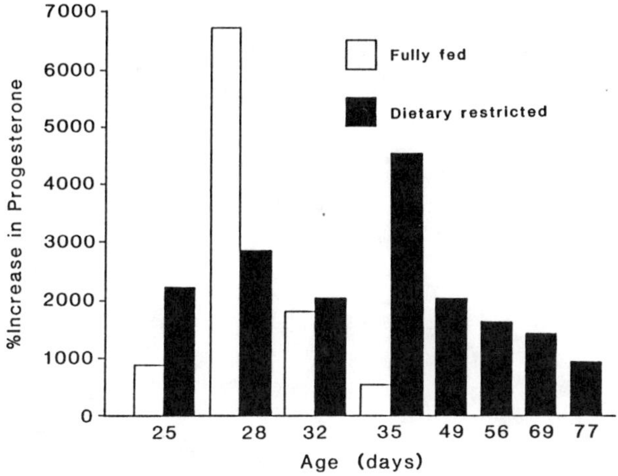

Reprinted with permission from Merry and Holehan (1985)

FIG. 10.2. PERCENTAGE INCREASE IN SERUM PROGESTERONE FOR SUPEROVULATED PREPUBERTAL FEMALE RATS COMPARED TO SALINE INJECTED CONTROLS WHEN MAINTAINED ON FULL FEEDING OR A RESTRICTED DIET

increased age the proportion of fully fed females with regular estrous cycles decreased and an increased frequency of irregular cycles was recorded. The most common irregularities were an extension in the period of cornification (persistent estrus) or an increased frequency of recurrent pseudopregnancy. Underfeeding resulted in a much later onset of these age-related irregularities.

Measurement of serum LH and FSH in fully fed and diet-restricted rats showing persistent estrus or recurrent pseudopregnancy revealed no significant differences between groups, with the exception of diet-restricted females in recurrent pseudopregnancy which had significantly lower FSH levels compared to control animals (Fig. 10.3). Recurrent pseudopregnant diet-restricted animals had significantly lower serum prolactin values than recurrent pseudopregnant fully fed females, with the values seen in both groups being significantly lower than in persistent estrus rats (Fig. 10.4). This reduction in serum prolactin values in recurrent pseudopregnant rats was associated with significantly higher values for serum progesterone.

Binding kinetics determined for the uterine estradiol-17β receptor present in a high-speed cytosol preparation showed no significant effect of diet at all ages analyzed. However, in both fully fed and diet-restricted animals, a significantly lower keq ($P < 0.05$) was recorded in constant estrus rats (Merry *et al.* 1985).

It was concluded that restricted feeding sufficient to significantly extend lifespan in the rat did not inhibit sexual maturation, but could retard reproductive aging. Although these findings do not support the suggestion that restricted feeding operates through a dietary pseudo-hypophysectomy, they do not contradict the idea that the

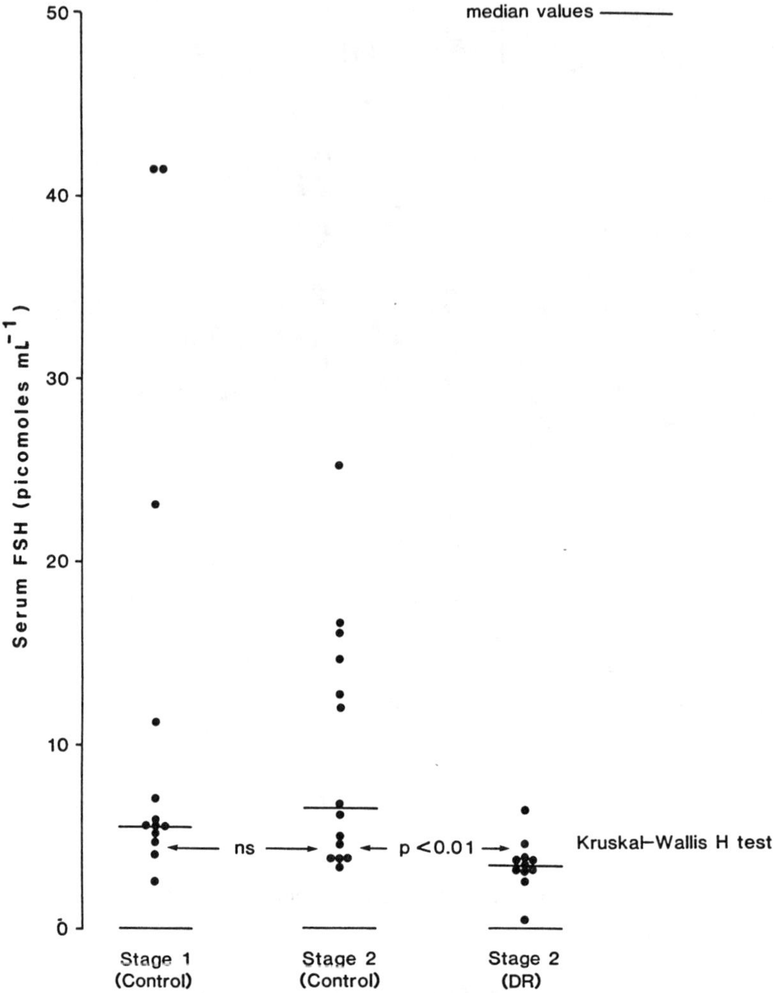

FIG. 10.3. SERUM LEVELS OF FSH IN FULLY FED OR DIET-RESTRICTED RATS IN STAGE 1 (PERSISTENT ESTRUS) OR STAGE 2 (RECURRENT PSEUDOPREGNANCY) REPRODUCTIVE AGING

process of aging may be under neural and endocrine control. The neuroendocrine axis provides for the control of gene expression, the regulation of cellular metabolism and immune function, and provides a critical link between the timing and expression of the genetic program and its modification by environmental influences (Everitt and Porter 1976; Segall 1979). Many theoretical attempts to explain the action of diet on longevity have invoked a central role for the neuroendocrine system (Everitt and Porter 1976; Segall 1979; Meites *et al.* 1987). These proposals were assessed in a series of studies on the endocrine response of rats to restricted feeding (Merry and Holehan 1985a, 1988). Particular emphasis was placed on studying the endocrine

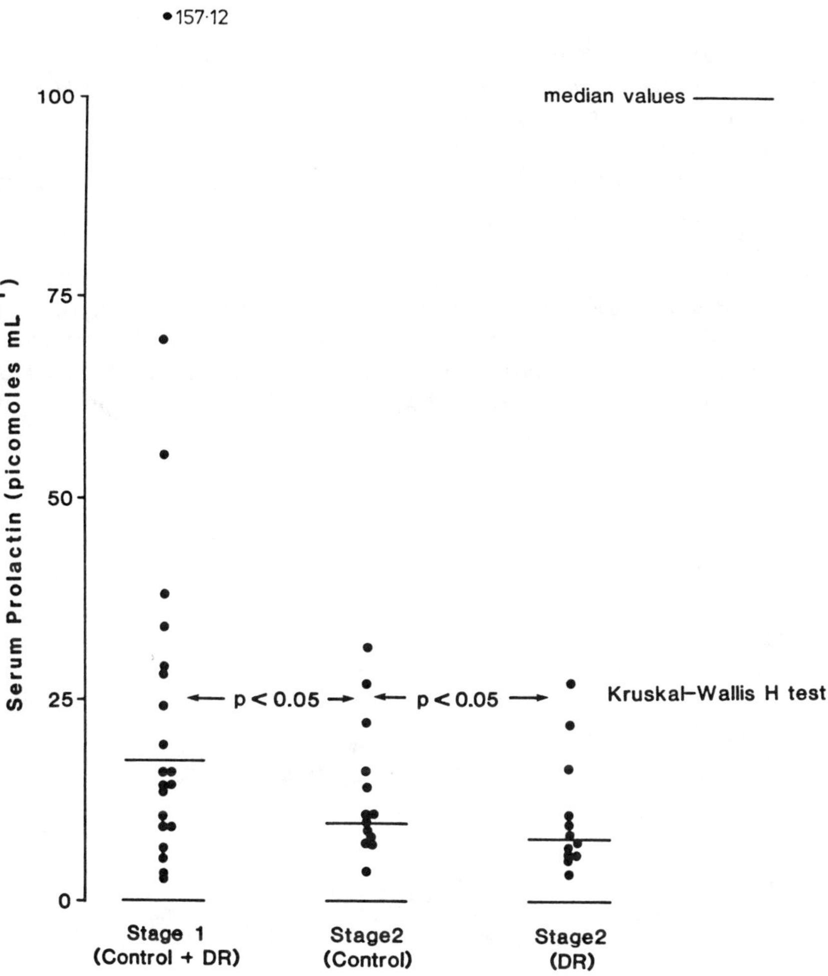

FIG. 10.4. SERUM LEVELS OF PROLACTIN IN FULLY FED OR DIET-RESTRICTED RATS IN STAGE 1 (PERSISTENT ESTRUS) OR STAGE 2 (RECURRENT PSEUDOPREGNANCY) REPRODUCTIVE AGING

control of delayed reproductive aging, intrinsic to which is the functional retention of an integrated system involving many tissues and organs.

Estrous Cycle Hormone Profiles

The irregularities in estrous cyclicity with aging have been attributed to changes in ovarian endocrine secretion and reduced capacity of the hypothalamic-pituitary system to respond to gonadal hormone feedback (Lu 1983). A series of studies were undertaken to evaluate this proposal in the diet-restricted rat.

The hormonal profile of the estrous cycle of underfed rats was compared with that of fully fed animals at an age (180–200 days) when over 75% of rats in each group showed regular estrous cycles, but when control animals were indicating from vaginal cytology the first age-induced increase in cycle length. The serum levels of luteinizing hormone (LH), follicle-stimulating hormone (FSH), progesterone and estradiol-17β were determined by radioimmunoassay across the 5-day cycle at 3-h intervals. A significantly higher level of FSH was observed in the diet-restricted rats which was associated with a smaller, but earlier preovulatory peak of LH. The LH peak was released approximately 6.5 h earlier on the afternoon of proestrus, and there was a delay of 6 h in the rise of serum estradiol-17β (Fig. 10.5). The total amount of estradiol-17β and progesterone released over the cycle in underfed females was reduced, but the profiles recorded were similar in both dietary groups (Holehan and Merry 1985b). Associated with extended estrous cycles in aging fully

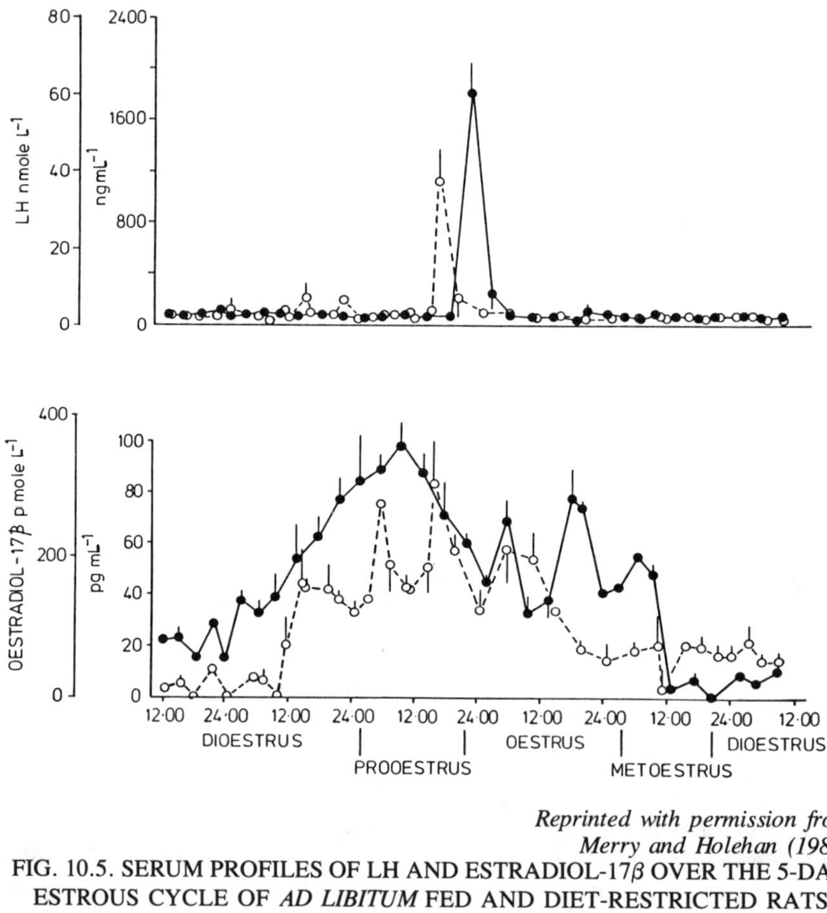

Reprinted with permission from Merry and Holehan (1985)

FIG. 10.5. SERUM PROFILES OF LH AND ESTRADIOL-17β OVER THE 5-DAY ESTROUS CYCLE OF *AD LIBITUM* FED AND DIET-RESTRICTED RATS

Mean ± s.e.m. for 5 animals at each time point and group are shown, *ad libitum* (●), diet-restricted (○).

fed animals is an early rise in serum estradiol-17β and a delayed preovulatory LH peak (van der Schoot 1976; Cooper *et al.* 1980). Lu (1983) suggests that the progressive cessation of regular estrous cycles is preceded in middle-aged female rats by advanced follicular growth and an increased ovarian estrogen production. Repeated exposure to higher levels of circulating estrogen may eventually reduce hypothalamic responsiveness to ovarian steroid feedback and result in a progressive delay and decrease in the LH surge. Such a process may affect follicular maturation and ovulation during the estrous cycle. The serum LH and estradiol-17β profiles from 6 month, diet-restricted rats suggest a retardation in this aspect of endocrine aging.

Follicular Steroidogenesis

The altered steroidogenic pathways in the ovary which result in the modified hormonal profiles seen in diet-restricted animals were investigated *in vitro* by the method of Uilenbroek *et al.* (1981). Individual follicles were collected from the ovaries of fully fed and diet-restricted rats on each day of the estrous cycle and incubated in medium 199 for 4 h under an atmosphere of 95% O_2/5% CO_2. The follicular content and release of estradiol-17β, progesterone, testosterone, androstenedione and 20 α-dihydroprogesterone were determined by radioimmunoassay. Follicles were also incubated with 50 ng/mL testosterone or 20 μg/mL bovine LH to selectively stimulate the steroidogenic pathway.

Effects of Age and Diet. Comparisons were made between follicles obtained from fully fed animals of 4 and 12 months and diet-restricted animals of 12 and 20 months. Ovarian follicles from both diet-restricted and fully fed animals which were incubated with testosterone (a precursor for aromatization to estrogen) showed increased estradiol-17β synthesis and release. The presence of testosterone and LH in the incubation media had the greatest effect in stimulating estradiol-17β release on proestrus and estrus follicles from young rats (4 months, fully fed and 12 months, diet-restricted), but on estrus and metestrus follicles from older animals (12 months fully fed and 20 months, diet-restricted). With increasing age, follicles from fully fed animals showed an increased release of progesterone after LH stimulation and enhanced aromatization of available androgen resulting in a greater activity of the delta-4 pathway to estradiol-17β and reduced activity of the pathway of progesterone metabolism (Fig. 10.6). This age effect in follicles from control rats was confirmed from data on the release of the progesterone metabolite 20 α-dihydroprogesterone where a significant reduction across all stages of the estrus cycle was seen. Follicular androgen content and release (androstenedione and testosterone) were similarly significantly reduced with age. The follicular release of estradiol-17β was not only significantly increased in one year, fully fed animals but was associated with all stages of the cycle in contrast to the profile of estrogen release in 4 month old follicles where enhanced estradiol-17β release was observed only at diestrus 2 and proestrus (Holehan and Merry 1985d, 1986). Thus, a loss of synchronization of hormone release is seen with age under *in vitro* and *in vivo* conditions.

These age-related changes in follicular steroid synthesis were retarded by chronic diet restriction in agreement with the observations on estradiol-17β serum levels.

There was no difference in follicular steroid content or release between follicles from 4 month, fully fed and 12 month, diet-restricted animals. At 20 months follicles from diet-restricted rats did show some age-related changes but the effects were intermediate between those observed from 4 and 12 month follicles removed from fully fed animals. The elevation in estradiol-17β was restricted to the estrus and metestrus phases of the cycle, and the decrease in progesterone metabolism (reduction in 20α-dihydroprogesterone levels) was not as marked (unpublished data). It is possible, therefore, to demonstrate retarded aging of the steroid synthetic pathways at the level of the individual follicle in diet-restricted animals, but it is not clear from these studies whether the retarded changes observed are intrinsic to the follicles.

Ovarian Transplantation. To determine the controlling factors resulting in the retardation of aging in the steroid synthetic pathways of ovarian follicles from diet-restricted females, bilateral orthotopic ovarian transplantations were performed by adapting the method developed for mice of Jones and Krohn (1960). The animal group combinations were the same as reported above for the original studies on follicular steroidogenesis, i.e., 2 fully fed groups of 6 and 14 months were contrasted with diet-restricted animals of 14 and 24 months (Fig. 10.7). The 16 transplantation combinations were established in 160 animals which were allowed 50 days to recover from surgery. Estrus cycles were determined by vaginal cytology for 30 days from day 50 following surgery. Follicular steroidogenesis for the transplanted ovaries in different stages of the estrous cycle and transplantation combination were assessed *in vitro* by the method of Uilenbroek *et al.* (1981), as described above. Follicular estradiol-17β synthesis at estrus, following orthotopic transplantation between animals of the same age and dietary group, showed no significant differences when compared with estradiol-17β synthesis from nontransplanted follicles. The ef-

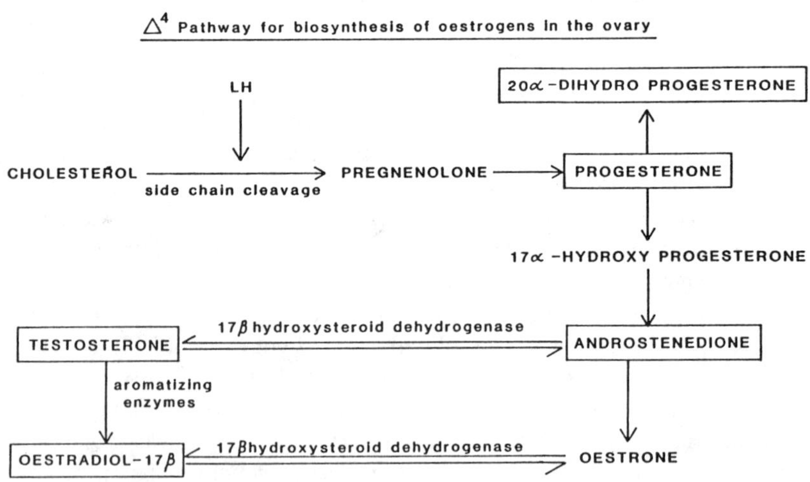

FIG. 10.6. Δ^4 PATHWAY FOR THE BIOSYNTHESIS OF ESTROGENS IN THE OVARIAN FOLLICLE

fects of aging and restricted feeding on estradiol-17β synthesis were maintained in these control transplantations.

In spite of the large interfollicular variance, the results of the transplantation study were clear. The release of estradiol-17β at estrus for follicles from 14 month, fully fed and 24 month, diet-restricted ovaries transplanted into 6 month, fully fed or 14 month diet-restricted animals was significantly reduced. The release of estradiol-17β from these follicles returned to the levels observed in young ovaries transplanted into young fully fed and diet-restricted hosts. While it was possible to reverse the age changes observed in estradiol-17β release in old ovaries, a more complex response was observed when 6 month, fully fed or 14 month, diet-restricted ovaries were transplanted into old hosts. Significantly enhanced estradiol-17β release was observed in follicles from 14 month, diet-restricted ovaries transplanted into 14 month, fully fed hosts. No significant difference in hormone release was observed when the 14 month, diet-restricted ovary was transplanted into a 24 month, diet-restricted host. Increased estradiol-17β release was recorded for follicles from 6 month, fully fed ovaries transplanted into 14 month, fully fed hosts, but the variance of the response was large, and thus no significant difference could be demonstrated. Transplanting

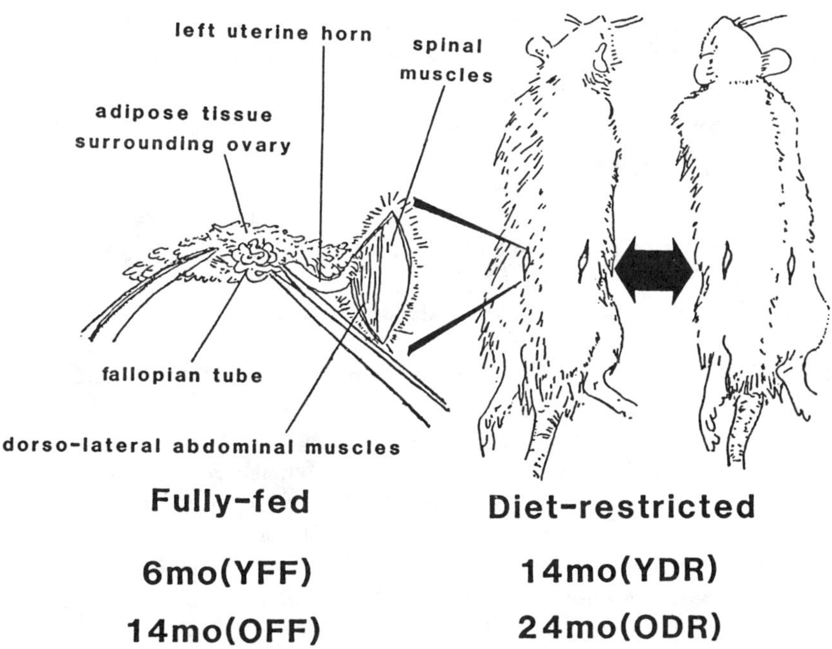

FIG. 10.7. EXPERIMENTAL DESIGN FOR BILATERAL ORTHOTOPIC OVARIAN TRANSPLANTATIONS

The 16 possible combinations between 6 mo fully-fed, 14 mo fully-fed and diet-restricted animals and 24 mo diet-restricted rats were performed. Ten replicate transplant combinations were established for each diet and age combination. Follicular steroidogenesis was assessed *in vitro* 80 days after surgery in the 160 animals.

6 month, fully fed ovaries into 24 month, diet-restricted animals had no effect on hormone release (unpublished data).

The conclusion from this study was that age changes in the follicle steroidogenic pathway were reversible and dependent upon the hypothalamic-pituitary axis of the host animal. The transplantation of young ovaries into old animals was only partially successful in enhancing estradiol-17β release. It is not clear whether premature aging of the endocrine component of the follicle can be induced by orthotopic transplantation.

Refeeding. A study was undertaken to determine if the delay in the age-related changes observed for follicular steroidogenesis in 12 month, diet-restricted rats could be reversed by a return to full feeding. Twelve month, diet-restricted animals were returned to *ad libitum* feeding for either 28 or 56 days prior to assessing *in vitro* follicular steroidogenesis. No reversal of the estradiol-17β profile, with respect to either follicle content or release, was observed. When either testosterone (50 ng/mL) or oLH (20 μg/mL) were included in the incubation media, the increase in estradiol-17β release was significantly less in comparison with follicles from either 12 month, diet-restricted or fully fed animals. The pattern of testosterone and 20 α-dihydroprogesterone release did, however, revert to that characteristic of 12 month, fully fed animals. The response of follicular steroidogenesis to short periods of full feeding in 12 month, diet-restricted animals is therefore complex and data on serum levels of FSH and LH will be required to fully understand the response observed.

Reproductive Lifespan

In the studies of Merry and Holehan (1979), Holehan (1984) and Merry *et al.* (1985), it was reported that rats maintained on a restricted diet throughout the post-weaning period were fertile, bearing multiple live litters to an age far exceeding that of the fully fed control females. Extended reproductive lifespans for rodents had been achieved in earlier studies by refeeding calorie-restricted or underfed animals (Ball *et al.* 1947; Carr *et al.* 1949; Berg and Simms 1960; Segall and Timiras 1975). Diet-restricted rats were unable to maintain a pregnancy until 8–9 months of age. Maximum fertility was achieved at 17 months, an age when fully fed animals have ceased to breed. Female CFY diet-restricted virgin females can be induced to breed and rear multiple litter as late as 28–31 months. Overall fertility and litter size were significantly reduced in diet-restricted females, but they did not demonstrate the decline in litter size observed in fully fed mothers with age (Holehan 1984; Holehan and Merry 1985c). The age-related decline in litter size could be reinitiated in underfed mothers by a return to full feeding but, irrespective of the timing of refeeding (350, 530 or 760 days), a maximum of only three litters were produced (Holehan and Merry 1985c). The longer the period of restricted feeding, the better was the fertility on return to full feeding. Animals returned to full feeding at 760 days had a reproductive performance equal to that of females maintained on a restricted diet throughout their lifespan (last litter produced when the mother was 32 months).

It has been shown that a short (10 weeks), acute phase of underfeeding followed by subsequent refeeding delayed the age-related loss in cycling (Quigley *et al.* 1987). At the start of the study, 100% of the young and 41% of the middle-aged rats were showing normal cycles, but during underfeeding all rats ceased to cycle and lost body weight. When placed on *ad libitum* feeding at the end of the 10 week underfeeding period, 100% of both young and middle-aged rats resumed cycling and rapidly regained body weight. With age, the proportion of animals continuing to cycle remained significantly higher in the underfed groups compared to their continuously *ad libitum* fed controls. During underfeeding both estrogen and prolactin levels declined but subsequent to refeeding enhanced LH release was observed.

NONREPRODUCTIVE ENDOCRINOLOGY

It is well documented that the rate of protein synthesis declines with age in many cell types from a wide range of organisms (Makrides 1983). Despite the decline in protein synthesis, there is evidence against a general decline in protein content of tissues with age (Richardson 1985). It can therefore be predicted that the rate of protein degradation must also decline with age at a rate similar to that seen for protein synthesis. The consequence of both a decreased rate of protein synthesis and degradation with aging would be an increase in the half life or "dwell time" of proteins and a decrease in the rate of protein turnover. Data to support this hypothesis has been published by Rothstein (1981) and Richardson and Cheung (1982). The turnover of two liver enzymes (ornithine decarboxylase and aldolase) decline significantly with age in C57BL/6J mice, and this may be an important factor in the increased proportion of altered proteins which have been identified in older organisms (Jacobus and Gershon 1980; Reznick *et al.* 1981; Adelman and Dekker 1985).

It has been proposed that the decrease in protein turnover could be the molecular basis for many of the physiological manifestations of aging (Richardson and Cheung 1982). Metabolic response to hormone signals would be less efficient with loss of enzyme regulation and impaired homeostasis. In rodents in which aging is retarded by controlled underfeeding, enhanced rates of protein turnover at advanced chronological age have been demonstrated for both the whole animal and for particular tissues under *in vitro* and *in vivo* assay conditions (Lewis *et al.* 1985; Goldspink *et al.* 1986; Richardson and Cheung 1982; Richardson and Birchenall-Sparks 1983; Richardson *et al.* 1984; Richardson 1985; Birchenall-Sparks *et al.* 1985). The response of protein turnover in individual tissues to chronic underfeeding is much more variable when measured under *in vivo* conditions. Although the various types of skeletal muscle respond to differing degrees, they generally show a fall in protein turnover which, while similar to that of the lung, was more prolonged (El Haj *et al.* 1986; Goldspink *et al.* 1987; Goldspink and Merry 1988). The heart and small intestine exhibit increased rates of protein turnover in response to chronic underfeeding. Hence, it is clear that different tissues do not respond uniformly to changes in nutritional status.

At least six hormones are recognized to affect the rate of protein synthesis and degradation: insulin, growth hormone (GH), somatomedins, glucagon, thyroid hormones, corticosteroids and prostaglandins (Buttery 1983). A series of investigations was initiated to document the changes induced by restricted feeding on such hormones and their effects on protein synthesis.

Growth Hormone. It has been proposed that at least part of the reduction in the ability to synthesize protein with age may be due to a decline in GH secretion. Restoration of GH pulse amplitude and GH mean plasma concentrations to that of young animals can be achieved by the administration of L-dopa, a precursor of brain catecholamines, and protein synthesis can be restored by GH administration in the skeletal muscle of old *ad libitum* fed rats (Sonntag *et al.* 1985). Growth hormone release and serum values in the rat are characterized by an endogenous ultradian rhythm with an episodic release of approximately 3.3 h (Tannenbaum *et al.* 1978). This periodicity of release is maintained in young diet-restricted male rats (4–5 months), but, although the frequency of release is unaffected by underfeeding, peak duration is reduced (Merry and Holehan 1985a). It was not possible to accelerate the rate of growth in 4 month, diet-restricted male rats by the daily administration of growth hormone, (500 μg/day ovine GH). No significant difference in growth rate was observed over the experimental period between GH and saline-injected, diet-restricted rats. A steady accelerated rate of growth of GH injected compared to saline-injected, fully fed animals was, however, seen over the 3 week period (Merry and Holehan 1985a). Growth hormone, either directly or by stimulating the release of somatomedins, increases amino acid uptake and initiates DNA transcription through the synthesis of poly-A+RNA and the synthesis of protein.

Somatomedins. Serum somatomedin-C measured in Lobund-Wistar rats was depressed by 3–5 months of age when this strain was maintained from 6 weeks on 12 g of diet per day. With age, the serum somatomedin-C levels fell in fully fed rats and by 30 months were not significantly different from those in underfed animals. This form of restricted feeding was considered to become restrictive at 8 weeks and results in a 30% reduction in food intake in adult rats. Survival of the last decile in this study was increased by approximately 19% (D'Ercole and Prewitt 1988; Snyder 1988).

Thyroid Hormones. Low protein or diets restricted in energy are known to be associated with reduced circulating levels of thyroxine (T_4) and triiodothyronine (T_3) resulting from depressed pituitary release of thyroid-stimulating hormone (TSH) (Campbell *et al.* 1977). Depressed serum levels of T_4 were seen from 7 days of restricted feeding until approximately 15 months, although the individual animal response was somewhat variable. After this age no significant differences were observed between serum T_4 in control and restricted rats because of the age-related depression of T_4 levels recorded in fully fed animals (Fig. 10.1). A period of *ad libitum* feeding of 7 days returned circulating T_4 levels to or above age-matched control values (Merry and Holehan 1985a).

In comparison with T_4, the levels of T_3 were much more sensitive to the regime of underfeeding. Serum levels were depressed to 40% those of control animals within 3–4 days of restricting the diet (Fig. 10.1), (Merry and Holehan 1985b). The serum peaks of T_3 and T_4 observed at puberty in fully fed rats were seen in the diet-restricted animals but appeared 20 days after those in control animals in agreement with the findings for serum testosterone (Fig. 10.1) (Merry and Holehan 1981; Holehan and Merry 1986). Although T_4 is the principal secretory product of the thyroid gland, the intrinsic biological activity of T_4 probably contributes only a small proportion (10–15%) of the overall thyroidal status of target tissues, with T_3 being the major biologically active component (Oppenheimer and Dillman 1978). The monodeiodination of T_4 to T_3 at the peripheral conversion sites is decreased under conditions of calorie restriction (van Doorn *et al.* 1984; unpublished data). Therefore, in this model, there is a greater effect of diet on the peripheral conversion of T_4 to T_3, than on a central neuroendocrine depression of T_4 release through TSH.

Protein and RNA synthesis are both stimulated by T_3 in the rat (Bernal *et al.* 1978), and a direct effect of T_3 on the rate of elongation of nascent peptides in the liver has been demonstrated (Mathews *et al.* 1973). It has been proposed that the decreased rate of protein synthesis observed with age in many organisms results, in part, from decreased rates of peptide elongation. This is supported by observations recorded in brain, kidney, liver and skeletal muscle of mice (Blazejowski and Webster 1984).

In our studies of *in vivo* protein synthesis and turnover in the diet-restricted rat, both total protein synthesis and the fractional rate of synthesis were significantly depressed during the first year of life (Merry *et al.* 1987). We therefore initiated a study utilizing the method of Mathews *et al.* (1973) to determine the effect of chronic underfeeding on the rate of elongation during *in vivo* liver protein synthesis. The time course of relative incorporation of labelled amino acids into completed and total polypeptides (i.e., completed and nascent chains) was determined at short intervals, (10–105 s), after an intravenous injection into the hepatic portal vein. The measured translation time is the average of the individual translation times for a wide spectrum of proteins being synthesized. The effect of T_3 on the rate of polypeptide synthesis appears independent of mitochondrial activity (Carter *et al.* 1975).

Restricted feeding significantly increased the time required to assemble the average polypeptide in 4 month animals from 76.4 to 177.3 s when measured under *in vivo* conditions (Holehan and Merry 1986). With age, the transit time increased in fully fed control rats (96.9 s at 24 months) but in diet-restricted animals a decrease was seen (81.6 s at 24 months). The significantly increased transit time recorded in 4 month, diet-restricted rats could be returned to nearly control values by 3 days of T_3 administration (40 μg/100 body weight, s.c., 177.3 to 96.2 s), without increasing food intake (Holehan and Merry 1986). When the transit time in 4 month, diet-restricted rats was measured 2 h after feeding, no effect was observed although the rate of hepatic protein synthesis had significantly increased. Refeeding previously diet-restricted, 4 month rats was not accompanied by an immediate return of transit time values to control levels. A period of approximately one month was required before the rate of elongation during polypeptide synthesis was equal to or less than that observed for control animals (Merry and Holehan 1985b). Refeeding did accelerate hepatic protein synthesis, and this was associated with a significant increase in cellular RNA. This was interpreted to be mainly ribosomal RNA which would allow for a high rate of initiation complexes to be formed, offsetting the retarded rate of peptide elongation during protein synthesis. Although T_4 serum levels rise to or above normal within 2 h of refeeding, the peripheral monodeiodination of T_4 to T_3 remains impaired for 2 or more weeks (unpublished data).

SUMMARY

It is not possible in the available space to document all the endocrine changes which are induced in rodents by chronic caloric restriction of the type known to extend survival and retard physiological aging. Such data have been reviewed elsewhere (Merry and Holehan 1985a; Holehan and Merry 1986). What we have attempted is an evaluation of some of the hypotheses which invoke a central role for the endocrine system to explain the effect of diet on aging. We have also explored the role of the endocrine system in modifying protein synthesis with age in rodents with delayed aging induced by controlled underfeeding. Enhanced protein turnover at advanced chronological age has been postulated as an explanation of delayed aging in diet-restricted rodents (Richardson and Cheung 1982; Birchenall-Sparks *et al.* 1985), and some experimental data exists to support this proposal. Whether the endocrine system plays a major role in determining the rate of protein turnover at advanced age in these animals is not known. Unquestionably, the rate of elongation of hepatic peptides during synthesis on the ribosome is very sensitive to the hormonal status of the tissue, whereas the initiation of protein synthesis appears much more directly dependent on the dietary status of the animal.

Although many studies in different physiological systems have confirmed that caloric restriction in rodents will delay physiological aging, the biochemical mechanism(s) by which this is achieved is still unresolved. The neuroendocrine axis does provide for the intricate control of gene expression which is required during development and for the maintenance of homestasis. Since the neuroendocine axis is central to other ontogenetic processes and is subject to environmental influences, it may also play a basic role in the timing and induction of age changes. Support for this view is provided by the work of Richardson *et al.* (1987) on the expression of the α_{2u}-globulin genes in hepatocytes from diet-restricted rats. The synthesis of α_{2u}-globulin is under complex multihormonal control with the levels of α_{2u}-globulin mRNA and the transcription of α_{2u}-globulin genes in isolated liver nuclei falling by 80–85% between 5 and 24 months of age. The synthesis, mRNA levels and transcription of α_{2u}-globulin were 1.8–3 fold higher in liver tissue from 18 month rats on a restricted diet (40% restriction of total calories), when compared with their fully fed, age-matched controls.

Whether the age-related expression of other genes is similarly modified by restricted feeding is unknown. Although the basic changes induced in serum levels for many hormones have been determined in diet-restricted rats, much of the detail regarding the control of immune function with age, multihormone interaction and the regulation of gene expression awaits to be determined.

ACKNOWLEDGMENTS

Parts of the work presented were supported by grants from the Nuffield Foundation (AGE/56) and the Medical Research Council (G7810908SB and G7810910SB).

REFERENCES

ADELMAN, R. C. and DEKKER, E. E. 1985. Modification of Proteins During Aging. Modern Aging Research, Vol. *7*. Alan R. Liss, New York.

ANDREWS, W. W. and OJEDA, S. R. 1977. On the feedback actions of estrogen on gonadotropin and prolactin release in infantile female rats. Endocrinology *101*, 1517–1523.

BALL, Z. B., BARNES, R. H. and VISSCHER, M. B. 1947. The effects of dietary caloric restriction on maturity and senescence, with particular reference to fertility and longevity. Am. J. Physiol. *150*, 511–519.

BERG, B. N. and SIMMS, H. S. 1960. Nutrition and longevity in the rat. 1. Food intake in relation to size, health and fertility. J. Nutr. *71*, 242–254.

BERNAL, J., CLEONI, A. H. and DE GROOT, L. J. 1978. Triiodothyronine stimulation of nuclear protein synthesis. Endocrinology *102*, 452–459.

BIRCHENALL-SPARKS, M. C. *et al.* 1985. Effect of dietary restriction on liver protein synthesis. J. Nutr. *115*, 110–116.

BLAZEJOWSKI, C. A. and WEBSTER, G. C. 1984. Effect of age on peptide chain initiation and elongation in preparations from brain, liver, kidney and skeletal muscle of the C57BL/6J mouse. Mech. Age. Dev. *25*, 323–333.

BUTTERY, P. J. 1983. Hormonal control of protein deposition in animals. Proc. Nutr. Soc. *42*. 137–148.

CAMPBELL, G. A., KURCZ, M., MARSHALL, S. and MEITES, J. 1977. Effects of starvation in rats on serum levels of follicle stimulating hormone, luteinising hormone, thyrotropin, growth hormone and prolactin: response to LH releasing hormone and thyrotropin releasing hormone. Endocrinology *100*, 580–587.

CARR, C. J., KING, J. T. and VISSCHER, M. B. 1949. Delay of senescence infertility by dietary restriction. Fed. Proc. *8*, 22.

CARTER, W. J., FAAS, F. H. and WYNN, J. 1975. Demonstration of thyroxine-stimulated incorporation of amino acid into peptide linkage in mitochondria-free system. J. Biol. Chem. *250*, 3588–3594.

COMFORT, A. 1979. The Biology of Senescence. Churchill Livingstone, Edinburgh and London.

COOPER, R. L., CONN, M. and WALKER, R. F. 1980. Characterization of the LH surge in middle-aged female rats. Biol. Reprod. *23*, 611–615.

D'ERCOLE, J. and PREWITT, E. 1988. Effect of modest dietary restriction on serum somatomedin-C levels in young, mature and old Lobund-Wistar rats. Presented at the Symposium on the Effects of Dietary Restriction on Aging and Disease in Germfree and Conventional Lobund-Wistar Rats, March 27–29, Notre Dame.

EL HAJ, A. J. *et al.* 1986. The effect of chronic and acute dietary restriction on the growth and protein turnover of fast and slow types of rat skeletal muscle. Comp. Biochem. Physiol. *85A*, 281–287.

EVERITT, A. V. 1976. Hypophysectomy and aging in the rat. *In* Hypothalamus, Pituitary and Aging, A. V. Everitt and J. A. Burgess (eds.). Charles C. Thomas, Springfield.

EVERITT, A. V. and PORTER, B. 1976. Nutrition and aging. *In* Hypothalamus, Pituitary and Aging, A. V. Everitt and J. A. Burgess (eds.). Charles C. Thomas, Springfield.

FRISCH, R. E. 1972. Weight at menarche: Similarity for well-nourished and undernourished girls at differing ages, and evidence for historical constancy. Pediatrics (Springfield) *50*, 445–450.

FRISCH, R. E. 1980. Pubertal adipose tissue: is it necessary for normal sexual maturation? Evidence from the rat and human female. Fed. Proc. *39*, 2395–2400.

GOLDSPINK, D. F. *et al.* 1987. The influence of chronic dietary intervention on protein turnover and growth of the diaphragm and extensor digitorum longus muscles of the rat. Exp. Gerontol. *22*, 67–78.

GOLDSPINK, D. F., LEWIS, S. E. M. and MERRY, B. J. 1986. The effects of ageing and chronic dietary intervention on protein turnover and the growth of ventricular muscle in the rat heart. Cardiovasc. Res. *XX*, 672–678.

GOLDSPINK, D. F. and MERRY, B. J. 1988. Changes in protein turnover and growth of the rat lung in response to ageing and long-term dietary restriction. Mech. Age. Dev. *42*, 253–262.

HOLEHAN, A. M. 1984. The effect of ageing and dietary restriction upon reproduction in the female CFY Sprague-Dawley rat. Ph.D. Thesis, University of Hull, UK.

HOLEHAN, A. M. and MERRY, B. J. 1985a. The control of puberty in the dietary restricted female rat. Mech. Age. Dev. *32*, 179–191.

HOLEHAN, A. M. and MERRY, B. J. 1985b. Modification of the oestrous cycle hormonal profile by dietary restriction. Mech. Age. Dev. *32*, 63–76.

HOLEHAN, A. M. and MERRY, B. J. 1985c. Lifetime breeding studies in fully fed and dietary restricted female CFY Sprague-Dawley rats. I. Effect of age, housing conditions and diet on fecundity. Mech. Age. Dev. *33*, 19–28.

HOLEHAN, A. M. and MERRY, B. J. 1985d. Follicular steroidogenesis in diet restricted rats with delayed reproductive ageing. Presented at the XIIIth International Congress of Gerontology, July 12–17, New York.

HOLEHAN, A. M. and MERRY, B. J. 1986. The experimental manipulation of ageing by diet. Biol. Res. *61*, 329–368.

JACOBUS, S. and GERSHON, D. 1980. Age-related changes in inducible mouse liver enzymes: ornithine decarboxylase and tyrosine aminotransferase. Mech. Age. Dev. *12*, 311–322.

JONES, E. C. and KROHN, P. L. 1960. Orthotopic ovarian transplantation in mice. J. Endocrinol. *20*, 135–146.

LEWIS, S. E. M. *et al.* 1985. The effects of ageing and chronic dietary restriction on whole body growth and protein turnover in the rat. Exp. Gerontol. *20*, 253–263.

LU, J. K. H. 1983. Changes in ovarian function and gonadotropin and prolactin secretion in aging female rats. *In* Neuroendocrinology of Aging, J. Meites (ed.). Plenum Press, New York.

MAKRIDES, S. C. 1983. Protein synthesis and degradation during aging and senescence. Biol. Rev. *58*, 343–422.

MATHEWS, R. W., ORONSKY, A. and HASCHEMEYER, A. E. V. 1973. Effect of thyroid hormone on polypeptide chain assembly kinetics in liver protein synthesis *in vivo*. J. Biol. Chem. *248*, 1329–1333.

McCAY, C. M., MAYNARD, L. A., SPERLING, G. and BARNES, L. L. 1939. Retarded growth, lifespan, ultimate body size and age changes in the albino rat after feeding diets restricted in calories. J. Nutr. *18*, 1–13.

MEITES, J., GOYA, R. and TAKAHASHI, S. 1987. Review article. Why the neuroendocrine system is important in aging processes. Exp. Gerontol. *22*, 1–15.

MERRY, B. J. 1988. The retardation of ageing by diet: an animal model. *In* Comparative Nutrition, K. Blaxter and I. Macdonald (eds.). John Libbey, London.

MERRY, B. J. and HOLEHAN, A. M. 1979. Onset of puberty and duration of fertility in rats fed a restricted diet. J. Reprod. Fert. *57*, 253–259.

MERRY, B. J. and HOLEHAN, A. M. 1981. Serum profiles of LH, FSH, testosterone and 5α-DHT from 21 to 1000 days of age in *ad libitum* fed and dietary-restricted rats. Exp. Gerontol. *16*, 431–444.

MERRY, B. J. and HOLEHAN, A. M. 1985a. The endocrine response to dietary restriction in the rat. *In* The Molecular Biology of Aging, Vol. 35, Basic Life Sciences, A. D. Woodhead, A. D. Blackett and A. Hollaender (eds.). Plenum Press, New York.

MERRY, B. J. and HOLEHAN, A. M. 1985b. Action of life-prolonging food restriction on the endocrine system and on protein biosynthesis. Presented at the XIIIth International Congress of Gerontology, July 12–17, New York.

MERRY, B. J. and HOLEHAN, A. M. 1988. Dietary restriction and the neuroendocrinology of aging. *In* Regulation of Age Changes along the Hypothalamic-Pituitary Axis. Monograph Series: Interdisciplinary Topics in Gerontology, A. V. Everitt and J. R. Walton (eds.). S. Karger, Basel.

MERRY, B. J., HOLEHAN, A. M., LEWIS, S. E. M. and GOLDSPINK, D. F. 1987. The effects of ageing and chronic dietary restriction on *in vivo* hepatic protein synthesis in the rat. Mech. Age. Dev. *39*, 189–199.

MERRY, B. J., HOLEHAN, A. M. and PHILLIPS, J. G. 1985. Modification of reproductive decline and lifespan by dietary manipulation in CFY Sprague-Dawley rats. *In* Current Trends in Comparative Endocrinology, B. Lofts and W. N. Holmes (eds.). Hong Kong University Press, Hong Kong.

MULINOS, M. G. and POMERANTZ, L. 1940. Pseudo-hypophysectomy produced by malnutrition. J. Nutr. *19*, 493–504.

OPPENHEIMER, J. H. and DILLMAN, W. H. 1978. Nuclear receptors for triiodothyronine: A physiological perspective. *In* Receptors and Hormone Action, Vol. III, L. Birnbaumer and B. W. O'Malley (eds.). Academic Press, New York.

QUIGLEY, K., GOYA, R. and MEITES, J. 1987. Rejuvenating effects of 10-week underfeeding period on estrous cycles in young and old rats. Neurobiol. Aging *8*, 225–232.

REZNICK, A. Z., LAVIE, L., GERSHON, H. E. and GERSHON, D. 1981. Age-associated accumulation of altered FDP aldolase B in mice. Conditions of detection and determination of aldolase half-life in young and old animals. FEBS Lett. *128*, 211–224.

RICHARDSON, A. 1985. The effect of age and nutrition on protein synthesis by cells and tissues from mammals. *In* Handbook of Nutrition in the Aged, R. R. Watson (ed.). CRC Press, Boca Raton.

RICHARDSON, A. and BIRCHENALL-SPARKS, M. C. 1983. Age-related changes in protein synthesis. *In* Review of Biological Research in Aging, Vol. 1., M. Rothstein (ed.). Alan R. Liss, New York.

RICHARDSON, A. *et al.* 1987. Effect of age and dietary restriction on the expression of α_{2u}-globulin. J. Biol. Chem. *262*, 12821–12825.

RICHARDSON, A. and CHEUNG, H. T. 1982. The relationship between age-related changes in gene expression, protein turnover, and the responsiveness of an organism to stimuli. Life Sci. *31*, 605–613.

RICHARDSON, A., ROBERTS, M. S. and BIRCHENALL-SPARKS, M. C. 1984. The possible role of protein synthesis in the aging process. Mod. Aging Res. *4*, 47–68.

ROTHSTEIN, M. 1981. Posttranslational alteration of proteins. *In* Handbook of Biochemistry in Aging, J. R. Florini (ed.). CRC Press, Boca Raton.

SAMUELS, L. T. 1946. The relation of the anterior pituitary hormones to nutrition. Recent Prog. Horm. Res. *1*, 147–171.

SEGALL, P. E. 1979. Interrelations of dietary and hormonal effects in aging. Mech. Age. Dev. *9*, 515–525.

SEGALL, P. E. and TIMIRAS, P. S. 1975. Age-related changes in thermoregulatory capacity of tryptophan deficient rats. Fed. Proc. *34*, 83–85.

SNYDER, D. 1988. Design of the Lobund aging project and growth and survival characteristics of the Lobund-Wistar rat. Presented at the Symposium on the Effects of Dietary Restriction of Aging and Disease in Germfree and Conventional Lobund-Wistar Rats. March 27–29, Notre Dame.

SONNTAG, W. E., HYLKA, V. W. and MEITES, J. 1985. Growth hormone restores protein synthesis in skeletal muscle of old male rats. J. Gerontol. *40*, 689–694.

TANNENBAUM, G.S. *et al.* 1978. Antiserum to somatostatin reverses starvation-induced inhibition of growth hormone but not insulin secretion. Endocrinology *102*, 1909–1914.

UILENBROEK, J. T. J., VAN DER SCHOOT, P. and WOUTERSEN, P. J. A. 1981. Changes in steroidogenic activity of preovulatory rat follicles after blockage of ovulation with Nembutal. *In* Dynamics of Ovarian Function, N. B. Schwartz and M. Hunzicker-Dunn (eds.). Raven Press, New York.

VAN DOORN, J., VAN DER HEIDE, D. and ROELFSEMA, F. 1984. The influence of partial food deprivation on the quantity and source of triiodothyronine in several tissues of athyreotic thyroxine-maintained rats. Endocrinology *115*, 705–711.

VAN DER SCHOOT, P. 1976. Changing pro-oestrous surges of luteinizing hormone in ageing 5-day cyclic rats. J. Endocrinol. *69*, 287–288.

CHAPTER 11

MECHANISM OF FOOD RESTRICTION: CHANGE OF RATE OR CHANGE OF SET POINT?

ARLAN RICHARDSON, Ph.D.
Department of Chemistry
Illinois State University
Normal, Illinois
and
ROGER McCARTER, Ph.D.
Department of Physiology
The University of Texas
Health Science Center at San Antonio
San Antonio, Texas

INTRODUCTION

The nutritional status of an organism is of importance in gerontological research because food restriction or undernutrition (but not malnutrition) is the most effective method for increasing the life expectancy of an organism, and it is the only strategy known to consistently increase the survival of mammals (Rose 1976; Bertrand 1983; Yu 1985, 1987; Masoro 1988). Although it is well established that dietary restriction dramatically increases the survival of laboratory rodents, the biological mechanism responsible for the increase in survival is not currently known. In this chapter we describe two models of how dietary restriction might act at the molecular level. In both models dietary restriction would result in an increase in survival, which is characteristic of dietary restriction (Masoro 1988). In the "rate model," we propose that dietary restriction retards the rate at which biological processes change with age. This model is consistent with the view that dietary restriction acts by retarding the rate of aging. In the second model, the "set point model," we propose that dietary restriction does not alter the rate at which biological processes change with age but alters the level of the processes. In this model, dietary restriction would not retard the rate of aging. Rather, the physiological status of the organism would be altered by dietary restriction in such a way that the levels of those biological processes involved in survival are enhanced.

A REVIEW OF THE EFFECTS OF DIETARY RESTRICTION

The classic experiments by McCay *et al.* (1935) showed that a drastic restriction of total calories increased the survival of Osborn-Mendel rats. Later studies by Berg (1960) demonstrated that the longevity of rats could be increased by dietary restriction procedures less severe than those used by McCay *et al.* (1935). In addition to increasing the life expectancy of rodents, dietary restriction has been shown to affect the processes listed below:

(1) The maximum survival of rodents is consistently increased (Bertrand 1983; Yu 1985).

(2) A variety of physiological processes that change with age are altered, e.g., the decrease in hormone responsiveness of adipocytes (Masoro *et al.* 1980; Yu *et al.* 1980); impaired cold tolerance (Talan and Ingram 1985); bone loss (Kalu *et al.* 1984); the onset of reproductive senescence (Merry and Holehan 1979); changes in serum lipids (Liepa *et al.* 1980); the decrease in protein synthesis (Birchenall-Sparks *et al.* 1985; Ricketts *et al.* 1985; Ward 1988); proteinuria (Fujita *et al.* 1984; Ricketts *et al.* 1985); the decline in the immune response (Fernandes *et al.* 1978; Weindruch *et al.* 1979); changes in the eye, i.e., loss of lens gamma crystallins (Leveille *et al.* 1984) and loss of cells in the corneal endothelium (Nadakavukaren *et al.* 1987).

(3) The incidence of a variety of age-related diseases is retarded and/or reduced, e.g., the incidence of tumors (Ross and Bras 1973; Sakar *et al.* 1982; Yu *et al.* 1982; Weindruch and Walford 1982; Cheney *et al.* 1983; Maeda *et al.* 1985), nephropathy (Fernandes *et al.* 1983; Fujita *et al.* 1984; Maeda *et al.* 1985; Rhem *et al.* 1985), cardiomyopathy (Berg and Simms 1960; Sakar *et al.* 1982; Maeda *et al.* 1985), periarteritis (Berg and Simms 1960) and bile duct hyperplasia (Sakar *et al.* 1982).

(4) The change in rodent behavior with aging is altered, e.g., maze performance is better for animals fed a restricted diet (Goodrick 1984), and dietary restriction attenuates the age-related loss of behavioral responsiveness to various drugs (Joseph *et al.* 1983).

Because dietary restriction increases the maximum survival of rodents and produces profound effects on a variety of physiological and pathological processes, it has been proposed that the aging process is altered in animals fed a calorie-restricted diet (Masoro 1988). In other words, a decrease in the rate of aging is responsible for the reduction in the incidence of disease and the increase in survival observed in rodents fed a restricted diet.

MODELS OF DIETARY RESTRICTION: RATE VERSUS SET POINT

Over the past decade, gerontologists have used the paradigm of dietary restriction to elucidate the biological mechanism underlying the aging process. It is generally accepted that the biological process(es) controlling the survival of an organism will be altered by dietary restriction. If dietary restriction alters the rate of aging, it would follow that the rate of change in the biological process(es) responsible for the death of the animal would also be altered by dietary restriction. This concept is graphically presented in Fig. 11.1. The effect of dietary restriction on a hypothetical biological process that is responsible for the age-related decrease in survival is shown in Fig. 11.1. We will assume that the hypothetical process declines with age; however, an increase in the process also would fit this model. At some point (C) a threshold is reached where any further decline or change in the process would result in the death of the animal. In this model, dietary restriction would alter the rate of decline in the hypothetical process so that the age when the threshold is reached would be extended. Thus, animals fed the restricted diet would live to an older age, i.e., an increase in the mean and maximum survival would be observed. In this model, which would be in agreement with the view that dietary restriction reduces the rate of aging, one need not assume that dietary restriction has altered the physiological status of the animals. The animals fed *ad libitum* and the restricted diet could go through

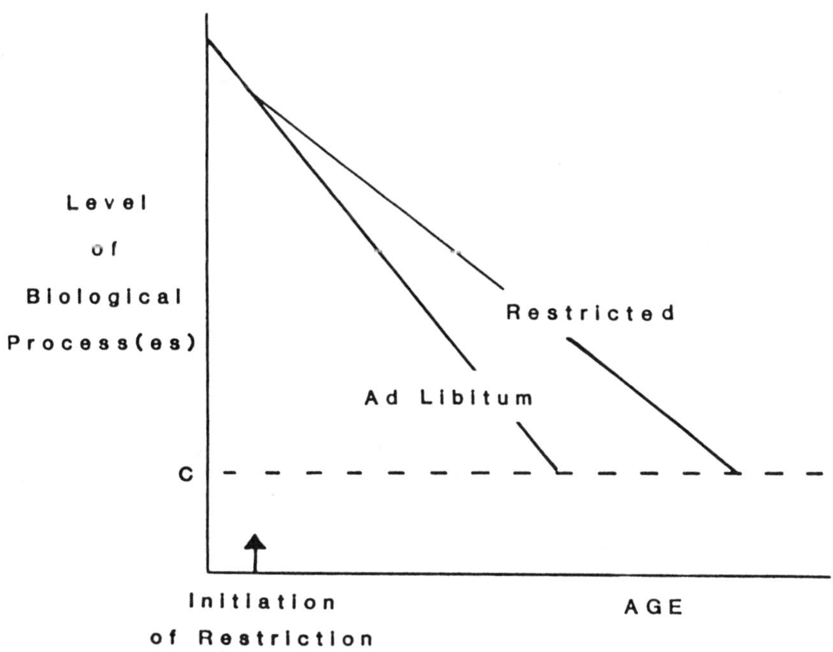

FIG.. 11.1. RATE MODEL OF DIETARY RESTRICTION

the same physiological changes with increasing age. The only difference would be the rate at which these physiological changes would occur.

In Fig. 11.2, we present the set point model. In this model, dietary restriction has no effect on the rate of change in the hypothetical biological process responsible for the death of the animals. However, dietary restriction alters the physiological status of the organism in such a way that the set point or the level of the biological process is altered. One could envision dietary restriction altering the set point in two ways. As shown in Fig. 11.2, this could occur by an induction in the process or by a delay in the decline of the process. One might argue that this delay would be analogous to a retardation in the rate of change in the process, which would be similar to the rate model shown in Fig. 11.1. However, the retardation in the rate of the process would only be transient in the set point model. Figure 11.2 shows that even though the rate of change in the hypothetical biological process is not affected by dietary restriction, the age at which the threshold (C) is reached is extended compared to animals fed *ad libitum*. Thus, the animals fed the restricted diet would live to an older age. In this model, the effect of aging on the hypothetical process would be identical in the rats fed *ad libitum* or the restricted diet, i.e., the rate of aging would be the same. The increase in the longevity of the animals would be due to the initial alteration in the process, not an alteration in the rate of aging.

An example of this phenomenon in gerontology is the incidence of osteoporosis in white and black females (Garn 1975). The delayed incidence of osteoporosis in

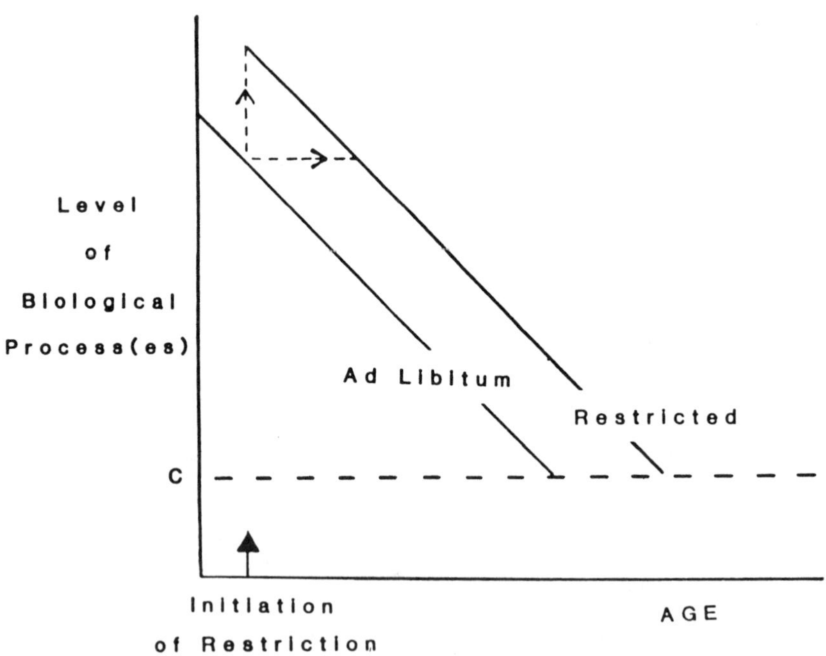

FIG. 11.2. SET POINT MODEL OF DIETARY RESTRICTION

black women is probably not due to a decrease in the rate of bone loss. Both black and white women show loss of bone with age due to hormonal changes. The difference in the incidence of osteoporosis appears to be due primarily to a difference in bone mass at maturity, i.e., a difference in set point. Because black women have a greater peak bone mass, it will take more time for the black women to lose bone mass to the point that fractures will occur.

EXPERIMENTAL EVIDENCE ON SUPPORT OF MODELS

Because the process(es) that is responsible for the increase in the survival of rodents is not known, it is impossible to determine if dietary restriction is increasing survival by altering the rate or set point of such a process(es). However, it is possible to determine if dietary restriction alters the rate or set point of biological processes that change with age by comparing the age-related changes in various biological processes that have been measured in rats fed *ad libitum* and a restricted diet.

During the past five years, there have been several reports describing the effect of dietary restriction on protein synthesis. Figure. 11.3 compares data from two studies in which liver protein synthesis was measured. In both studies, the level of protein synthesis was higher in the restricted rats. However, in the first study (left

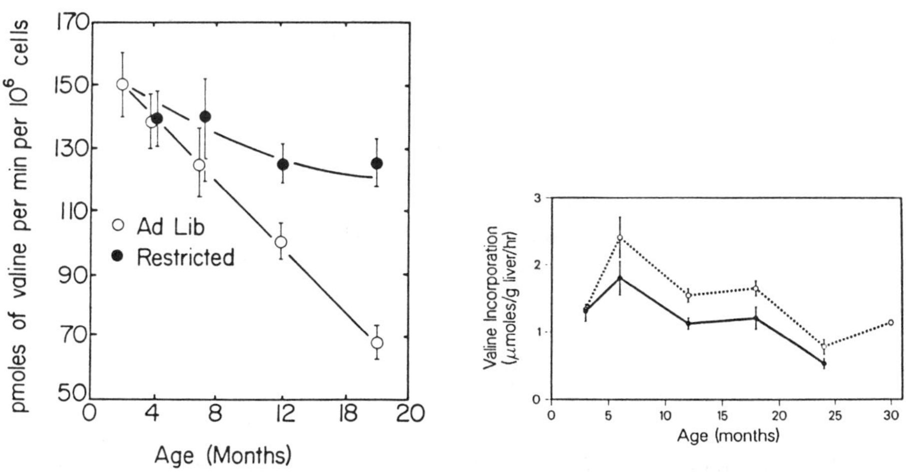

From Birchenall-Sparks et al. (1985) *From Ward (1988)*

FIG. 11.3. EFFECT OF DIETARY RESTRICTION ON THE AGE-RELATED DECLINE IN LIVER PROTEIN SYNTHESIS

The data shown in the left graph give the rate of incorporation of radioactive valine into protein by suspensions of hepatocytes isolated from male rats of various ages. The data shown in the right graph give the rate of incorporation of radioactive valine into protein by perfused liver from male rats of various ages.

graph) it appears that dietary restriction alters the rate of decline in protein synthesis, while in the second study (right graph) the age-related decline in protein synthesis in the restricted rats was parallel to the decline observed in the rats fed *ad libitum*. More recently, Pahlavani *et al.* (1989) showed that dietary restriction also alters the age-related decline in protein synthesis in mitogen-stimulated lymphocytes. As noted in Fig. 11.4, dietary restriction initially reduced the level of protein synthesis; however, the level remained the same until 12 months of age. After 12 months of age, the level of protein synthesis declined with increasing age at similar rates in rats fed *ad libitum* and the restricted diet.

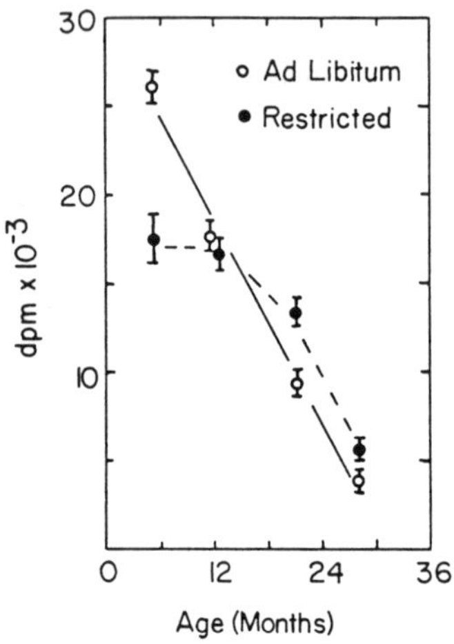

From Pahlavani et al. (1989)

FIG. 11.4. EFFECT OF DIETARY RESTRICTION ON THE AGE-RELATED DECLINE IN PROTEIN SYNTHESIS BY LYMPHOCYTES

The rate of valine incorporation into protein by concanavalin A stimulated lymphocytes isolated from the spleen of male rats of various ages is shown.

Because the early studies by Walford's laboratory showed that dietary restriction altered the immunological status of rodents (Weindruch *et al.* 1979), several investigators have studied the effect of dietary restriction on various immunological processes. Figure 11.5 illustrates the effect of dietary restriction on mitogen-induced proliferation by lymphocytes isolated from the spleen of mice. The left graph shows that concanavalin A induced proliferation by mice fed *ad libitum* and a restricted diet decreased in parallel with increasing age. Mitogenesis was consistently higher in the restricted mice. The right graph shows that mitogenesis induced by either concanavalin A or phytohemagglutinin was higher in lymphocytes isolated from mice fed a restricted diet, which was initiated after midlife. However, a similar age-related

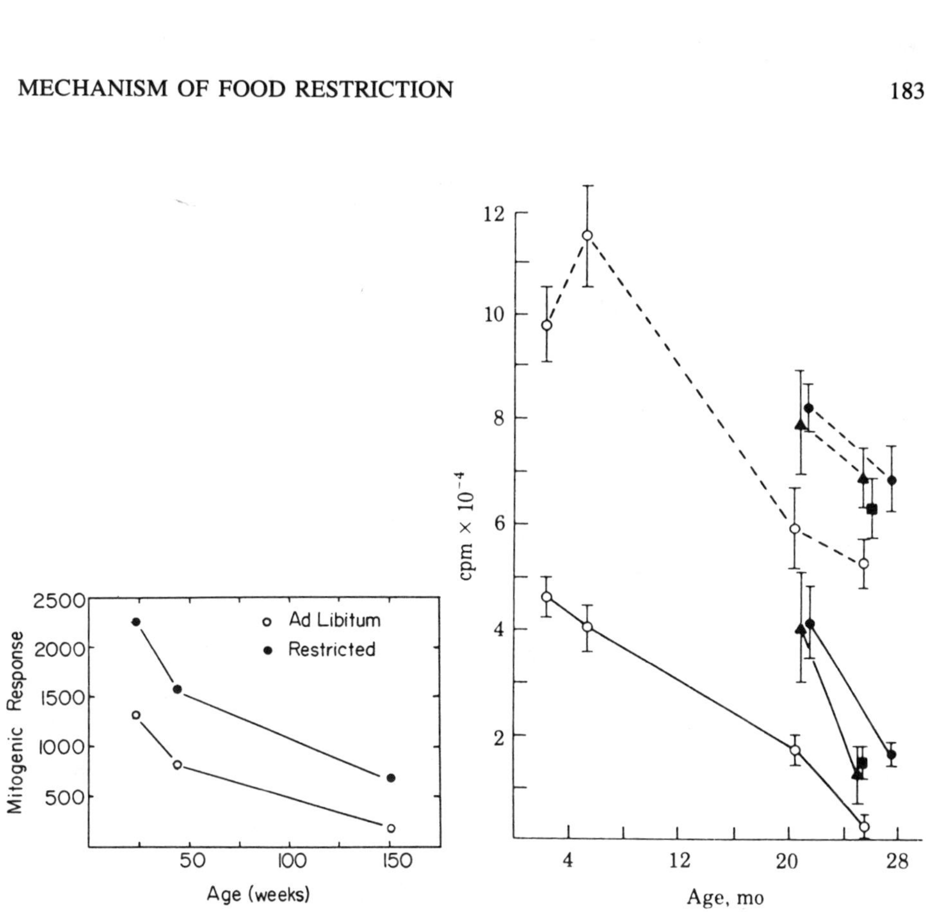

From Cheney et al. (1983) *From Weindruch et al. (1982)*

FIG. 11.5. EFFECT OF DIETARY RESTRICTION ON IMMUNE FUNCTION
The left graph shows concanavalin A induction of lymphocyte proliferation by female mice fed *ad libitum* or a restricted diet, which was initiated post-weaning. The right graph shows concanavalin A (---) or phytohemagglutinin (——) induction of lymphocyte proliferation by female mice fed *ad libitum* (○) or a restricted diet initiated at 12 (●), 17 (▲), or 21 (■) months of age.

decline in lymphocyte proliferation was observed for mice fed *ad libitum* and the restricted diet for both mitogens.

Figure 11.6 provides examples of two processes in which dietary restriction has altered the rate of change with age. The upper graph shows that the rate at which the postabsorptive serum free fatty acid concentrations decreases with age was altered by dietary restriction. The lower graph suggests that the rate of progression of renal disease was altered by dietary restriction. The severity of chronic nephropathy lesions increased steadily with age for all rats; however, the rate of increase was lower for the rats fed the restricted diets.

Figures 11.7, 11.8 and 11.9 offer examples of three biological processes that are altered by dietary restriction but show a similar rate of change with age. Figure 11.7 shows the age-related decrease in the lipolytic response of fat cells to glucagon. In restricted rats, there was no decline in the response until 12 months of age. However,

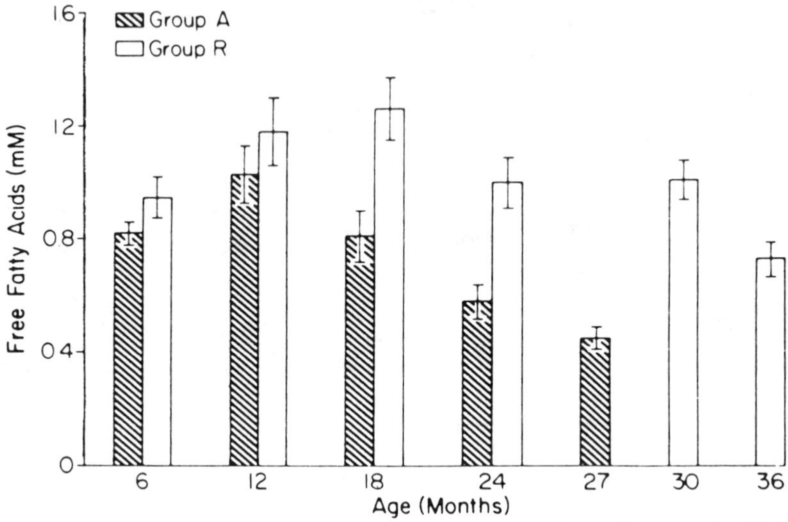

From Liepa et al. (1980)

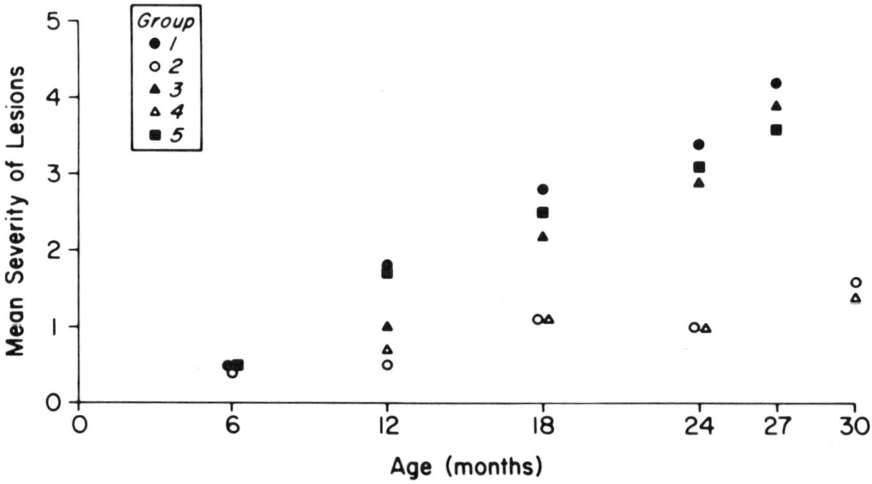

From Kalu and Masoro (1990)

FIG. 11.6. EXAMPLES OF DIETARY RESTRICTION ALTERING THE RATE OF CHANGE

The upper graph shows the postabsorptive serum free fatty acid concentrations in male rats fed *ad libitum* (group A) and a restricted diet (group R). The lower graph shows the effect of age and diet on the severity of chronic nephropathy lesions in male rats. Solid symbols (groups 1, 3, and 5) represent rats fed *ad libitum* and open symbols (group 2 and 4) represent rats fed a restricted diet over most of the life span.

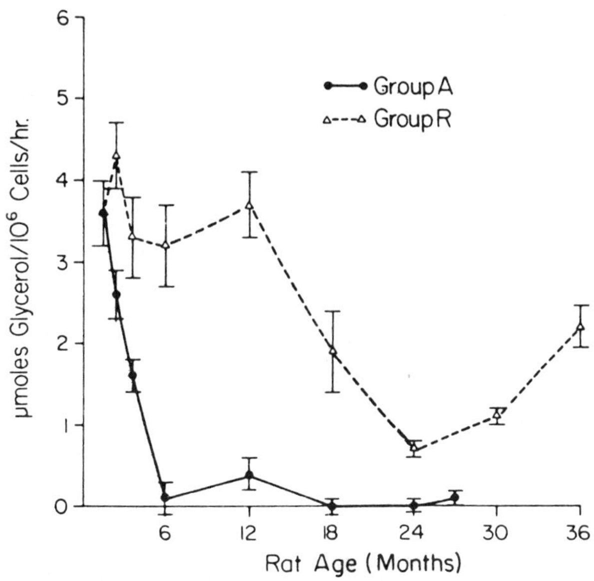

From Masoro et al. (1980)

FIG. 11.7. EFFECT OF DIETARY RESTRICTION ON THE AGE-RELATED DECREASE IN THE LIPOLYTIC RESPONSE TO GLUCAGON

The lypolytic response of adipocytes isolated from male rats fed *ad libitum* (group A) or a restricted diet (group R) is shown.

the rate of decline in this response, which occurs after 12 months of age, is similar to the rate of decline observed earlier in the rats fed *ad libitum*. Figure 11.8 depicts the level of endogenous lipid hydroperoxides in liver mitochondria and microsomes. In both cell fractions, lipid hydroperoxides increased with age; however, the hydroperoxides were consistently lower in the restricted rats, and the age-related changes were parallel in the rats fed *ad libitum* and the restricted diet. Figure 11.9 illustrates the effect of dietary restriction on the age-related decline in UV-induced DNA repair in isolated hepatocytes. The rate of decline in DNA repair was essentially the same in the rats fed *ad libitum* and the restricted diet; however, the level of DNA repair was consistently higher in the restricted rats.

Thus, the data in Fig. 11.3 through 11.9 show examples of dietary restriction altering both the rate of change and the set point of biological processes. We were surprised to find in our preliminary review of the literature that dietary restriction altered the set point of so many processes, i.e., the age-related changes in the processes were parallel in rats fed *ad libitum* and the restricted diet. In a recent study, Kalu *et al.* (1988) showed that in the same tissue dietary restriction altered the rate of change of one process while altering the set point of another process. Figure 11.10 shows that the increase in thyroid calcitonin (upper graph) was reduced in restricted rats. However, the number of C-cells (calcitonin-producing cells) in the thyroid

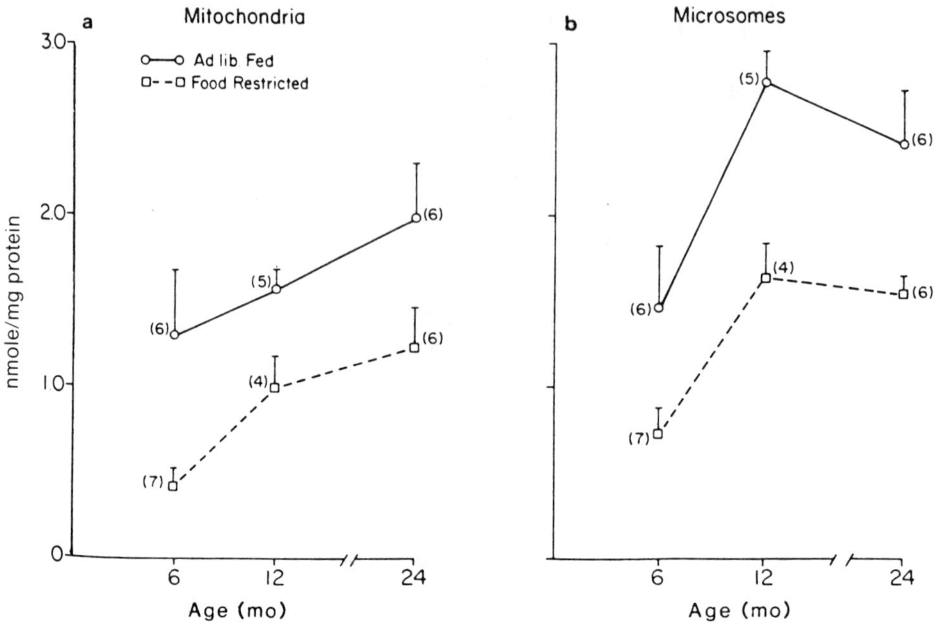

From Laganiere and Yu (1987)

FIG. 11.8. EFFECT OF DIETARY RESTRICTION ON LIPID HYDROPEROXIDES
Endogenous lipid hydroperoxides were measured in mitochondria (a) and microsomes (b) from liver tissue isolated from male rats.

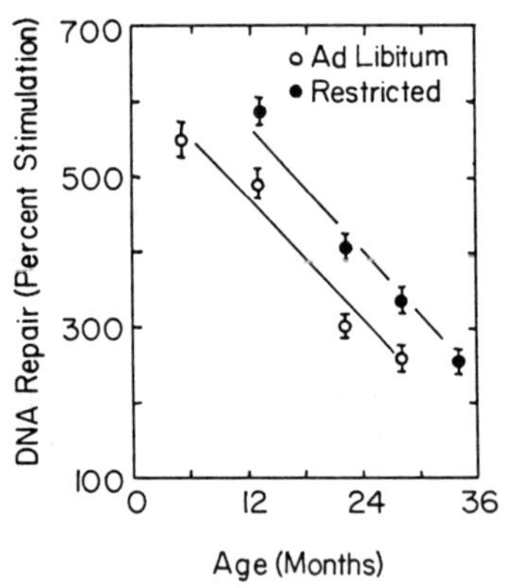

From Weraarchakul et al. (1989)

FIG. 11.9. EFFECT OF DIETARY RESTRICTION ON DNA REPAIR
The induction of unscheduled DNA synthesis by UV-irradiation was measured in suspensions of hepatocytes isolated from male rats.

showed an age-related increase that was parallel for rats fed *ad libitum* and a restricted diet; rats fed the restricted diet consistently had fewer C-cells (lower graph).

SUMMARY

We have described two models of how dietary restriction might increase the survival of laboratory rodents. The rate model is consistent with the view that dietary restriction exerts its effect by retarding the rate of aging. In contrast, the rate of aging would not be retarded in the set point model. In the set point model, the physiological status of an organism would be altered by dietary restriction in such away that the level of the process is altered; the rate of change in the process is not affected. Currently there are examples of biological processes in which either the rate of the process or the set point of the process has been altered by dietary restriction. However, the majority of studies on dietary restriction do not allow one to judge between these two models because only one or two, at most, ages have been compared. When only one age is studied, it is not possible to determine if dietary restriction has had any effect on the rate of change in the process; it is only possible to determine if dietary restriction has altered the process. In the future, we would hope that more investigators would use a range of ages when studying dietary restriction.

Although it is not possible at the present time to determine which of the two models accurately describes the molecular mechanism underlying dietary restriction, it is important to do so because the two models would have different biological consequences. For example, if dietary restriction were acting through a set point mechanism, it would mean that the only experimental manipulation (i.e., dietary restriction) that has been shown to increase the longevity of mammals does not retard the rate of aging. Instead it acts by inducing or changing the level of a process(es) that protects the organism from death. The aging process would still occur at the same rate; however, it would take longer before the biological process(es) reaches a level where death would occur. Thus, aging at the molecular level might be inevitable, and only the level of the process(es) that results in death can be changed, not the rate at which the process(es) changes.

A second consequence of the mechanism of action of dietary restriction would be the number of biological processes that could be affected. Dietary restriction could affect more biological processes through a set point mechanism than a rate mechanism. For example, in the rate model, dietary restriction would not alter processes that are unchanged with age or processes in which the age-related change has occurred before the imposition of the restriction procedure. In contrast, dietary restriction could alter these two types of processes through a set point mechanism. Figure 11.11 shows an example of dietary restriction altering a process that has changed before the restriction is initiated. In this example, glucagon induction of lipolysis was studied in adipocytes from rats in which dietary restriction was in-

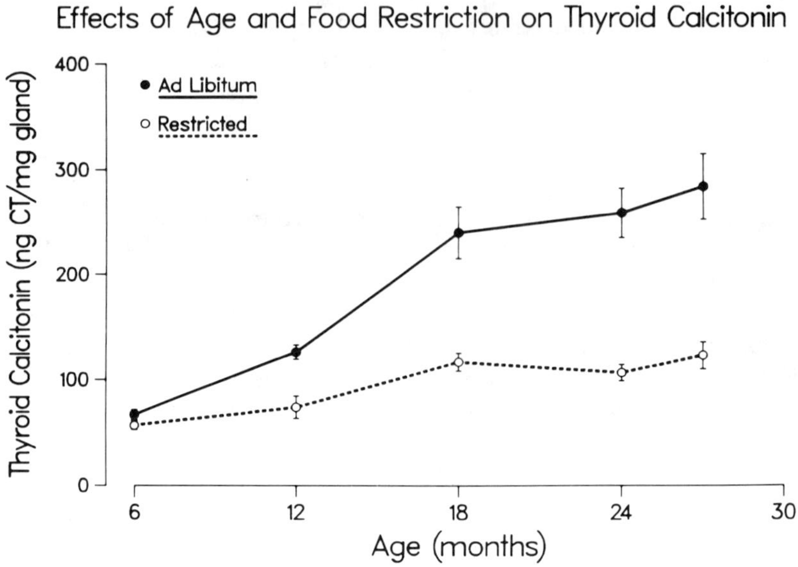

From Kalu et al. (1988)

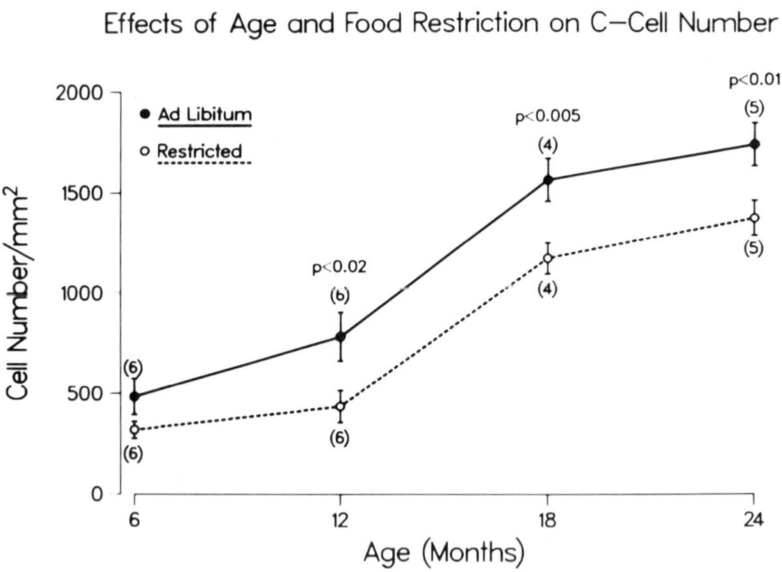

From Herbert and Kalu (1989)

FIG. 11.10. EFFECT OF DIETARY RESTRICTION ON CALCITONIN
The concentration of calcitonin (upper graph) and the number of calcitonin-producing cells (lower graph) in the thyroid gland of male rats are shown.

itiated at six months of age. At this age, the decline in glucagon-induced lypolysis has already occurred, and lipolysis is very low (see Fig. 11.10). However, Fig. 11.11 shows that dietary restriction initiated at six months of age eventually restored the lipolytic action of glucagon on adipocytes. In this case, the action of dietary restriction on lipolysis could only occur through a set point type of mechanism; if dietary restriction was changing only the rate of lipolysis, one would not expect the initiation of dietary restriction at six months of age to have any effect on lipolysis.

A third important consequence of the set point model is that it focuses attention on the importance of events immediately following the initiation of food restriction. This is the time that the signal for the change in the physiological status of the animal would occur. If dietary restriction were acting through a set point mechanism, it should be possible to measure changes in the physiological status of animals soon after the initiation of the restriction. Unfortunately, there is a dearth of information on the immediate effect of dietary restriction on most biological processes. This is probably because most investigators have assumed that dietary restriction is changing the rate of the process, and therefore, any change would be more pronounced and easier to demonstrate in older animals. Recently, McCarter and McGee (1988) showed that the rates of whole body metabolism in rats fed *ad libitum* and a restricted

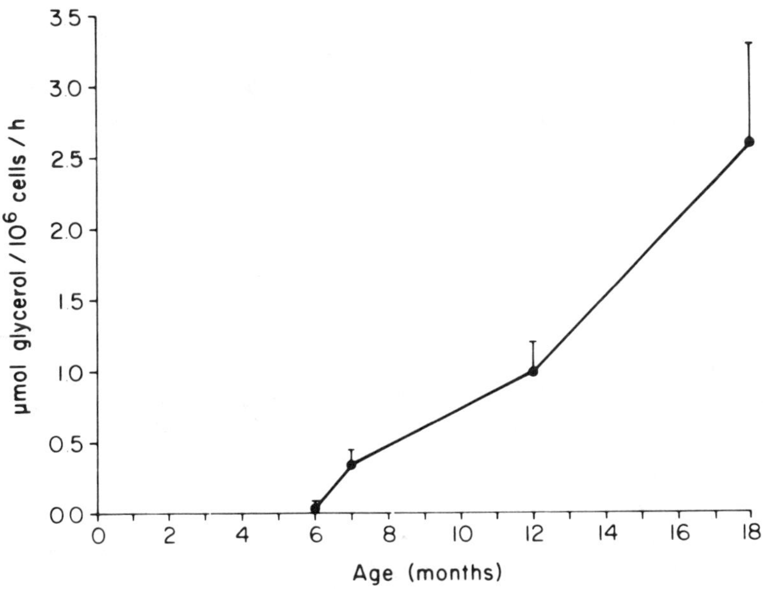

From Masoro (1985)

FIG. 11.11. EFFECT OF MIDLIFE DIETARY RESTRICTION ON LIPOLYSIS

The glucagon stimulated lipolytic response is shown for adipocytes isolated from rats fed a restricted diet from six months of age.

diet were strikingly similar throughout life even though the restricted rats received 40% less calories. The animals had adapted to the reduced dietary intake. Only during the first four weeks after the initiation of the restriction was there any significant difference in the rates of whole body metabolism in rats fed *ad libitum* and the restricted diet. Future studies on dietary restriction should begin to focus on the immediate actions of restriction because these events might provide important information on the mechanism by which dietary restriction alters biological processes and survival.

A utility of the set point mechanism would be the potential to study the effectiveness of dietary restriction in long-lived organisms. Currently, the vast majority of data available on the effect of dietary restriction on survival come from studies with laboratory rodents, which are short lived. It is very difficult, if not impossible, to conduct studies on dietary restriction with animals that have an average life expectancy of 20 or more years. If dietary restriction were occurring though a set point mechanism, one should be able to predict early in the restriction procedure if the procedure would be effective, i.e., if the level of the biological process(es) responsible for increased survival was altered. Thus, scientists would be able to study the efficacy of applying dietary restriction to humans.

ACKNOWLEDGMENTS

The authors were supported by grants AG01548, AG06819, and AG01188 awarded by the National Institute on Aging.

REFERENCES

BERG, B. N. 1960. Nutrition and longevity in the rat. I. Food intake in relation to size, health and fertility. J. Nutr. *71*, 242–254.

BERG, B. N. and SIMMS, H. S. 1960. Nutrition and longevity in the rat. II. Longevity and onset of disease with different levels of intake. J. Nutr. *71*, 255–263.

BERTRAND, H. A. 1983. Nutrition-aging interactions: Life-prolonging action of food restriction. *In* Review of Biological Research in Aging, Vol. 1, M. Rothstein (ed.). Raven Press, New York.

BIRCHENALL-SPARKS, M. C. *et al.* 1985. Effect of dietary restriction on liver protein synthesis in rats. J. Nutr. *115*, 944–950.

CHENEY, K. E. et al. 1983. The effect of dietary restriction of varying duration on survival, tumor patterns, immune function, and body temperature in B10C3F$_1$ female mice. J. Gerontol. *38*, 420–430.

FERNANDES, G., FRIEND, P., YUNIS, E. J. and GOOD, R. A. 1978. Influence of dietary restriction on immunologic function and renal disease in (NZB × NZW)F1 mice. Proc. Natl. Acad. Sci. USA *75*, 1500–1504.

FERNANDES, G. *et al.* 1983. Influence of diet on vascular lesions in autoimmune-prone B/W mice. Proc. Natl. Acad. Sci. USA *80*, 874–877.

FUJITA, Y., ICHIKAWA, M., KURIMOTO, F. and RIKIMARU, T. 1984. Effect of feed restriction and switching the diet on proteinuria in male Wistar rats. J. Gerontol. *39*, 531–537.

GARN, S. M. 1975. Bone loss and aging. *In* The Physiology and Pathology of Human Aging, R. Goldman and M. Rockstein (eds.). Academic Press, New York.

GOODRICK, C. L. 1984. Effects of lifelong restricted feeding on complex maze performance in rats. Age *7*, 1–2.

HERBERT, D. and KALU, D. 1989. Personal communication.

JOSEPH, J. A., WHITAKER, J., ROTH, G. S. and INGRAM, D. K. 1983. Lifelong dietary restriction affects striatally-mediated behavioral responses in aged rats. Neurobiol. Aging *4*, 191–196.

KALU, D. N. *et al.* 1984. Lifelong food restriction prevents senile osteopenia and hyperparathyroidism in F344 rats. Mech. Age. Dev. *26*, 103–112.

KALU, D. K. *et al.* 1988. Mechanism of dietary modulation of calcitonin levels in Fischer rats. J. Gerontol. Biol. Sci. *43*, B125–B131.

KALU, D. K. and MASORO, E. J. 1990. Undernutrition as a modulator of general and bone aging in the rat. *In* Nutrition and Bone Development, D. J. Simmons (ed.). Oxford Press, New York.

LAGANIERE, S. and YU, B. P. 1987. Anti-lipoperoxidation action of food restriction. Biochem. Biophys. Res. Commun. *145*, 1185–1191.

LEVEILLE, P. J. *et al.* 1984. Dietary restriction retards age-related loss of gamma crystallins in the mouse lens. Science *224*, 1247–1249.

LIEPA, G. U., MASORO, E. J., BERTRAND, H. A. and YU, B. P. 1980. Food restriction as a modulator of age-related changes in serum lipids. Am. J. Physiol. *238*, E253–E257.

MAEDA, H. *et al.* 1985. Nutritional influences on aging of Fischer 344 rats II. Pathology. J. Gerontol. *40*, 671–688.

MASORO, E. J. 1985. Metabolism. *In* Handbook of the Biology of Aging, C. E. Finch and E. L. Schneider (eds.). Van Nostrand Reinhold, New York.

MASORO, E. J. 1988. Food restriction in rodents: An evaluation of its role in the study of aging. J. Gerontol. Biol. Sci. *43*, B59–B64.

MASORO, E. J., YU, B. P., BERTRAND, H. A. and LYND, F. T. 1980. Nutritional probe of the aging process. Fed. Proc. *39*, 3178–3182.

McCARTER, R. and McGEE, J. 1988. Food restriction and metabolic rate: Different adaptive time courses of BMR and 24 hour metabolic rate. FASEB J. *2*, A1208.

McCAY, C., CROWELL, M. and MAYNARD, L. 1935. The effect of retarded growth upon the length of life and upon ultimate size. J. Nutr. *10*, 63–79.

MERRY, B. J. and HOLEHAN, A. M. 1979. Onset of puberty and duration of fertility in rats on a restricted diet. J. Reprod. Fertil. *57*, 253–259.

NADAKAVUKAREN, M. J., FITCH, K. L. and RICHARDSON, A. 1987. Dietary restriction retards age-related decrease in cell population of rat corneal endothelium. Proc. Soc. Exp. Biol. Med. *184*, 98–101.

PAHLAVANI, M. A., CHEUNG, H. T., CAI, N. S. and RICHARDSON, A. 1989. Influence of dietary restriction and aging on gene expression in the immune system of rats. *In* Biomedical Advances in Aging 1988, A. L. Goldstein (ed.). Plenum Publishing Corporation, New York.

REHM, S., RAPP, K. G. and DEERBERG, F. 1985. Influence of food restriction and body fat on life span and tumour incidence in female outbred Han:NMRI mice and two sublines. Z. Verrsuchstierkd. *27*, 249–280.

RICKETTS, W. G., BIRCHENALL-SPARKS, M. C., HARDWICK, J. P. and RICHARDSON, A. 1985. Effect of age and dietary restriction on protein synthesis by isolated kidney cells. J. Cell. Physiol. *125*, 492–498.

ROSS, M. H. 1976. Nutrition and longevity in experimental animals. *In* Nutrition and Aging, M. Winick (ed.). John Wiley & Sons, New York.

ROSS, M. H. and BRAS, G. 1973. Influence of protein under and overnutrition on spontaneous tumor prevalence in the rat. J. Nutr. *103*, 944–963.

SAKAR, N. H. et al. 1982. Low-calorie diet prevents the development of mammary tumors in C3H mice and reduces circulating prolactin level, murine mammary tumor virus expression, and proliferation of mammary alveolar cells. Proc. Natl. Acad. Sci. U.S.A. *79*, 7758–7762.

TALAN, M. I. and INGRAM, D. K. 1985. Effect of intermittent feeding on thermoregulatory abilities of young and aged C57BL/6J mice. Arch. Gerontol. Geriatr. *4*, 251–259.

WARD, W. F. 1988. Enhancement by food restriction of liver protein synthesis in aging Fischer 344 rat. J. Gerontol. Biol. Sci. *43*, B50–B53.

WEINDRUCH, R., KRISTIE, J. A., CHENEY, K. E. and WALFORD, R. L. 1979. Influence of controlled dietary restriction on immunologic function and aging. Fed. Proc. *38*, 2007–2016.

WEINDRUCH, R., GOTTESMAN, R. S. and WALFORD, R. L. 1982. Modification of age-related immune decline in mice dietarily restricted from or after midadulthood. Proc. Natl. Acad. Sci. USA *79*, 898–902.

WEINDRUCH, R. and WALFORD, R. L. 1982. Dietary restriction in mice beginning at 1 year of age: Effect on life span and spontaneous cancer incidence. Science *215*, 1415–1418.

WERAARCHAKUL, N., STRONG, R., WOOD, W. G. and RICHARDSON, A. 1989. The effect of aging and dietary restriction on DNA repair. Exp. Cell Res. *181*, 197–204.

YU, B. P. 1985. Recent advances in dietary restriction and aging. *In* Review of Biological Research in Aging, Vol. 2, M. Rothstein (ed.). Raven Press, New York.

YU, B. P. 1987. Update on food restriction and aging. *In* Review of Biological Research in Aging, Vol. 3, M. Rothstein (ed.). Raven Press, New York.

YU, B. P., BERTRAND, H. A. and MASORO, E. J. 1980. Nutrition-aging influence of catecholamine promoted lipolysis. Metabolism *29*, 438–444.

YU, B. P. *et al.* 1982. Life span study of SPF Fischer F344 male rats fed ad libitum or restricted diets: Growth, lean body mass and disease. J. Gerontol. *37*, 130–141.

CHAPTER 12

EFFECT OF CALORIC MODIFICATION ON AGING RATE IN NONHUMAN PRIMATES: A PROGRESS REPORT

GEORGE S. ROTH, Ph.D., DONALD K. INGRAM, Ph.D.
and
RICHARD G. CUTLER, Ph.D.
Molecular Physiology and Genetics Section
Laboratory of Cellular and Molecular Biology
Gerontology Research Center
National Institute on Aging
Francis Scott Key Medical Center
Baltimore, Maryland

INTRODUCTION

One of the first demonstrations that dietary restriction can extend the mean and maximum life span of laboratory rats was that of McCay *et al.* (1935). Since those initial studies, this observation has been confirmed and extended in numerous laboratories using various feeding regimens including reduced calories, proteins, specific nutrients or alternate day feeding (Weindruch and Walford 1988). Concommitant with life span extension, many investigators have reported that dietary restriction slows the rate of various age-associated structural and functional changes (Weindruch and Walford 1988). Among the most striking findings are decreased immunocompetance (Gerbase-DeLima *et al.* 1975), reduced collagen elasticity (Everitt 1971), altered enzyme activities (Ross 1969) and impaired endocrine/neuroendocrine regulation (Merry and Holehan 1985), such as loss of dopaminergic receptors and motor control (Joseph *et al.* 1983; Roth *et al.* 1984; Ingram *et al.* 1987).

The mechanisms by which dietary manipulation exerts such effects are still unclear. In fact, because of the difficulties in distinguishing normal from pathological aging, the extent to which reduced incidence of age-associated diseases influences life span and aging rate during dietary restriction has not been determined. Other possible explanations for dietary effects include regulation of metabolic rate and energy consumption (Ross 1985), control of gene expression (Lindell 1982), preservation of immune function (Walford *et al.* 1981), and neuroendocrine modulation (Everitt and Porter 1976).

Dietary restriction has been shown to extend life span in a number of animal models other than rodents. These include rotifers, *Tokophyra, Daphnia, Drosophila,* Nematodes, and fish (Weindruch and Walford 1988). However, to the best of our knowledge, this manipulation has never been attempted in a scientifically controlled manner for any species higher on the evolutionary scale than rats and mice. If indeed these findings are to be extrapolated to humans, it will first be necessary to test different dietary regimens in some higher species, preferably nonhuman primates.

PRIMATES MODELS OF AGING

For a number of reasons, most notably cost and relatively long life span, the use of primates as aging models has lagged considerably behind that of rodents and lower species. Only a few colonies contain sufficient numbers of aged and genetically/environmentally comparable younger primates for cross-sectional age analyses, let alone longitudinal studies over periods of time long enough to be meaningful. In addition, invasive studies or those requiring sacrifice are limited even more.

Nevertheless, several recent reports have revealed the very tempting potential of nonhuman primates as aging models with a great degree of relevance for humans. One of the most ambitious and comprehensive project has employed the pigtailed macaque, *Macaca nemestrina* (Short *et al.* 1987). Approximately 30 animals of each sex ranging from 4–28 years were examined over a 4–5 year period. Seventy-two different anatomical, biochemical and physiological measurements were performed. Of these, 23 exhibited significant main effects of age. Some of these are listed in Table 12.1. Although sex differences in age effects can be noted in a few cases, most exhibit fairly consistent patterns across gender. Particularly robust age changes have been reported for rectal body temperature, blood albumin, immunoglubulin A, fingernail growth rate, bone thickness and blood calcium (Short *et al.* 1987). It must be emphasized, however, that not all of these cross-sectional age differences prove predictive of longitudinal changes and vice versa (Bowden 1989).

It is interesting to note that T-lymphocyte mitogenic stimulation failed to show significant age effects in pilot studies and was eliminated from the above investigation. However, a very recent examination of 92 rhesus monkeys (*Macaca mulatta*) of both sexes ranging from 2 to more than 20 years of age indicates that lymphocyte stimulation by concanavalin A, phytohemagglutinin and pokeweed mitogen all significantly decline with age (Ershler *et al.* 1988). Greatest decrement in these im-

TABLE 12.1
BIOLOGICAL INDICES OF AGING IN *Macaca nemestrina*

Variables	Female: Y to M[1]	Female: M to O[2]	Male: Y to M[1]	Male: M to O[2]
Immunoglobulin A	↑	↑	↑	↑
Triglycerides (L)[3]	↑	—	↑	—
Testosterone			↑	↓
Tactile corpuscles	↓	↓	↓	—
Activated suppressor T-cells	—	↑	↑	↑
Fingernail growth rate	↓	↓	↑	↓
Heart rate	—	↓	↑	↓
Follicle stimulating hormone	—	↑	—	—
Blood chloride	↓	↓	—	—
Blood calcium	↓	—	↓	↓
Bone thickness	↓	↓	—	↓
Blood albumin	↓	↓	↓	↓
Blood platelets	—	↓	—	↓
Rectal body temperature	↓	↓	↓	↓
Estradiol	—	↓		
Hemoglobin	—	—	—	↑
Blood glucose	↑	↑	—	↑
Blood potassium	↓	↑	—	—
Apolipoprotein-A1 (H)[3]	↓	↑	↑	—
Very low-density lipoprotein	↑	—	—	—

Source: Adapted from reference Short *et al.* (1987)
Note: ↑ and ↓ indicate, respectively, an increase or decrease in age-group means with increasing age: — indicates no apparent difference, and blanks indicated not tested.
[1]Y to M stands for between the young and middle age groups.
[2]M to O stands for between the middle and old age groups.
[3]H = high-density fraction; L = low-density fraction.

munological responses occurs between midlife (11–17 years) and senescence (> 20 years) in all cases. In addition, a roughly progressive 70–80% decline in natural killer cell function was observed in the same study.

Changes in bone thickness, particularly in females, are another important manifestation of aging reported in *Macaca nemestrina* (DeRousseau 1985a). Complementary observations of age-related osteopenia (DeRousseau 1985a) and degenerative joint disease (DeRousseau 1985b; Kessler *et al.* 1986) have been noted for *Macaca mulatta*. Taken together, these findings further emphasize the similarity of skeletal aging in monkey and humans.

Neurological degeneration represents still another area in which nonhuman primates may serve as useful models for human aging. For example, squirrel monkeys (*Saimiri sciurius*) were recently reported to exhibit senile plaques in the brain that are quite similar to those occurring in aged rhesus monkeys and humans (Walker *et al.* 1987). Although this phenomenon may be more representative of age-associated disease than normal aging, the parallels with the human situation are impressive. If it is indeed possible to separate pathological and nonpathological aging, a striking marker appears to be the loss of striatal dopamine receptors. This phenomenon has now been observed in rats, mice, rabbits, humans and, most recently, rhesus monkeys (Roth *et al.* 1986; Lai *et al.* 1987).

It should be recognized that several of the age-related changes reported for subhuman primates are similar to those which have been affected by reduced feeding in rodents. Perhaps best known are the reductions in immunological function, body temperature and striatal dopamine receptor concentrations. Thus, these primate models not only exhibit many parallels with human aging processes, but also may be ideal systems with which to compare dietary modulation of aging rate with studies performed in rodents.

DIETARY RESTRICTION IN PRIMATES

In their recent examination of biological markers of aging in the pig-tailed macaque, Short *et al.* (1987) attempted to assess the effects of a diet rich in liquid, cholesterol, sugar, and salt on the parameters under study. Although this protocol simulated the average diet of the U.S. population, it did not attempt to mimic the studies of reduced intake relative to *ad libitum* feeding shown to extend life span in rodents.

Having ascertained the need for the latter type of investigation in primates to determine relevance to human aging, we selected two monkey species for study, rhesus (*Macaca mulatta*) and squirrel (*Saimiri sciurius*) monkeys. The selection considered the length of life span, documentation of age-related changes similar to those of rodents and humans, resistance to disease, adaptability to a captive environment, availability of nutritional information and availability of sufficient quantities of animals over a broad age range for a statistically meaningful study.

Initially 30 males of each species were housed at the NIH Animal Center at Poolesville, MD, and divided into the age and diet groups shown in Table 12.2. Semisynthetic diets based on established nutritional requirements for the two species (NIH open formula nonhuman primate diets) were formulated (Tables 12.3 and 12.4) and supplemented with 40% greater vitamin and mineral contents to allow for a 30% reduction in overall intake without reduction in trace nutrients. All animals were fed *ad libitum* for the first month at Poolesville, then experimental groups sequentially received 10% less food (bases an *ad libitum* intake of body weight matched controls) each month for 3 months, at which point (30% reduction) they have been maintained to date.

Data in Table 12.5 indicate that this dietary manipulation successfully reduced the absolute rate of body weight gain to 48 and 29% in juvenile and adult rhesus monkeys, respectively. The corresponding figures for juvenile and adult squirrel monkeys were 35 and 24% compared to their respective control groups. Relative

TABLE 12.2
ASSESSMENT OF PRIMATE AGING: EFFECTS OF CALORIC MODIFICATION
EXPERIMENTAL DESIGN FOR STUDY

Species	Approximate Age at Incorporation Into Study (Years)	Control	Experimental
Saimiri sciurius	1–4	7	6
	5–9	7	6
	> 10	4	—
Macaca mulatta	1–4	6 (10)[1]	6 (10)
	5–9	6 (10)	6 (10)
	> 20	6 (10)	— (10)

[1]Numbers in parentheses reflect total animals in respective groups after the 1988 expansion of the rhesus population.

TABLE 12.3
RHESUS MONKEY DIET

Ingredient	Amount (% by Weight)
Ground whole winter wheat	34.00
Alfalfa meal (17%)	3.00
Oat byproduct	11.50
Soybean meal (48%)	8.00
Fish meal (65%)	5.50
Brewer's dried yeast	2.00
Dried whey	3.00
Ground whole #2 corn	21.00
Soybean oil	3.10
Sugar	4.00
Dicalcium phosphate	1.00
Calcium carbonate	1.30
Salt	0.60
Vitamin premix	1.00
Mineral premix	1.00
	100.00
Protein	15%
Fat	5%
Fiber	7%

growth rates for each monkey were also calculated by dividing absolute weight gain by baseline weight (mean of the first two monthly weighings prior to dietary restriction). Table 12.5 indicates that dietary restriction reduced relative body weight

TABLE 12.4
SQUIRREL MONKEY DIET

Ingredient	Amount (% by Weight)
Fish meal (60% protein)	10.00
Soybean (48% protein)	12.00
High fat milk solids	6.50
Corn flour	25.50
Casein	6.40
Glucose	17.90
Apple pomace	10.00
Beet pulp	5.00
Soybean oil	1.90
Soybean lecithin	0.60
Dicalcium phosphate	1.00
Calcium carbonate	0.60
Salt	0.60
Mineral premix	1.00
Vitamin premix	1.00
	100.00
Protein	20%
Fat	7%
Fiber	5%

TABLE 12.5
EFFECT OF AGE AND DIET ON RATES OF WEIGHT GAIN[1]

	Absolute Body Weight Gain (g/week)			
	Rhesus Monkeys		Squirrel Monkeys	
Age Group	Control	Experimental	Control	Experimental
Juvenile	15.81 ± 1.90	7.49 ± 1.45	1.62 ± 0.28	0.56 ± 0.48
Adult	37.82 ± 10.3	11.00 ± 3.48	2.63 ± 0.27	0.63 ± 0.90
Old	31.66 ± 10.20		2.97 ± 0.37	

	Relative Body Weight Gain (% of baseline weight/week)			
	Rhesus Monkeys		Squirrel Monkeys	
Age Group	Control	Experimental	Control	Experimental
Juvenile	0.81 ± 0.13	0.37 ± 0.085	0.38 ± 0.72	0.12 ± 0.089
Adult	0.81 ± 0.25	0.40 ± 0.065	0.38 ± 0.041	0.08 ± 0.106
Old	0.34 ± 0.098		0.36 ± 0.045	

[1]Values represent mean ± standard errors for the numbers of animals indicated in Table 12.2.

TABLE 12.6
THYMIC LYMPHOCYTE MITOGENESIS IN RHESUS MONKEYS[1]

	ID	CON A	PHA	PWM
Control	1–4 Years			
	47Z	157771	20106	17158
	77Z	306226	32427	62940
	164Z	258916	46498	127586
	199Z	109083	40371	42525
	19Z	209072	31364	4944
	65Z	94392	20900	21287
	Mean	189,410	31,944	46,073
Experimental	1–4 Years			
	83Z	114066	41437	37746
	113Z	203835	27634	28555
	52Z	209483	32221	78879
	99Z	68001	34224	36756
	28Z	155012	23425	38127
	120Z	219082	136683	55043
	Mean	161,580	49,271	45,851
Control	5–9 Years			
	CH16	61499	8812	20242
	CH48	94336	16125	30999
	CH113	22189	15221	8661
	CH152	28070	4747	10794
	CH119	140924	16719	31311
	CH170	186308	28964	55030
	Mean	88,888	15,098	26,173
Experimental	5–9 Years			
	CH83	16489	5528	5018
	CH159	120301	27882	41282
	CH77	111912	12914	34087
	CH98	40502	9087	20001
	CH178	81528	12254	16539
	CH79	30572	7294	16850
	Mean	66,884	12,493	22,296
Control	> 20 Years			
	C58	53845	4504	14315
	P959	49041	7270	12576
	833	61048	9246	9105
	H2	60472	16841	21219
	W270	25472	9091	1402
	V295	21351	4444	4837
	Mean	45,205	8,566	10,576

[1]Rhesus T-lymphocyte mitogenesis (pm) for April 1988, Ershler and Klopp (1988), Thymic lymphocyte mitogenesis was determined as described Ershler *et al.* (1988). Values are for the individual monkies identified by I.D.

gain to 46 and 49% for rhesus and 32 and 20% for squirrel monkey juvenile and adult groups, respectively. Both absolute and relative body weight gains were statistically significant between control and experimental groups of each species/age (Ingram *et al.* in press).

In addition to monitoring rates of body weight gain in the monkeys under study, various biological indices of aging were examined. Table 12.6 reveals typical data for thymic lymphocyte mitogenesis in response to concanavalin A, phytohemagglutin and pokeweed mitogen in *ad libitum* fed and dietarily restricted rhesus monkies of several ages. A general decline with increasing age is evident in agreement with Ershler *et al.* (1988). However, at the time of this assessment (April 1988), no differences between the different diet groups could be observed.

Serum thyroxine levels were determined in both rhesus and squirrel monkeys. Table 12.7 gives the mean values over the entire year of 1987 (6 determinations for each animal). As with lymphocyte mitogenesis, a progressive age-related decline is observed, but no significant effects of diet are detectable.

TABLE 12.7
MEAN 1987 SERUM T_4 (ng/dL)[1]

	Rhesus Monkeys	Squirrel Monkeys
JC	5.8 ± 0.5 (6)	3.7 ± 0.2 (7)
JE	7.0 ± 0.7 (6)	3.7 ± 0.4 (5)
AC	5.2 ± 0.6 (6)	3.0 ± 0.3 (7)
AE	5.8 ± 0.7 (6)	3.1 ± 0.3 (6)
OC	2.0 ± 0.2 (6)	2.7 ± 1.0 (4)

[1]Serum thyroxine (T_4) levels were determined by RIA as previously described (Blackman *et al.* 19____). Values are the means ± standard errors for the annual means (6 determinations) of the numbers of individual monkeys indicated in parenthesis (Blackman 1987, personal communication). The effect of age is significant ($P < 0.01$) as analyzed by analysis of variance of individual values.

To monitor the health status of the monkeys, we have also examined a number of blood chemistry and cellular parameters. Most striking age-related changes are observed for serum alkaline phosphatase (Fig. 12.1) and albumin-globulin ratio (Fig. 12.2) in both species. No significant effect of diet was observed for these parameters during the first year of study. Several of these standard clinical parameters may emerge as candidates for assessing the impact of diet manipulation on aging processes.

SUMMARY AND CONCLUSIONS

Rhesus and squirrel monkeys have been administered a semisynthetic, *ad libitum* or 30% reduced intake, diet for more than 15 months and continue to be in good health as determined by physical examinations, hematology, and blood chemistry. Rates of body weight gain in the restricted animals have been substantially reduced.

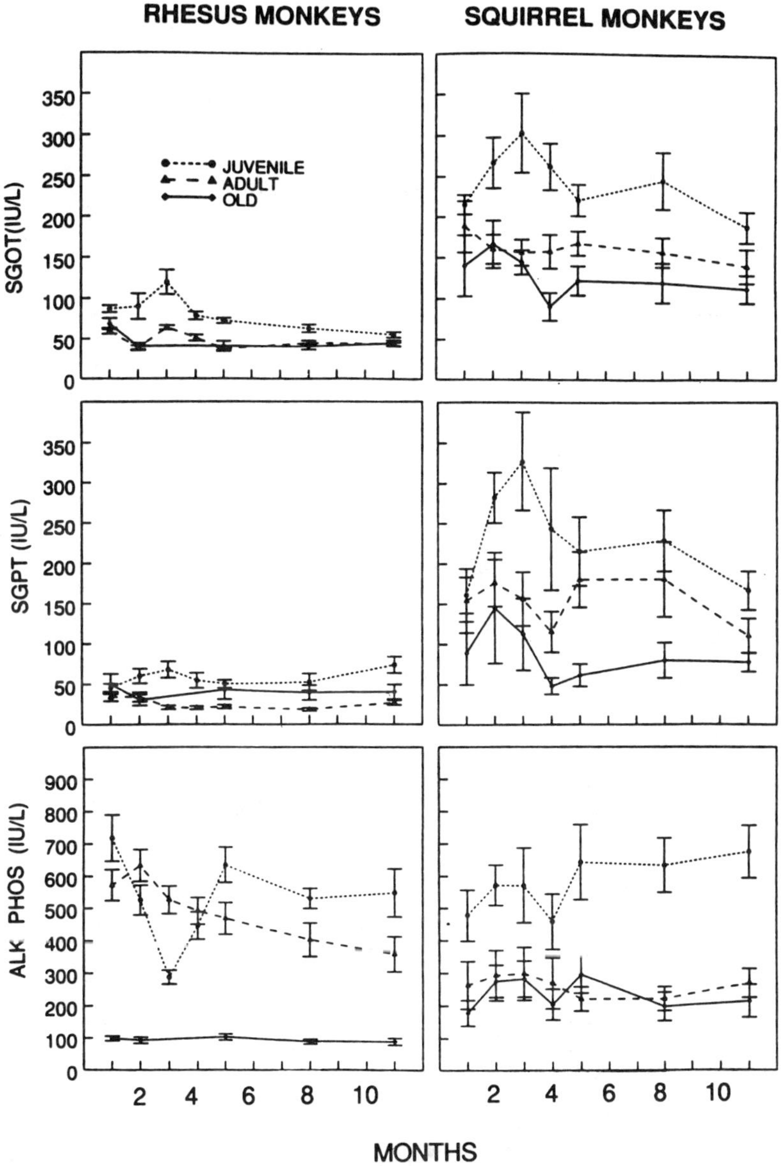

FIG.12.1. MEAN (± SEM) VALUES OBTAINED FOR SERUM GLUTAMIC OXALACETIC TRANSAMINASE (SGOT), SERUM GLUTAMIC PYRUVIC TRANSAMINASE (SGPT), AND ALKALINE PHOSPHATASE (ALK PHOS) FROM SERA OF MONKEYS AS A FUNCTION OF AGE AND MEASUREMENT OCCASION

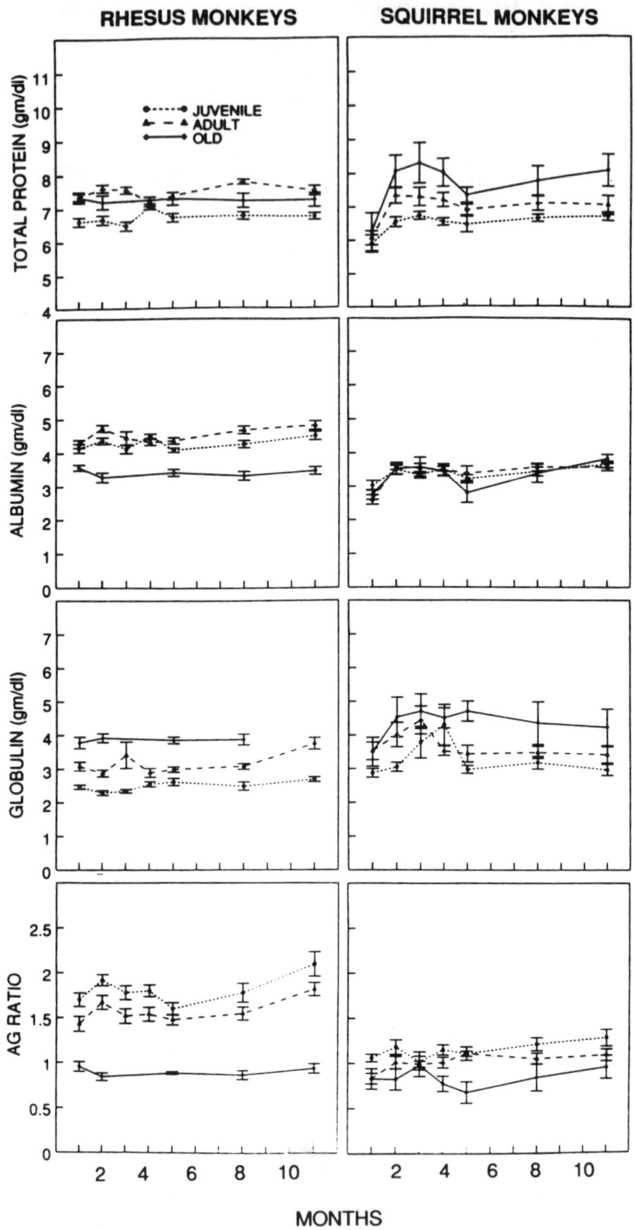

FIG. 12.2. MEAN (± SEM) VALUES OBTAINED FOR TOTAL PROTEIN, ALBUMIN, GLOBULIN, AND THE ALBUMIN/GLOBULIN (AG) RATIO FROM SERA OF MONKEYS AS A FUNCTION OF AGE AND MEASUREMENT OCCASION

At the same time, a number of anatomical, biochemical and physiological measurements of parameters that are correlated with age have been identified. Although significant cross-sectional age differences have been documented for many of these measurements, no significant effects of diet on parameters other than body weight have been detected to date. Nevertheless, with the recent expansion of the study to 90 monkeys and the relatively robust age differences already documented, it should be possible within the next 5–7 years to detect dietary effects if they do indeed occur.

ACKNOWLEDGMENTS

Thanks are due to the staff of the NIH Animal Center in Poolesville, MD, for their excellent maintenance of the animals described herein. They include Drs. David Renquist and Milton April, Mssrs. Claude Belcher and Charles Hatcherson and Ms. Margaret Clark. We also gratefully acknowledge the assistance of Dr. Joseph Knapka of the Div. of Res. Services, NIH, for formulating the primate diets, Ms. Sharon Davison for data processing and analysis, a multitude of other collaborators and advisors, including Drs. Marc Blackman, William Ershler, Douglas Bowden, Edward Masoro and David Harrison, without whose assistance many of the data presented here would not exist and Mrs. Rita Wolferman for superb clerical assistance.

REFERENCES

BLACKMAN, M. R., INGRAM, D. K., CUTLER, R. C. and ROTH, G. S. 19____. Effect of age and dietary restriction on thyroxine, triodothyronmine and testosterone levels in rhesus and squirrel monkey. (Submitted).

BOWDEN, D. 1989. Personal communication.

DEROUSSEAU, C. J. 1985a. Aging in the musculoskeletal system of rhesus monkeys. III. Bone loss. Am. J. Phys. Anthropol. *68*, 157–167.

DEROUSSEAU, C. J. 1985b. Aging in the musculoskeletal system of rhesus monkeys. II. Degenerative joint disease. A. J. Phys. Anthropol. *67*, 177–184.

ERSHLER, W. B. *et al.* 1988. Aging and immunity in nonhuman primates. I. Effects of age and gender on cellular immune function in rhesus monkeys (*Macaca mulatta*). Am. J. Primatol. *15*, 181–188.

ERSHLER, W. and KLOPP, R. 1988. Personal communication.

EVERITT, A. V. 1971. Food intake, growth and the ageing of collagen in rat tail tendon. Gerontologia *17*, 98–104.

EVERITT, A.V. and PORTER, B. 1976. Nutrition and aging. *In* Hypothalamus, Pituitary and Aging, A. V. Everitt and J. A. Burgess (eds.). Charles C Thomas, Springfield, IL.

GERBASE-DELIMA, B. *et al.* 1975. Immune function and survival in a long-lived mouse strain subjected to undernutrition. Gerontologia *21*, 184–202.

INGRAM, D. K. *et al.* 1987. Dietary restriction benefits learning and motor performance of aged mice. J. Gerontol. *42*, 78–81.

INGRAM, D. K. *et al.* 19____. Dietary restriction and aging: The initiation of a primate study. J. Gerontol. (In press).

JOSEPH, J. A., WHITAKER, J., ROTH, G. S. and INGRAM, D. K. 1983. Life-long dietary restriction affects striatally-mediated behavioral responses in aged rats. Neurobiol. Aging *4*, 191–196.

KESSLER, M. J., TURNQUIST, J. E., PRITZKER, K. P. H. and LONDON, W. T. 1986. Reduction of passive extension and radiographic evidence of degenerative knee joint diseases in cage-raised and free-ranging aged rhesus monkeys (*Macaca mulatta*). J. Med. Primatol. *15*, 1–9.

LAI, H., BOWDEN, D. M. and HORITA, A. 1987. Age-related decreases in dopamine receptors in the caudate nucleus and putamen of the rhesus monkey (*Macaca mulatta*). Neurobiol. Aging *8*, 45–49.

LINDELL, T. J. 1982. Molecular aspects of dietary modulation of transcription and enhanced longevity. Life Sci. *31*, 625–635.

McCAY, C. M., CROWELL, M. F. and MAYNARD, L. A. 1935. The effect of retarded growth upon the length of the life span and upon the ultimate body size. J. Nutr. *10*, 53–79.

MERRY, B. J. and HOLEHAN, A. M. 1985. The endocrine response to dietary restriction in the rat. *In* molecular Biology of Aging, A. D. Woodhead, A. D. Blackett and A. Holleander (eds.). Plenum Publishing Corp., New York.

ROSS, M. H. 1969. Aging, nutrition and hepatic enzyme activity patterns in the rat. J. Nutr. *97*, 565–601.

ROSS, M. H., LUSTBADER, E. D. and BRAS, G. 1985. Dietary habits and the prediction of life span of rats: a prospective test. Am. J. Clin. Nutr. *41*, 1332–1359.

ROTH, G. S., INGRAM, D. K. and JOSEPH, J. A. 1984. Delayed loss of striatal dopamine receptors during aging of dietarily restricted rats. Brain Res. *300*, 27–32.

ROTH, G. S., HENRY, J. M. and JOSEPH, J. A. 1986. The striatal dopaminergic system as a model for modulation of altered neurotransmitter action during aging: effects of dietary and neuroendocrine manipulation. Prog. Brain Res. *70*, 473–484.

SHORT, R., WILLIAMS, D. D. and BOWDEN, D. M. 1987. Cross-sectional evaluation of potential biological markers of aging in pigtailed-macaques: effect of age, and diet. J. Gerontol. *42*, 644–654.

WALFORD, R. L., TAM, C. F. and WEINDRUCH, R. H. 1981. Alterations in cyclic nucleotide metabolism in aging. Abstracts of the XII Intl. Congr. Gerontol. p. 173.

WALKER, L. C. *et al.* 1987. Senile plaques in aged squirrel monkeys. Neurobiol. Aging *8*, 291–296.

WEINDRUCH, R. and WALFORD, R. L. 1988. The Retardation of Aging and Disease by Dietary Restriction. Charles C Thomas, Springfield, IL.

SECTION IV

The Involvement of Specific Nutrients in Aging Processes

CHAPTER 13

THE ROLE OF DIETARY MINERALS IN BONE AGING

H. H. DRAPER, Ph.D.
Department of Nutritional Sciences
College of Biological Science
University of Guelph
Guelph, Ontario, Canada

Although its predominantly structural function implies that the adult skeleton has a low level of metabolic activity, it undergoes continual renewal and serves as a vital reservoir of minerals which are transferred to the extracellular fluid, and hence to the blood plasma and other tissues, where they have pervasive physiological roles. Bone renewal is generally referred to as remodelling, a term that reflects a difference from the biochemical concept of turnover, which entails the replacement of one molecule with an identical molecule. Bone remodelling involves the resorption of aged cells and their replacement with cells which differ morphologically and physiologically from their predecessors. It is a complex process, in the course of which a small quantum of bone is resorbed by bone-resorbing cells, the osteoclasts, and is replaced through the action of bone-forming cells, the osteoblasts. This process is necessary for the removal of aged, biomechanically fatigued bone tissue. The main stimulator of bone resorption is parathyroid hormone, which at moderately increased serum levels enhances remodelling with no net loss of bone (and possibly a net gain) but at high levels (clinical hyperparathyroidism) causes bone loss. In women, estrogen is necessary for the replacement of resorbed bone, and hence postmenopausal women are subject to a progressive loss of bone mass.

The central interest of nutritionists in bone aging has lain in the possibilities for modulating the loss of bone mass that predisposes to osteoporotic bone fractures in the elderly. This loss affects both cortical bone, which is predominant in the appendicular skeleton, and trabecular bone, which is characteristic of the axial skeleton and the ends of the long bones. Cortical bone mass peaks in the latter part of the fourth decade and begins to decline in the fifth decade in both men and women (Melton *et al.* 1988). Trabecular bone mass peaks in the early part of the fourth decade and begins to decline soon thereafter. A progressive loss of trabecular and cortical bone occurs in both sexes at an average rate of about 3% per annum. Loss sufficient to pose a risk of bone fractures results in a clinical condition termed senile osteoporosis.

Superimposed on this loss there is, in women, an increment beginning with the cessation of estrogen production at the menopause and lasting 10–15 years. During the first half of this period the rate of trabecular bone loss is about 9% per annum; that of cortical bone has been variously estimated at up to 10%. Thereafter the rate of bone loss in women again resembles that in men.

Because of this additional postmenopausal increment in bone loss, elderly women may lose 40–50% of their peak trabecular bone mass and 20% of their peak cortical bone, compared to 10–25% and less than 5%, respectively, in men (Melton *et al.* 1988). Some investigators classify postmenopausal bone loss as a condition distinct from senile osteoporosis that is due specifically to estrogen deficiency (Riggs and Melton 1983). This loss entails a reduction as much as 50% in the thickness of cortical bones as well as an increase in porosity. Trabecular bone loss is marked by thinning, perforation and dissolution of the trabecular plates, predisposing to fractures of the spine and hip (Melton *et al.* 1988). An estimated quarter of a million women are admitted to hospitals in the United States each year for treatment of a hip fracture (Conference Report 1987). In postmenopausal women, osteoporosis is the main cause of bone fractures.

The nutrients of primary interest in research on nutrition and aging bone loss have been calcium, phosphorus, protein, vitamin D and (to a lesser extent) fluoride. Their influence on bone homeostasis will be discussed individually; however, their interactions are of greater significance than their isolated effects.

CALCIUM

Defining the relationship between calcium intake and aging bone loss has turned out to be one of the most difficult problems in the history of human nutrition. There are several reasons for this difficulty. Young adults are capable of establishing calcium balance over a wide range of intakes. This adaptation entails an increase in the efficiency of dietary calcium absorption at low levels of intake mediated by a protein synthesized in the epithelial cells of the intestine in response to the genomic action of $1,25(OH)_2D$ (1,25-dihydroxyvitamin D), the metabolically active form of vitamin D. The renal synthesis of this metabolite is stimulated by PTH (parathyroid hormone), the synthesis of which is increased in response to a small decrease in serum calcium that occurs when the intake of calcium is reduced. This adaptive mechanism is mainly responsible for the ability of young adults to maintain overall calcium homeostasis at various levels of intake, but it is obviously incapable of preventing the chronic negative calcium balance associated with aging. In the classical studies of Malm (1958) which first demonstrated this adaptive capacity, the time required for restoration of calcium balance in men after a reduction in calcium intake ranged from days to months, and some individuals never adapted completely. The question arises whether a decline in the fractional absorption of calcium observed in the aged is due to impairment of this adaptive mechanism.

A major complication in research on the role of calcium intake in the prevention of osteoporosis is the protracted period of time over which intake must be monitored quantitatively. Retrospective estimates of calcium intakes are of little value, and it is usually impractical to monitor ongoing intake over the period (up to 5 years) necessary to detect a change in bone loss of a magnitude sufficient to be quantified using densitometry. A further complication is that osteoporotic subjects given a calcium supplement frequently exhibit a positive calcium balance, or a diminution of negative balance, for periods of up to a year, then lapse into their previous pattern of calcium loss. Time constraints on the duration of controlled feeding studies also create uncertainty regarding the long term significance of any short term change observed in calcium homeostasis.

Under these circumstances, the question whether a high calcium intake has any effect on aging bone loss within a given population is best determined by means of controlled intervention studies on free living subjects consuming their habitual diets, in which bone density is monitored in subjects given a calcium supplement versus placebo over several years. The results of such studies have generally been negative. In a double-blind controlled clinical study, Riis *et al.* (1987) monitored bone mineral loss from the proximal forearm and the lumbar spine over 2 years in early postmenopausal Danish women given 2000 mg of calcium per day versus placebo or estradiol. Although loss of mineral from the cortex of the forearm was somewhat reduced by calcium administration, loss from the trabecular bone of the spine was similar to that in the controls. Estrogen prevented bone loss at both sites. Similar results were obtained in a 4-year intervention study on Wisconsin women; a small reduction was observed in the rate of thinning of the long bones in subjects given a supplement of 1500 mg calcium per day, but there was no change in the loss of bone from the vertebrae (Freudenheim *et al.* 1986). These studies indicate that calcium supplementation may have a small effect on the loss of cortical bone but not on the loss of trabecular bone from the central skeleton, which is the site of most osteoporotic fractures.

A negative epidemiologic relationship between calcium intake and bone loss was found among a group of postmenopausal Nebraska women consuming self-selected diets (Heaney *et al.* 1978). From linear regression analysis of individual intakes ranging from 205–1412 mg/day with a mean of 659 mg, it was calculated that postmenopausal bone loss could be prevented by an average intake of 1500 mg per day. However, subsequent epidemiologic studies carried out in Denmark, the Netherlands and Switzerland have failed to detect a significant correlation between chronic calcium intake and bone density. In a cohort of 107 U.S. women up to 88 years of age whose bone density was monitored over 4.3 years, no relationship with calcium intake was found over an estimated range of 269–2000 mg/day (Riggs *et al.* 1987). Bone loss in a subgroup which consumed less that 500 mg/day was similar to that in another subgroup which consumed more than 1400 mg/day. A lower fracture rate was observed among Yugoslavian goat herders with a high calcium intake (approximately 1000 mg/day) than in a reference population with less than half this intake, but there was no difference in the rate of bone loss (Matkovic *et al.* 1979). The lower fracture rate in the herders was attributable to a greater bone mass of undetermined origin achieved in early adulthood, the predominant factor affecting the risk of fractures in late life.

The calcium content of national food supplies varies over at least a 2-fold range, from $\leqslant$500 mg per capita per day in countries with a cereal-based food economy, to 1000 mg in countries with a highly developed dairy industry. In the absence of a reliable estimate of the calcium requirement, recommended intakes in different countries reflect the application of Parkinson's Law, i.e., the intake recommended rises to meet the supply available. There is no evidence that these differences in recommended intakes are negatively related to the prevalence of osteoporosis in national populations. Indeed, the reported prevalence of hip fractures is greater in countries with a rich supply of calcium (Hegsted 1986). Garn (1967) observed that cortical bone loss was similar in Central American women and in women residing in Ohio, despite a 2-fold difference in calcium intake. He concluded that bone loss is a universal accompaniment of human aging. Aging osteopenia also has been documented in several species of animals, and is illustrated in Fig. 13.1 for mice fed a diet high in calcium and adequate in other osteogenic nutrients (Krishnarao and Draper 1969).

Although it can be inferred from the foregoing findings that the calcium requirement of adults does not exceed the 400–500 mg/day recommended by the WHO/FAO, or not more than half the intake of 800 mg/day recommended in the 1980 edition of the *U.S. Recommended Dietary Allowances* (Food and Nutrition Board 1980), cross-cultural comparisons can be misleading. It does not necessarily follow that if 500 mg of calcium per day is adequate for adults consuming a low protein, low phosphorus, neutral ash cereal-based diet, the same amount is also adequate for adults consuming the high protein, high phosphorus, acid-producing Western diet. The case for increasing the recommendation from 800 to 1000 mg/day, as proposed by the committee for the 1985 edition of the RDAs, has been undercut by the results of subsequent intervention trials, but until such time as reliable information is available on the calcium requirement of elderly subjects consuming the mixed diet of industrialized societies, they should be encouraged to avail themselves of the liberal supply of calcium that is obtainable from the modern food supply. The report of the European consensus development conference on osteoporosis (Conference Report 1987) includes a recommendation that physicians prescribe a high calcium intake for menopausal women diagnosed as being at high risk of a bone fracture, if only as a prudent measure.

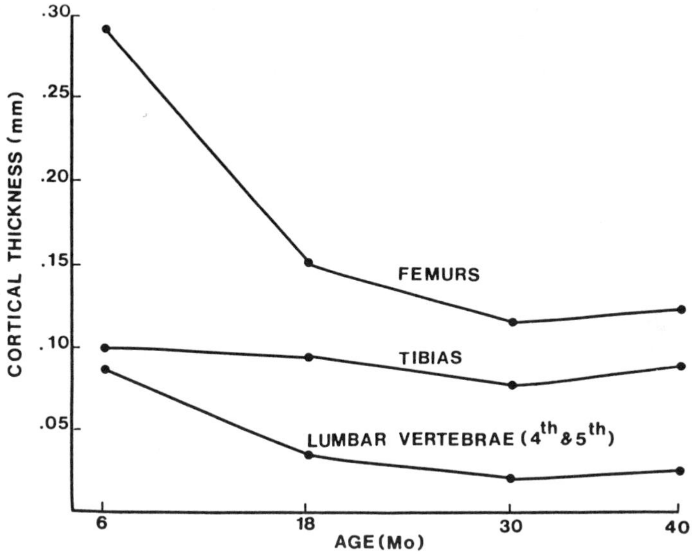

From Krishnarao and Draper (1969)

FIG. 13.1. CORTICAL THINNING IN MICE AS A FUNCTION OF AGING

PHOSPHORUS

All normal diets appear to provide sufficient phosphorus to meet the needs of adults. Even populations with a cereal-based food economy, in which the phosphorus present in phytin and hemicelluloses is only partially available, show no evidence of a deficiency. A natural association between phosphorus and protein assures an adequate intake of phosphorus from the high protein diet of industrialized societies. This natural supply is augmented by the use of phosphate food additives, which provide U.S. adults with about 300 mg of phosphorus per capita per day compared to a total intake of approximately 1400 mg (Draper and Scythes 1980). In fact, most research on the effect of phosphorus intake on bone aging has dealt with the question whether excess phosphorus in the modern diet has an adverse effect on bone homeostasis.

In animal nutrition it is an established principle that bone development in growing animals, and bone homeostasis in adults, is impaired by either a deficiency of calcium or a relative excess of phosphorus. During rapid growth, the phosphorus requirement of animals, determined experimentally and expressed as a percentage of diet, is half of that for calcium, reflecting the dominant influence of the 2:1 ratio of these elements in the mineral being deposited in new bone. Following skeletal maturation, the requirement for calcium decreases more than the requirement for phosphorus, and the ratio of their requirements shifts in favor of phosphorus, reflecting its greater requirement in the metabolism of soft tissues. Rats simultaneously offered a series of diets containing a constant, adequate level of calcium, but ranging from deficient to excess concentrations of phosphorus, self-regulate their phosphorus intake in accordance with physiological needs with remarkable consistency, i.e., in a calcium to phosphorus ratio of 2:1 during growth and of 1:1.2 as adults (Draper and Scythes 1980). These self-determined ratios are the same as those that have been determined experimentally. Other studies also indicate that a homeostatic mechanism exists which regulates the relative concentrations of calcium and phosphorus in the blood and extracellular tissues. This mechanism appears to be activated by a depression of serum calcium in the presence of excess phosphorus and to be expressed in part by a suppression of appetite for phosphorus.

The calcium and phosphorus requirements of animals, and sometimes of humans, are expressed in terms of a desirable ratio between the intakes of these elements, but this expression is not generally useful because the optimal ratio changes with the absolute intake of both nutrients. This is due to a progressive difference in the fractional absorption of the two elements at increasing levels of intake. Whereas the fractional absorption of phosphorus remains relatively constant at 70–75% over a wide range of phosphorus intakes, the absorption of calcium declines at intakes beyond about 8 mg/kg/day.

Excess dietary phosphorus leads to a rise in serum phosphorus, a decrease in serum calcium and a consequent increase in the synthesis of PTH, producing a so-called secondary hyperparathyroidism. The most dramatic example of this phenomenon in human nutrition is the hypocalcemic tetany seen in infants fed unmodified bovine milk, which contains 6 times as much phosphorus as does human milk. The calcium lost from the serum is secreted into the intestine, presumably as a phosphate complex, from which it is partially reabsorbed and partially excreted in the feces. Urinary loss of calcium is decreased as a result of PTH stimulation of renal reabsorption of calcium.

Serum calcium is more readily depressed by a high intake of dietary phosphorus than by a low intake of dietary calcium, a fact that is explained by the increase in fractional absorption of calcium at low intakes and the lack of regulation of phosphorus absorption. Phosphorus intake is an important determinant of urinary cyclic AMP (adenosine monophosphate) excretion, which is frequently measured as an indicator of renal PTH activity.

Feeding high phosphorus diets to adult dogs, cats, rodents and farm animals results in a decrease in bone mass that can be prevented, at least in part, by increasing calcium intake. Whether excess phosphorus in the human diet increases the calcium requirement for bone homeostasis has been a subject of lengthy speculation. Controlled studies on adults have shown that a high phosphorus intake induces a rise in serum phosphorus, a depression of serum calcium, an increase in urinary cyclic AMP (indicative of enhanced renal parathyroid function) and an increase in hydroxyproline excretion (indicative of enhanced bone resorption) (Bell *et al.* 1977; Zemel and Linkswiler 1981). However, an increase in bone resorption does not necessarily result in an increase in bone loss. Controlled experiments on young adults indicate that they are capable of maintaining calcium balance, in the presence of increased bone resorption, at phosphorus intakes up to 2500 mg/day (Hegsted *et al.* 1981). The loss of calcium from the skeleton associated with an increase in bone resorption evidently is offset by an increase in new bone formation, i.e., osteoclastic bone resorption remains closely coupled to osteoblastic bone formation. This also has been found to be true in postmenopausal women fed a high protein, high phosphorus diet, indicating that it is not estrogen-dependent (Draper and Piche, unpublished data). It has also been speculated that the renal 25OHD-1α-hydroxylase, which is stimulated by hypophosphatemia, may be inhibited by excess phosphate. In animals, however, the activity of the enzyme increases in response to the depression in serum calcium associated with a high phosphorus intake (Fig. 13.2) (Siu and Draper 1981).

The impact of a rise in serum iPTH (immunoreactive PTH) with age (Fig. 13.3) on aging bone loss is obscure. There has been uncertainty whether this rise reflects PTH bioactivity, but this ambiguity has been allayed by the recent development of assay methods specific for the intact hormone. Some investigators believe that the increase is a contributing factor in aging bone loss (Forero *et al.* 1987). However, this conclusion is not readily reconcilable with the finding that there is no net loss of calcium associated with the parathyroid stimulation caused by excess dietary phosphorus, nor with the finding that bone loss is not decreased by giving calcium supplements, the purpose of which is to raise serum calcium and thereby suppress parathyroid activity. There is evidence that increased bone remodelling induced by PTH or phosphate administration has a homeostatic effect on bone. Bone remodelling may promote mineral homeostasis by replacing damaged aged bone with new bone (Parfitt 1988). Until the role of PTH in bone metabolism is more clearly delineated, it will be difficult to understand fully the effect of the dietary minerals which influence its synthesis on the processes of bone aging.

There is no epidemiological evidence of a relationship between phosphorus intake and bone loss within populations. While the greater incidence of bone fractures reported in industrialized countries is positively correlated with a higher intake of available phosphorus, a similar correlation can be derived with calcium intake and various other nutritional and nonnutritional factors. An unusually rapid rate of bone loss in Alaskan and Canadian Eskimos (Mazess and Mathur 1974; Mazess and Mathur 1975) consuming a semicarnivorous diet very high in phosphorus and low in calcium is noteworthy, particularly in view of their physically active lifestyle. In the national nutrition survey carried out in Canada in the 1970's, higher phosphorus and lower calcium levels were found in the serum of Eskimos than in the general population (Health and Welfare Canada 1975). This finding is characteristic of animals and humans fed a high phosphorus diet. Eskimos appear to be resistant to osteoporotic fractures, however, because of a high resistance to trauma conferred by their short, thick bones. Another aspect of the Eskimo diet which has been of interest because of its possible relevance to their rapid bone loss is its very high protein content.

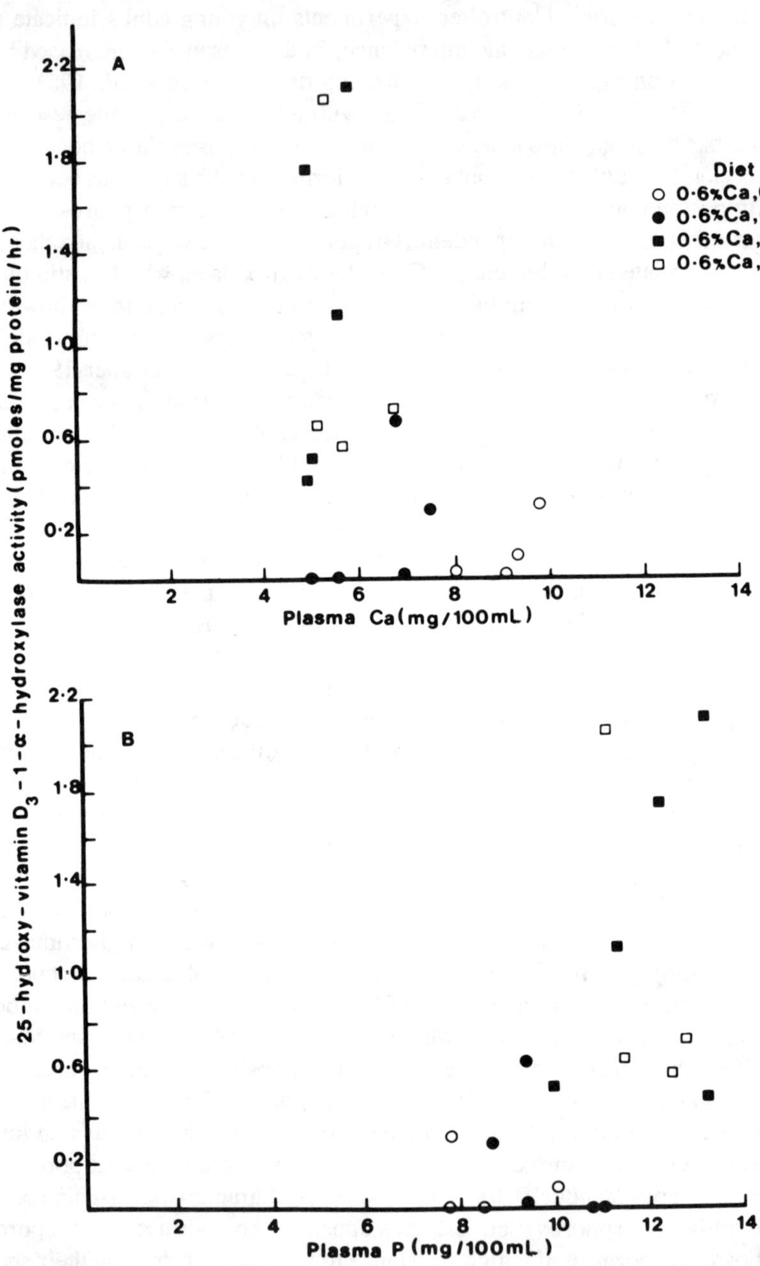

From Siu and Draper (1981)

FIG. 13.2. STIMULATION OF RENAL 25OHD-1α-HYDROXYLASE ACTIVITY IN RATS BY DIETARY PHOSPHATE

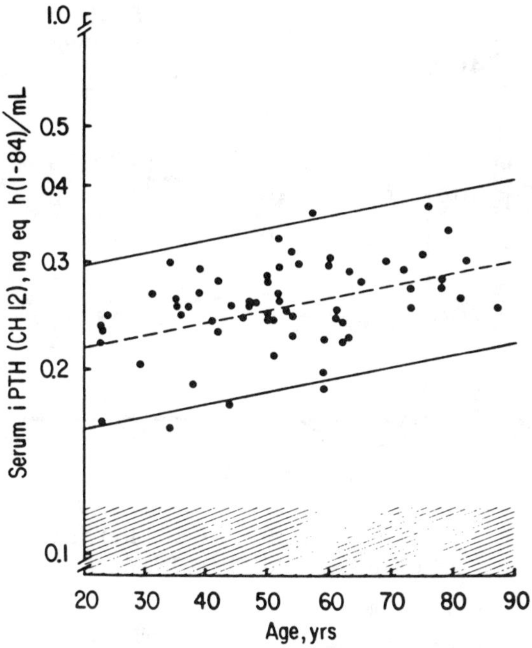

From Gallagher et al. (1980)

FIG. 13.3. RELATIONSHIP BETWEEN SERUM iPTH LEVEL AND AGE IN WOMEN

PROTEIN

Consumption by adults of excess protein in the form of a mixture of purified proteins results in an increased loss of calcium in the urine (Fig. 13.4) and an increase in the intake of calcium required to restore calcium balance (Fig.13.5) (Linkswiler *et al.* 1974). Calciuria is associated with a decrease in the renal fractional tubular reabsorption of calcium and a small increase in glomerular filtration rate. The calciuretic effect of proteins varies according to their content of sulfur amino acids. Oxidation of a mole of excess methionine or cystine yields (in addition to a mole of pyruvate) two moles of hydrogen ions and one mole of sulfate (i.e., one mole of sulfuric acid). Excretion of the hydrogen ions as ammonium and dihydrogen phosphate increases net acid excretion in the urine and reduces the efficiency of parathyroid-dependent reabsorption of calcium by the renal tubules. The pH of urine produced on high protein diets is characteristically acid, whereas that excreted on low protein diets is nearly neutral or slightly alkaline. The effect of a high protein intake on endogenous acid production and excretion by adults is illustrated in Fig. 13.6 (Yuen *et al.* 1984). Consequently, the question has arisen whether the high

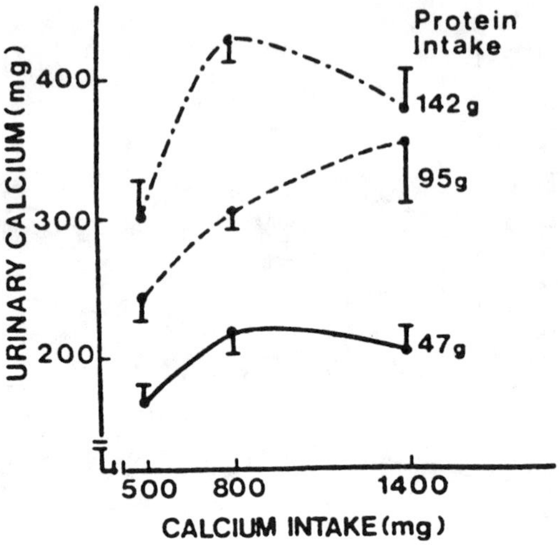

From Linkswiler et al. 1974

FIG. 13.4. EFFECT OF PROTEIN INTAKE ON URINARY CALCIUM IN MEN

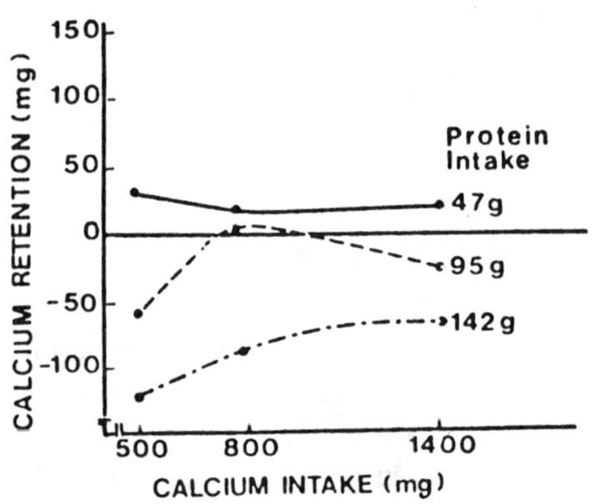

From Linkswiler et al. 1974

FIG. 13.5. EFFECT OF PROTEIN INTAKE ON CALCIUM BALANCE IN MEN

protein diet of industrialized societies increases the calcium requirement for the maintenance of bone homeostasis in adults.

When adults are fed a diet containing high protein foods (as opposed to a diet supplemented with purified proteins) different results are obtained (Fig. 13.7) (Spencer *et al.* 1983). No calciuria, and consequently no negative calcium balance, are observed. The explanation of these divergent findings apparently lies in a difference in the intake of phosphorus, which was held constant in studies on purified proteins (Linkswiler *et al.* 1974) but rose with the intake of high protein foods (Spencer *et*

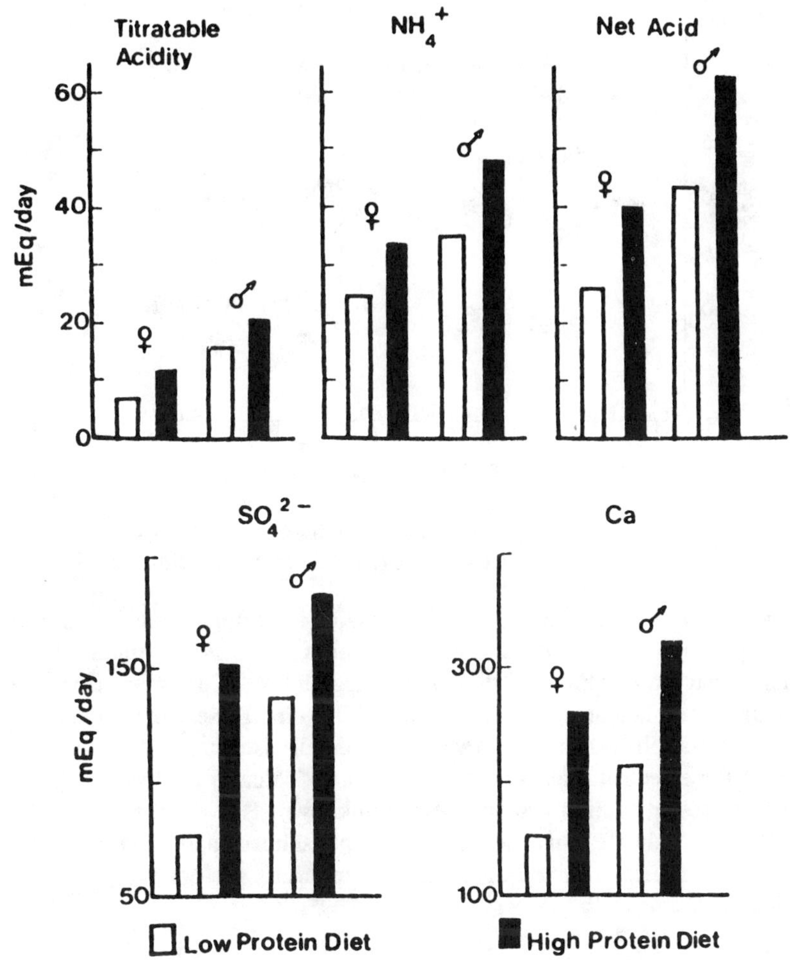

From Yuen et al. 1984

FIG. 13.6. EFFECT OF PROTEIN INTAKE ON ENDOGENOUS ACID PRODUCTION AND EXCRETION IN ADULTS

al. 1983). The PTH-mediated hypocalciuric effect of excess dietary phosphorus counteracts the calciuretic effect of excess dietary protein. Addition of phosphorus to a diet containing a high level of purified proteins reduces calcium excretion and restores calcium balance (Linkswiler *et al.* 1981).

THE PROTEIN-PHOSPHORUS-CALCIUM INTERACTION

The foregoing studies show that at high protein intakes there is an increase in the amount of phosphorus required to maintain calcium balance. The interaction be-

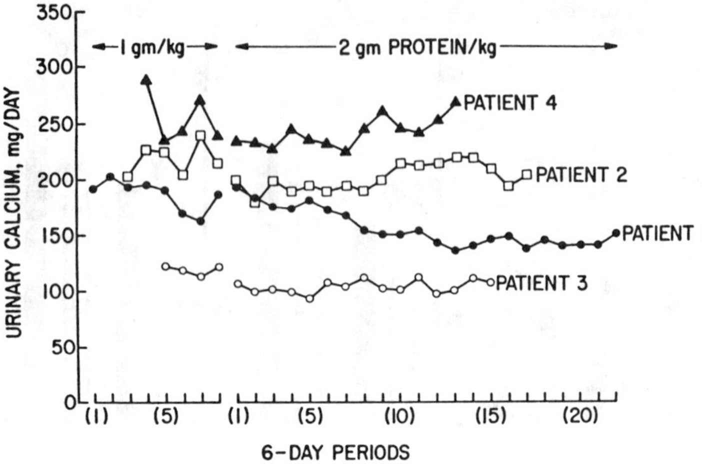

From Spencer et al. 1983

FIG. 13.7. EFFECT OF A DIET HIGH IN PROTEIN AS MEAT ON URINARY CALCIUM EXCRETION

tween dietary protein and phosphorus is of major importance in calcium nutrition, particularly in populations with a food supply high in protein. Stimulation of PTH-dependent renal reabsorption of calcium by a high intake of phosphorus is necessary to maintain calcium balance at a high intake of protein. The effect of dietary protein on calcium metabolism has been reviewed in detail elsewhere (Yuen *et al.* 1984).

Whether the effect of excess protein on urinary calcium is always offset by the phosphorus present in high protein diets is unknown. However, the evidence currently available indicates that the amounts of phosphorus and protein provided by typical North American mixed diets are not important factors in the loss of bone associated with aging.

VITAMIN D

The plasma level of 25OHD (25-hydroxyvitamin D) declines progressively with adult age (Fig.13.8) (Baker *et al.* 1980). Under normal conditions this hepatic metabolite consists mainly of $25OHD_3$, the product of vitamin D_3 synthesized in the skin, and therefore its plasma concentration is determined primarily by the level of exposure to solar radiation.

Plasma 25OHD concentration is the best indicator of vitamin D status, but the clinical setpoints have not been clearly defined. Levels below 10 ng/mL are generally regarded as reflecting low tissue stores of vitamin D, but 5 ng/mL appears to be sufficient to prevent rickets and osteomalacia. Plasma 25OHD levels vary according to season, climatic conditions and food fortification practices. Mean values reported for young adults in Britain and Denmark (9 and 12 ng/mL, respectively)

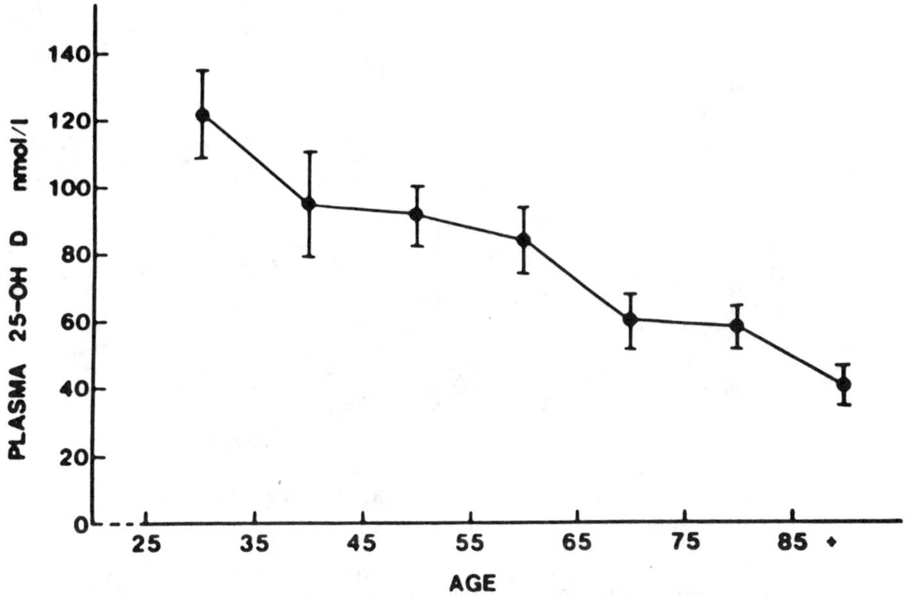

From Baker et al. (1980)

FIG. 13.8. RELATIONSHIP BETWEEN PLASMA 25-OHD LEVEL AND AGE IN NORMAL WOMEN

(Lester *et al.* 1980) are lower than those observed in the United States and Canada (approximately 25 ng/mL) (Chesney 1981). In Britain, where there is less food fortification and sunlight than in North America, biochemical and clinical evidence of low vitamin D status and osteomalacia is prevalent in the elderly (Fraser 1983).

Even in countries with liberal sunlight, surveys of plasma 25OHD levels have revealed low levels ($\leqslant$ 10 ng/mL) in a significant fraction of older adults. The levels found for a cohort of 96 noninstitutionalized Canadian postmenopausal women aged 58–89 years are typical (Fig. 13.9) (Gibson *et al.* 1986). Eleven percent of the total sample (mean value 16.5 ng/mL) had values below 10 ng/mL, but none was below 5 ng/mL.

The main cause of low plasma 25OHD levels in elderly adults is limited exposure to sunlight associated with a predominantly indoor existence. Although it has been proposed that the efficiency of vitamin D synthesis in the skin is reduced in the elderly, following ultraviolet irradiation under controlled conditions elderly adults exhibited increases in plasma 25OHD similar to those seen in young adults (Davie and Lawson 1980). It has been estimated that at least 12.5 μg of dietary vitamin D (500 IU) per day are necessary to maintain serum 25OHD within the normal range for adults in the absence of sunlight (MacLennan and Hamilton 1977; Somerville *et al.* 1977). Adults with limited exposure to sunlight obtain a smaller fraction of their vitamin D requirement from endogenous sources and therefore must obtain a larger fraction from the diet. The fact that elderly adults generally receive less exposure to solar

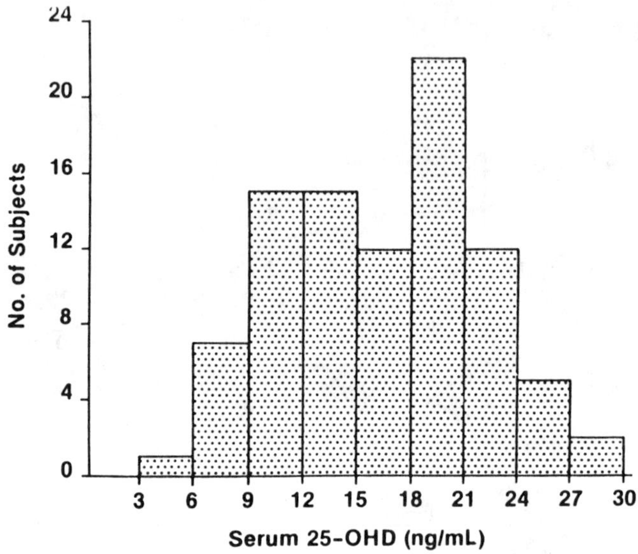

From Gibson et al. (1986)

FIG. 13.9. FREQUENCY DISTRIBUTION OF SERUM 25-OHD LEVELS IN 96 NONINSTITUTIONALIZED CANADIAN POSTMENOPAUSAL WOMEN

radiation than young adults means that (unless this exposure is nevertheless adequate) they have a higher requirement for vitamin D in the diet. Data for plasma levels of 25OHD and 1,25$(OH)_2$D indicate that the vitamin D requirement of significant numbers of elderly adults currently is not being adequately met. Twenty percent of a cohort of Canadian postmenopausal women consumed less than 2.5 μg (100 IU) of vitamin D per day (Fig. 13.10) (Gibson *et al.* 1986). Over half of the intake was derived from fortified dairy products. The British experience indicates that casual sunlight exposure cannot be relied upon to prevent osteomalacia in elderly adults living in temperate climates.

The available strategies for improving the vitamin D status of the elderly are limited to increasing their exposure to sunlight, increasing the level of food fortification or providing a vitamin D supplement. The first option is the most physiological but the least practicable. Further food fortification is difficult to target for the elderly and may pose a risk of toxicity in the United States and Canada, where foods are already liberally fortified and where widespread publicity has been given to the purported value of fish oils, rich in vitamin D, in the prevention of heart attacks. Vitamin D supplementation has the advantage that it can be implemented selectively in the case of individuals with little exposure to sunlight. It has a precedent in the supplements given to infants for the same reason.

Plasma levels of 1,25$(OH)_2$D are under stringent homeostatic control and therefore do not reflect vitamin D status except in a state of deficiency. The plasma level remains stable during early and middle adulthood but appears to be lower in elderly

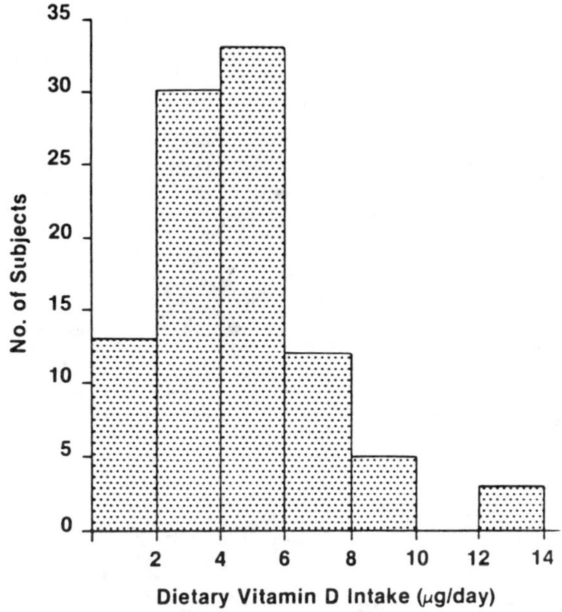

From Gibson et al. (1986)

FIG. 13.10. DIETARY INTAKE OF VITAMIN D BY A COHORT OF 96 NORMAL CANADIAN POSTMENOPAUSAL WOMEN CALCULATED FROM 3-DAY DIET RECORDS

adults (Fig.13.11) (Gallagher *et al.* 1979). It has also been inconsistently reported to be lower in osteoporotics than in age-matched controls.

Whether lower 1,25$(OH)_2$D levels in the aged reflect a state of deficiency or a decrease in renal 25OHD-1α-hydroxylase activity and whether they constitute a risk factor for aging bone loss is unclear. One hypothesis attributes aging bone loss to a decline in 1,25$(OH)_2$D synthesis caused by impaired 1α-hydroxylase activity resulting, sequentially, in decreases in calcium absorption and plasma calcium concentration and increases in PTH synthesis and bone remodelling, in the course of which new bone formation fails to keep pace with bone resorption because of impaired osteoblast activity (Eastell *et al.* 1988). A modification of this hypothesis attributes postmenopausal osteoporosis to increased bone resorption caused by cessation of estrogen production, a consequent rise in serum calcium and decrease in the synthesis of PTH, a potent agonist of 25OHD-1α-hydroxylase. According to this hypothesis, the decline in plasma 1,25$(OH)_2$D is a result, rather than a cause, of postmenopausal osteoporosis, and accounts for the decrease in calcium absorption in the aged.

In favor of this hypothesis, PTH infusions have been reported to increase 1,25$(OH)_2$D levels, although not as effectively in older as compared to younger adults (Tsai *et al.* 1984), and plasma iPTH has been found to be positively related to the

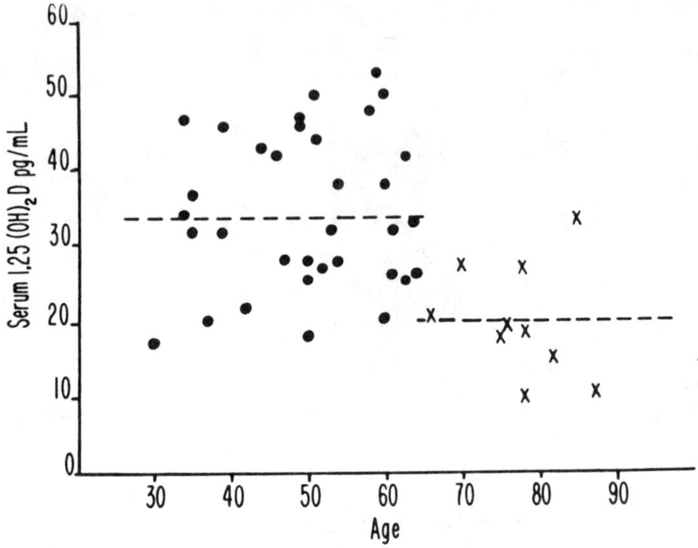

From Gallagher et al. (1979)

FIG. 13.11. SERUM 1,25$(OH)_2D_3$ LEVELS IN NORMAL ADULTS OF DIFFERENT AGES

fractional absorption of calcium. However, the failure of large supplements of calcium (which at high intakes is absorbed mainly by a passive, nonvitamin D-dependent process) to influence the rate of bone loss in older women militates against the hypothesis that impaired calcium absorption caused by 1,25$(OH)_2D$ deficiency is an important factor in the etiology of postmenopausal osteoporosis. The panel for a 1987 international consensus development conference concluded that "in the early postmenopausal period there is no evidence that vitamin D, its analogues, or its metabolites decrease the rate of bone loss or fracture" (Conference Report 1987).

FLUORIDE

Administration of pharmacological amounts of fluoride (about 20 mg daily) is the only known therapeutic measure that produces an increase in bone mass in osteoporotic patients. But there are negative side effects in some recipients, the fluorotic bone produced is more brittle than normal bone, and there is no clear evidence of a resulting decrease in bone fractures. Fluoride administration is not recommended for the prophylaxis of aging bone loss (Conference Report 1987). With the possible exception of geographic areas where the drinking water contains levels of fluoride which produce tooth mottling ($\geqslant$ 4 ppm), fluoride intake appears to have no effect on the rate of aging bone loss.

PROSPECTUS

Prospects for modulating the processes of bone aging by nutritional intervention currently are at a nadir. The main malnutritional theories of aging bone loss put forward over the last 25 years (calcium deficiency, phosphorus and/or protein excess, deficiency or impaired metabolism of vitamin D) have been tested to the extent necessary to conclude that they are not major factors in the etiology of osteoporotic bone disease.

There are, nevertheless, nutritional strategies that are worthy of implementing as precautionary measures. Despite the results of intervention trials which indicate that the current intake of calcium in industrialized societies is generally adequate, the decline in calcium absorption and vitamin D status in the elderly suggests that a liberal calcium intake may benefit some individuals. Compliance with the intake of 800 mg/day recommended for adults in the United States and Canada, as well as the intakes recommended during childhood and adolescence, should be encouraged. The evidence for suboptimal vitamin D status among some elderly adults justifies a supplement in the case of subjects receiving little exposure to sunlight. The calcium requirement of adults is still obscure and therefore remains a research priority. Obviously, there is some level of intake below which degenerative bone disease in the elderly is accelerated.

A full understanding of the role of dietary minerals in the processes of bone aging must await the results of ongoing research on the complex regulation of bone metabolism. The recent decline in evidence for a significant role of nutrition in aging bone loss has been followed by an increased interest in the role of physical activity. At present, however, the only fully effective measure for the prevention of postmenopausal osteoporosis, the main public health problem associated with bone aging, depends on identifying susceptible individuals at the time of the menopause and instituting estrogen and progestogen prophylaxis for at least a decade.

REFERENCES

BAKER, M. R., PEACOCK, M. and NORDIN, B. E. C. 1980. The decline in vitamin D status with age. Age Ageing *9*, 249–252.

BELL, R. R. *et al.* 1977. Physiological responses to foods containing phosphate additives. J. Nutr. *107*, 42–50.

CHESNEY, R. W. 1981. Current applications of vitamin D metabolite research. Clin. Orthop. *16*, 285–314.

Conference Report. 1987. Consensus development conference: prophylaxis and treatment of osteoporosis. Br. Med. J. *295*, 914–915.

DAVIE, M. and LAWSON, D. E. M. 1980. Assessment of plasma 25-hydroxyvitamin D response to ultraviolet irradiation over a controlled area in young and elderly subjects. Clin. Sci. *58*, 235–242.

DRAPER, H. H. and SCYTHES, C. A. 1980. Calcium, phosphorus and osteoporosis. Fed. Proc. *40*, 2434–2438.

EASTELL, R., HEATH, H., III, KUMAR, R. and RIGGS, B. L. 1988. Hormonal factors: PTH, vitamin D and calcitonin. *In* Osteoporosis. Etiology, Diagnosis and Management, B. L. Riggs and L. J. Melton III (eds.). Raven Press, New York.

Food and Nutrition Board, National Research Council. 1980. Recommended Dietary Allowances. National Academy of Sciences, Washington, D.C.

FORERO, M. S. *et al.* 1987. Effect of age on circulating immunoreactive and bioactive parathyroid hormone levels in women. J. Bone Miner. Res. *2*, 363–366.

FRASER, D. R. 1983. The physiological economy of vitamin D. The Lancet *i*, 969–971.

FREUDENHEIM, J. L., JOHNSON, N. E. and SMITH, E. L. 1986. Relationships between usual nutrient intake and bone-mineral content of women 35–65 years of age: longitudinal and cross-sectional analysis. Am. J. Clin. Nutr. *44*, 863–876.

GALLAGHER, J. C. *et al.* 1979. Intestinal calcium absorption and serum vitamin D metabolites in normal subjects and osteoporotic patients. J. Clin. Invest. *64*, 729–736.

GALLAGHER, J. C., RIGGS, B. L., JERPBAK, C. M. and ARNAUD, C. D. 1980. The effect of age on serum immunoreactive parathyroid hormone in normal and osteoporotic women. J. Lab. Clin. Med. *95*, 373–385.

GARN, S. M., ROHMANN, C. G. and WAGNER, B. 1967. Bone loss as a general phenomenon in man. Fed. Proc. *26*, 1729–1736.

GIBSON, R. S. *et al.* 1986. The vitamin D status of a cohort of postmenopausal non-institutionalized Canadian women. Nutr. Res. *6*, 1179–1187.

Health and Welfare Canada. 1975. Nutrition Canada. The Eskimo Survey Report. Information Canada, Ottawa.

HEANEY, R. P., RECKER, R. R. and SAVILLE, P. D. 1978. Menopausal changes in calcium balance performance. J. Lab. Clin. Med. *92*, 953–963.

HEGSTED, D. M. 1986. Calcium and osteoporosis. J. Nutr. *116*, 2316–2319.

HEGSTED, M. S., SCHUETTE, M., ZEMEL, M. B. and LINKSWILER, H. M. 1981. Urinary calcium and calcium balance in young men as affected by level of protein and phosphorus intake. J. Nutr. *111*, 553–562.

KRISHNARAO, G. V. G. and DRAPER, H. H. 1969. Age-related changes in the bones of adult mice. J. Geront. *24*, 149–151.

LESTER, E. *et al.* 1980. Serum 25-hydroxyvitamin D levels and vitamin D intake in healthy young adults in Britain and Denmark. Scand. J. Clin. Invest. *40*, 145–150.

LINKSWILER, H. M., JOYCE, C. L. and ANAND, C. R. 1974. Calcium retention of adult males as affected by level of protein and of calcium intake. Trans. New York Acad. Sci. Ser. II *36*, 333–340.

LINKSWILER, H. M., ZEMEL, M. B., HEGSTED, M. and SCHUETTE, S. A. 1981. Protein induced hypercalciuria. Fed. Proc. *40*, 2429–2433.

MacLENNAN, W. J. and HAMILTON, J. C. 1977. Vitamin D supplements and 25-hydroxy vitamin D concentration in the elderly. Br. Med. J. *ii*, 859–861.

MALM, O. J. 1958. Calcium Requirement and Adaptation in Adult Men. Oslo University Press, Oslo.

MATKOVIC, V. *et al.* 1979. Bone status and fracture rates in two regions of Yugoslavia. Am. J. Clin. Nutr. *32*, 540–549.

MAZESS, R. B. and MATHUR, W. 1974. Bone mineral content of northern Alaskan Eskimos. Am. J. Clin. Nutr. *27*, 916–925.

MAZESS, R. B. and MATHUR, W. 1975. Bone mineral content of Canadian Eskimos. Hum. Biol. *47*, 45–63.

MELTON, L. J., III, CHAO, E. Y. S. and LANE, J. 1988. Biomechanical aspects of fractures. *In* Osteoporosis. Etiology, Diagnosis and Management, B. L. Riggs and L. J. Melton, III (eds.). Raven Press, New York.

PARFITT, A. M. 1988. Bone remodelling: relationship to the amount and structure of bone, and the pathogenesis and prevention of fractures. *In* Osteoporosis. Etiology Diagnosis and Management, B. L. Riggs and L. J. Melton, III (eds.). Raven Press, New York.

RIGGS, B. L. and MELTON, J., III. 1983. Evidence for two distinct syndromes of involutional osteoporosis. Editorial. Am. J. Med. *75*, 899–901.

RIGGS, B. L. *et al.* 1987. Dietary calcium intake and rates of bone loss is women. J. Clin. Invest. *80*, 979–982.

RIIS, B., THOMSEN, K. and CHRISTIANSEN, C. 1987. Does calcium supplementation prevent postmenopausal bone loss? A double-blind controlled clinical study. N. Engl. J. Med. *316*, 173–177.

SIU, G. M. and DRAPER, H. H. 1981. Increased 1,25-dihydroxyvitamin D_3 synthesis in rats fed a high-phosphorus diet. Calcif. Tissue Intern. *33*, 667–672.

SOMERVILLE, P. J., LIEN, J. W. K. and KAYE, M. 1977. The calcium and vitamin D status in an elderly female population and their response to administered supplemental vitamin D_3. J. Gerontol. *32*, 659–663.

SPENCER, H. *et al.* 1983. Further studies on the effect of a high protein diet as meat on calcium metabolism. Am. J. Clin. Nutr. *37*, 924–929.

TSAI, K. S., HEATH, H., III, KUMAR, R. and RIGGS, B. L. 1984. Impaired vitamin D metabolism with aging in women. Possible role in pathogenesis of senile osteoporosis. J. Clin. Invest. *73*, 1668–1672.

YUEN, D. E., DRAPER, H. H. and TRILOK, G. 1984. Effect of dietary protein on calcium metabolism in man. Nutr. Abst. Rev., Rev. Clin. Nutr. *54*, 447–459.

ZEMEL, M. B. and LINKSWILER, H. M. 1981. Calcium metabolism in young adult males as affected by level and form of phosphorus intake and level of calcium intake. J. Nutr. *111*, 315–324.

CHAPTER 14

EFFECT OF DIETARY ZINC SUPPLEMENTATION ON IMMUNE FUNCTION IN AGING

NICOLA FABRIS, M.D., Ph.D., EUGENIO MOCCHEGIANI, Ph.D., MARIO MUZZIOLI, Ph.D. and MAURO PROVINCIALI, Ph.D.
Immunology Center
Department of Gerontology and Geriatric Research
Italian National Institute of Geriatrics (INRCA)
Ancona, Italy

INTRODUCTION

Among the more than 50 elements identified in mammalian tissues, some of them, called trace elements because they are present in minute amounts, play fundamental roles in various enzymatic and hormonal functions. Most relevant in this context are copper, iron, nickel, manganese, zinc, selenium and fluoride.

Since energy intake declines with advancing age and such a reduction is due to decreased food intake, as well as to qualitative modifications of alimentary habits, it may be expected, and it has been partially proven, that the intake of trace elements may also be reduced in the elderly. In fact, it has been shown that trace-element intake in old individuals is frequently lower than the Recommended Dietary Allowance (RDA) (Food and Nutrition Board 1980). Table 14.1 provides a general indication according to several major surveys performed in the last decade (DHEW 1979; USDA 1980; DHEW 1981).

The fact that most elderly consume trace elements in smaller quantities than the amount suggested in the RDA does not prove that their mineral intakes are inadequate to meet their needs. It simply pinpoints the fact that a large proportion of aged individuals may be at risk of consuming inadequate amounts of trace elements. This assumption has to be considered carefully because the present technology, largely

TABLE 14.1
RECOMMENDED DAILY ALLOWANCES (RDA) OR ESTIMATE SAFE AND ADEQUATE DAILY INTAKE OF SOME TRACE ELEMENTS AND ACTUAL INTAKE IN ELDERLY

Trace Elements	RDA (mg)	Daily Intake (mg)	References
Copper (RDA)	2–3	1.0–2.2	Gibson *et al.* (1983)
Zinc (RDA)	15	7.0–10	Wagner *et al.* (1983)
Manganese[1]	2.5–5.0	2.5–3.5	Gibson *et al.* (1983)
Chromium[1]	0.05–0.2	0.005–0.11	Levine *et al.* (1968)
Iron (RDA)	10	9.2–14.1	DHEW (1979)
Selenium[1]	0.05–0.2	0.05–0.2	Gibson *et al.* (1983)

[1]Estimated safe and adequate intake.

based on physicochemical determination of trace element concentration in different body fluids and tissues, does not indicate the quality of the mineral-bound proteins, their binding affinity, or the free-fraction of the mineral which may be of even greater relevance than the bound fraction. Due to these considerations, the determination of the total concentration of minerals may not reflect the real requirement. Thus, even marginal mineral deficiencies might play a relevant role in age-associated pathologies.

Since for the majority of trace elements such an analysis cannot be conducted at present, to evaluate whether a deficient mineral intake may have pathological consequences should be supported by clinical evidence. Similarly, the potentially beneficial effects of additional supplementation of trace elements should be proven on the same basis. A substantial number of investigations have been aimed in this direction during the last decade. These data offer insight into the role played by various trace elements in age-related pathologies. This presentation aims to review the relevance of trace elements for immune function and, particularly, for the immunological disorders associated with advancing age.

ROLE OF TRACE ELEMENTS IN IMMUNITY

The role of trace elements in immunological function has been achieved only recently and is still quite incomplete. Table 14.2 summarizes the major observations obtained regarding trace elements either in defective conditions or as possible toxicological agents.

Although several trace elements seem to influence immune functions, the role played by many of them is supported only by fragmentary and incomplete documentation. Thus, reduced antibody response has been reported in the course of selenium, nickel and arsenical deficiency (Chandra 1983). Interferon synthesis is also reduced

TABLE 14.2
EFFECT OF DEFICIENT AND/OR EXCESS TRACE ELEMENTS INTAKE IN DIFFERENT IMMUNOLOGICAL PARAMETERS

Trace Elements	Immunity	Cell-mediated Immunity	NK Activity
Deficiency			
Zinc	decreased	decreased	decreased
Iron	decreased	decreased	decreased
Copper	decreased	decreased	—
Selenium	decreased	decreased	—
Magnesium	decreased	normal/decreased	—
Excess			
Lithium	—	increased	—
Arsenic	decreased	normal	—
Nickel	decreased	decreased	decreased
Aluminum	decreased	decreased	—
Cobalt	decreased	—	—
Heavy metals (Pb, Ag, Au, Hg, Cd, Pt)	decreased	decreased	—

in nickel and arsenical deficiency (Chandra 1983). Lithium deficiency has been reported to increase mitogen responsiveness of lymphocytes (Chandra 1983). More convincing observations have been achieved with regard to iron, copper and zinc.

Iron

Iron may influence host resistance in several ways including direct effects on the immune system. Reductions in total lymphocytes and especially T-lymphocytes have been observed in the course of iron deficiency (Bhaskaram and Reddy 1975; Chandra and Saraya 1975). Also, the serum level of immunoglobulins has been found to be reduced in experimental animals (Nadler *et al.* 1972). In some cases, the impaired antibody production is not affected by iron availability directly, but it may be caused by concurrent infections (Chandra and Saraya 1975). Iron is, in fact, an essential nutrient for microbes, their ability to establish an infection being dependent on iron availability (Beisel 1982).

Conflicting data have been reported on cell-mediated immunity in iron deficiency, as either impaired or unaffected (Kulapongs *et al.* 1974; Suskind *et al.* 1977; Baliga *et al.* 1981; Bhaskaram and Reddy 1975; Joynson *et al.* 1972). Abnormalities in phagocitic cells related to iron deficiency have also been reported (Beard and Weintraub 1969).

Copper

Different immunological abnormalities have been reported in the course of copper deficiency. Congenital copper deficiency, such as in Menkes Syndrome (Solomons 1985), causes increased frequency and gravity of infectious diseases in the respiratory tract. Reduced antibody responses and decreased proliferative reactions to concanavalin A have also been reported to occur in copper-deficient individuals. Mitogen responsiveness to phytohemagglutinin does not seem, on the contrary, to be affected by copper deficiency.

Zinc

The involvement of zinc in immunocompetence in man and other animals is probably the best known at present. Zinc deficiency in laboratory animals causes thymic and lymphnode atrophy and impaired cell-mediated cutaneous hypersensitivity reactions. Lymphocytes isolated from zinc-deficient animals show impaired response to phytohemagglutinin (PHA) and depression of T-cell dependent antibody production. Furthermore, a zinc-deficient diet in experimental animals causes impaired T-helper and T-suppressor function, decreased T-killer and natural killer activity (Iwata 1979) (Table 14.3). Assessment of zinc involvement in development and function of different lymphoid cell populations indicates that this element has an effect predominantly on T-lymphocytes (Iwata 1979).

In humans the effect of zinc deficiency on immune function has been studied in congenital diseases such as acrodermatitis enteropathica, sickle cell anemia (Prasad 1985) and Down's syndrome (Fabris *et al.* 1984) and in conditions characterized by acquired altered zinc turnover, such as uremia (Travaglini *et al.* 1989) or during total parenteral nutrition. Depending on the severity and duration, zinc deficiency produces hypoplasia of the thymus, spleen, lymphnodes and Peyer's paches (McClain 1985). Alterations in lymphocyte population, including reduced helper-T lymphocyte function, reduced natural killer activity, decreased number of total T-lymphocytes with increased B-lymphocytes, are a common and constant aspect in zinc-deficiency diseases (Chandra 1985; Allen *et al.* 1981).

The mechanism by which zinc may affect the immune system is certainly multifaceted, due to the widespread action of zinc on different enzymes and hormones involved in various physiological steps of immune development and response. A direct effect of zinc on immune cells is supported by the evidence that zinc is a potent *in vitro* T-lymphocyte mitogen for both man and animals over a narrow range of concentrations (Fraker *et al.* 1977) and that zinc is required for the nucleoside phosphorylase, a purine enzyme which is required also by T-cell for its functioning (Underwood 1977).

In addition to a direct effect on lymphoid cells, zinc may influence the immune system through its action on the biological activity of thymulin. With regard to thymulin, it has been demonstrated that zinc is bound to the peptide in an equimolar ratio and that biological activity resides in the zinc-bound form (Dardenne *et al.*

TABLE 14.3
IMMUNOLOGICAL CONSEQUENCES OF ZINC DEPRIVATION

Hystology	Thymic atrophy
	Structural abnormalities of T-dependent areas
Thymus function	Reduced thymic hormone production
	Reduced peripheral activation of thymulin (Zn-FTS)
	Reduced proliferation and differentiation of T-lymphocytes
T-cell function	Impaired T-helper activity
	Impaired T-suppressor activity
	Reduced mitogen responsiveness
	Reduced T-killer activity
	Depressed Ab response to T-dependent antigens
B-cell function	Normal response to B-dependent antigens
NK functions	Decreased NK activity

1982); whereas, the zinc-unbound peptide is able to bind to target sites, but it is inactive and likely prevents the active form to exert its action (Fig. 14.1) (Fabris *et al.* 1984). The presence of inactive hormone molecules in biological fluids may be revealed by measuring their capacity to inhibit known amounts of synthetic active thymulin (Fabris *et al.* 1984; Bach and Beaurain 1979), and indirectly by measuring thymulin activity in biological samples before and after *in vitro* addition of zinc ions, which may unmask the presence of inactive hormone (Fabris *et al.* 1986).

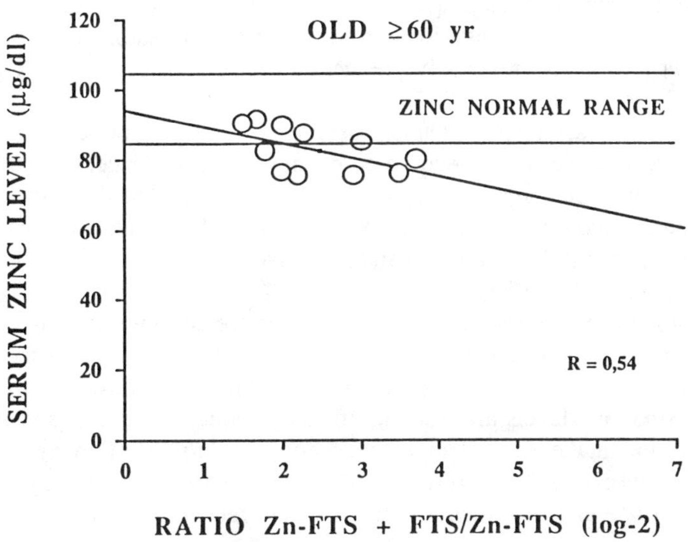

FIG. 14.1. ROLE OF HORMONES AND ZINC ON THYMULIN PRODUCTION AND ACTIVATION

It has been in fact demonstrated that in conditions characterized by more or less deep zinc deficiencies, such as those associated with physiological aging (Fabris *et al.* 1984), with congenital diseases such as acrodermatitis enteropathica, cystic fibrosis, Down's syndrome (Fabris *et al.* 1984) and Duchenne syndromes (Fabris *et al.* 1988b), or with infectious disease such as AIDS (Fabris *et al.* 1988a), a reduction of the circulating level of active thymulin is observed with a concomitant appearance of inactive zinc-unbound FTS molecules (Table 14.4). The *in vitro* addition to plasma samples of zinc ions is able to unmask inactive circulating FTS molecules, showing that the total amount of the thymic hormone (zinc bound + zinc unbound FTS) is frequently much higher than the active fraction in all the above reported zinc marginal deficiencies.

ZINC AND AGING

The possibility that trace elements may play a role in physiological aging processes had been originally hypothesized following the observation that with advancing age, at least in humans, alimentary habits consistently vary and defective intake of various micronutrients is almost unavoidable. With regard to zinc intake and turnover in old individuals, information is still incomplete. According to one of the major surveys performed by the USDA, zinc intake appears to be reduced in old age (USDA 1980). Plasma level of zinc was reduced; however, no definite information is available on intracellular zinc content. Nevertheless, it has been shown that zinc absorbtion is also reduced with advancing age. Also, zinc losses through urine and feces are reduced. This phenomenon has been considered as compensatory in nature, though not sufficient to prevent progressive reduction of zinc plasma levels (Turnlund *et al.* 1986) (Table 14.5).

The relevance of such age-dependent declines in plasma zinc levels is presently unknown. It does not seem, however, a pure temporal coincidence, particularly since some of the known zinc-dependent functions (such as wound healing, skin-cell turnover, taste acuity and immune efficiency) are all found depressed in older individuals and the age-dependent deterioration can be reversed in some instances, by zinc supplementation (Chandra 1985).

The hypothesis that alterations of zinc turnover are common findings in old age requires confirmation in species other than humans. In this context, very little data are available. Recent findings from our laboratory have demonstrated that in mice and rats plasma zinc levels are also significantly reduced with age and in spite of the fact that food intake is not changed when compared to that of young individuals. These observations would suggest that alterations in zinc turnover are a common finding in old age and that such a defect may be relevant for various age-related processes.

TABLE 14.4
ZINC SERUM LEVEL AND PLASMA LEVEL OF ACTIVE (Zn-FTS), INACTIVE (FTS) AND TOTAL THYMULIN (Zn-FTS + FTS) IN VARIOUS HUMAN PATHOLOGIES

Group	Zinc[1] (μg/dL)	Active Zn-FTS[2] (Log-2)	Inactive FTS[3] (pg/mL)	Total FTS[4] (Log-2)
Normal	113±2.4	5.3±0.4	0.3±0.1	5.8±0.5
Acrodermatitis enteropathica	58±1.3	1.4±0.3	65±4.3	5.4±0.4
Cystic Fibrosis	71±3.0	1.7±0.3	64±3.2	4.7±0.5
Down	86±3.9	1.0±0.2	45±4.6	4.8±0.4
Duchenne	67±9.4	1.2±0.2	40±3.5	3.5±0.5
AIDS	57±5.0	1.0±0.3	not done	5.7±0.4

[1]Measured by atomic absorption spectroscopy.
[2]Measured by conventional rosette inhibition assay (Bach *et al.* 1972).
[3]Measured by inhibitory activity on synthetic thymulin (Bach and Beaurain 1979).
[4]Measured by modified rosette inhibition assay (Fabris *et al.* 1986).

TABLE 14.5
ZINC TURNOVER IN YOUNG AND OLD HUMANS AND RATE OF ABSORPTION OF ZN^{67} AFTER SINGLE ADMINISTRATION

	Young	Old
Serum Zn (μg/dL)	105±4	78±3
Urinary Zn (mg/d)	0.92±0.11	0.67±0.13
Fecal Zn (mg/d)	15.3±0.7	14.2±0.9
% Zn^{67} Absorption[1]	29.9±3.4	17.3±4.1

[1]Rate of absorption of Zn^{67}, orally administered (mg10/day) evaluated 12 weeks later (redrawn from Turnlund *et al.* 1986).

EFFECT OF ZINC SUPPLEMENTATION IN OLD MICE

The observation of age-associated alterations in zinc turnover together with the knowledge of its involvement in immune efficiency has lead to investigations of the potential of zinc supplementation on the age-related decline of immune functions. Rodent experiments using dietary zinc supplemetation over the whole life span have demonstrated that many of the observed age-related immune modifications, including decreased thymic hormone production, reduced T-helper and T-suppressor activity and depressed NK cytotoxicity could be prevented by such treatments (Iwata *et al.* 1979).

Furthermore, when this regimen was given to autoimmune-susceptible NZB mice, the zinc supplementation was able to delay the time of appearance of autoaggressive reactions (Beach *et al.* 1981). These findings have been interpreted in the light of a possible prevention of age-related alterations. A major question suggested by these data has been whether age-related immune deterioration could be corrected, even after the immune alterations had occurred.

Trials performed in aged humans have shown that, in fact, zinc supplementation might be able to increase the cutaneous sensitivity to various antigens and the antibody response to tetanus toxoid (Ducheateu *et al.* 1981), and to improve thymic endocrine activity (Chandra 1990). Recent experiments from our laboratory have attempted to elucidate the mechanism of such an action. It has been demonstrated that oral zinc supplementation, even when applied to aged mice, is able to induce a regrowth of the thymus (Fig. 14.2) concomitant with increased thymic hormone production and an augmented percentage of thymulin-producing cells. In addition, complete recovery of the reduced number of Thy 1.2+ cells in the spleen and partial reconstitution of PHA response and NK cytotoxic activity of spleen cells was observed (Fabris *et al.* 1990).

The increased thymulin plasma level depends not only on the peripheral reactivation of zinc-unbound FTS, but on a central effect on the rate of production of thymic hormones. In fact, after oral zinc supplementation the total thymulin (Zn-FTS + FTS) increased over the values observed in age-matched controls.

Administration of zinc salts *in vitro* to spleen cells from old mice was unable to recover peripheral immune efficiency, whereas zinc-bound thymulin did. This last observation suggests that one of the major effects of zinc supplementation in old age is to recover thymic endocrine activity. This restoration appears to be responsible for the recovery of peripheral immune efficiency.

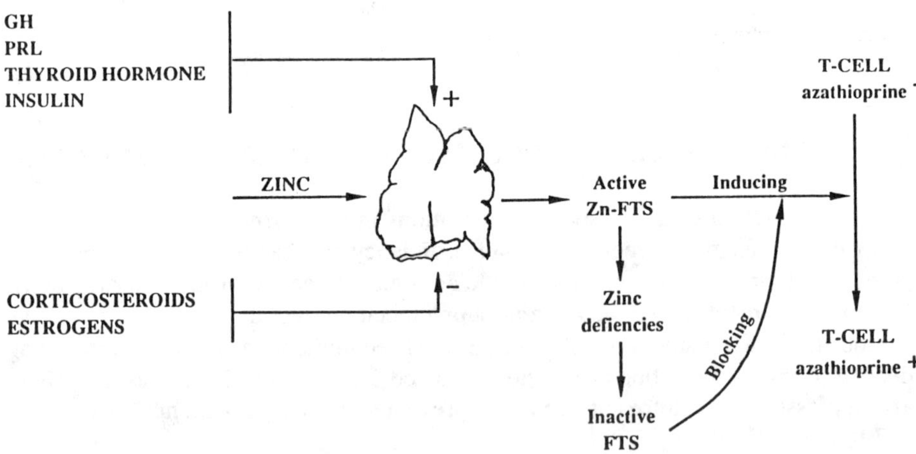

FIG. 14.2. CORRELATION BETWEEN SERUM ZINC LEVEL AND RATIO TOTAL (Zn-FTS + FTS)/ACTIVE (Zn-FTS) FRACTION OF THYMIC HORMONE IN ELDERLY SUBJECTS

That zinc supplementation may improve thymic endocrine activity has been recently supported by observations in old uremic patients treated with oral zinc for six months. In these conditions, patients showed, after only two weeks of treatment, an increase in the circulating level of thymulin which reached young-like values by the fourth week of treatment (Travaglini *et al.* 1988). Regarding the mechanism(s) by which zinc can exert its action on the thymus, the data available cannot yield substantial information. Due to the widespread action of zinc ions, it can be hypothesized that zinc supplementation may reactivate the enzyme cascade necessary for thymic peptide synthesis (Prasad 1982) or that it may correct the turnover of some hormones such as GH, TSH and thyroid hormones (Prasad 1985) which are of great relevance for optimal thymus function (Fabris and Mocchegiani 1985). Preliminary data from our laboratory have shown that zinc supplementation in old mice recovers the abnormally low serum level of triiodothyronine, a hormone which can directly modulate thymic peptide synthesis by the thymic epithelial cells (Mocchegiani and Fabris 1990a).

IMMUNOLOGICAL SIGNIFICANCE OF MARGINAL ZINC DEFICIENCY

According to the data presented here, there are two positions which may be taken concerning zinc. On one hand, zinc depletion seems to be present at older ages; however, the extent of zinc deficiency is relatively modest, and it is therefore difficult to accept the assumption that such a modest deficiency may cause the observed major defects in immune function. On the other hand, the demonstration of a recovery of various immune functions in old age, and in particular that of the thymus involution, through an oral supplementation with zinc at RDA physiological doses, supports the idea that even such a modest zinc supplementation is enough to exert an active and positive action on age-related immune disfunction.

It is difficult at present to reconcile these two points. However, it is to be noted that a quite similar picture with regard to marginal zinc deficiency and major immune defects have also been observed in physiological aging as well as in congenital diseases, such as Down's (Fabris *et al.* 1984), Duchenne (Fabris *et al.* 1988b), cystic fibrosis (Fabris *et al.* 1988b) syndromes, in infectious diseases, such as AIDS and AIDS related syndromes (Fabris *et al.* 1988a), and in neoplastic diseases, such as leukemia and solid tumors (Lightman *et al.* 1986; Ebadi and Swanson 1988). A possible explanation of this discrepancy might be suggested by consideration of the data presented in Fig. 14.2. If serum zinc level is plotted against the ratio of active/inactive plasma thymic hormone, i.e., zinc-bound/zinc-unbound thymic hormone, in blood samples from aged individuals, it appears that the ratio is markedly reduced in spite of the modest zinc deficiency. Furthermore, although the regression line is statistically significant, the majority of the points, as far as zinc level is concerned, fall within the range of normality. If the range of normality is taken as that usually considered in clinical laboratories, all the data fall in the normal range.

These patterns may be interpreted in light of these facts: (1) zinc is sequestered by various pools of proteins with different binding affinities for zinc (Gastinel *et al.* 1984). (2) it is the bioavailable pool of zinc, which cannot be determined with the actual technology employed, that plays the major role in activating low affinity proteins such as may occur for thymic hormone. This interpretation is further supported by the observation that in a serum-free system, zinc-deprived thymulin may be biologically activated by as low as 200 nM zinc concentration which is 1/100 of the concentration recorded in biological fluids.

CONCLUSIONS

The data presented here stress the following points:

(1) The age-related involution of the thymus does not appear to be due to intrinsic failure of the organ but to a functional alteration, likely related to age-associated modifications of microenvironmental factors which are important for optimum immune function, such as neuroendocrine factors and trace elements bioavailability.

(2) Among various nutritional factors zinc plays an important role in the maintenance of thymic efficiency. Age-associated marginal zinc deficiency is responsible for the low thymic endocrine activity. Zinc supplementation, at physiological doses, can completely restore impaired thymic function even when administered in old age, as well as various pheripheral immune functions. Thus zinc dietary supplementation represents an interesting physiological approach to immunological potentiation among the elderly.

(3) The determination of plasma zinc levels through atomic absorbtion spectroscopy or by means of chemical analysis does not offer a clear-cut picture of the quota of bioavailable element. The determination of zinc-bound active thymic hormone versus zinc-unbound fraction may be a much more suitable test to identify biologically significant marginal zinc deficiencies.

ACKNOWLEDGMENTS

This work was supported in part through the Italian National Research Council, Grant No. 86.01763.04 to Dr. Fabris and through the Italian Health Ministry INRCA-targeted program on Nutrition in Elderly. We thank Mr. Marzio Marcellini and Mrs. Clara Chesi for their excellent technical assistance.

REFERENCES

ALLEN, J. I., KAY, E. N. and McCLAIN, C. S. 1981. Severe zinc deficiency in humans. Association with a reversible T-lymphocyte dysfunction. Ann. Int. Med. *95*, 154–157.

BACH, J. F. and BEAURAIN, G. 1979. Respective influence of extrinsic and intrinsic factors on the age-related decrease of thymic secretion. J. Immunol. *122*, 2505–2507.

BACH, J. F. *et al.* 1972. Evidence for a serum thymic factor produced by the human thymus. Lancet *2*, 1056–1058.

BALIGA, B. S., KUVIVIDILA, S. and SUSKIND, R. M. 1981. The cytotoxic capacity of spleen and peritoneal cells from iron-deficient animal. Fed. Proc. Fed. Am. Soc. Exp. Biol. *40*, 918–925.

BEACH, R. S., GERSHWIN, M. E. and HURLEY, L. S. 1981. Nutritional factors and autoimmunity. 1. Immunopathology of zinc deprivation in New Zealand mice. J. Immunol. *126*, 1999–2006.

BEARD, M. E. J. and WEINTRAUB, L. R. 1969. Hypersegmented neutrophilic granulocytes in iron deficiency anaemia. Br. J. Haematol. *16*, 161–166.

BEISEL, W. R. 1982. Single nutrients and immunity. Am. J. Clin. Nutr. *35*, 417–424.

BHASKARAM, C. and REDDY, V. 1975. Cell-mediated immunity in iron- and vitamin-deficient children. Br. Med. J. *3*, 522–526.

CHANDRA, R. K. 1983. Trace elements and immune response. Immunol. Today *4*, 322–325.

CHANDRA, R. K. 1985. Trace element regulation of immunity and infection. J. Am. College Nutr. *4*, 5–16.

CHANDRA, R. K. 1990. Nutrition as a major determinant of immunocompetence in old age. *In* Biological Advances in Aging, A. L. Goldstein (ed.). Plenum Publishing Corp., New York.

CHANDRA, R. K. and SARAYA, A. K. 1975. Impaired immunocompetence associated with iron deficiency. J. Pediatr. *86*, 899–905.

DARDENNE, M. *et al.* 1982. Contribution of zinc and other metals to the biological activity of the serum thymic factor. Proc. Natl. Acad. Sci. USA *79*, 5370–5373.

DHEW. 1979. Dietary Intake Source Data. Health and Nutrition Examination Survey, United States, 1971–1974. DHEW Publ. No. (PHS) 1979, 79–1221. Dept. Health, Education and Welfare, U.S. Govt. Printing Office, Washington, D.C.

DHEW 1981. Health and Nutrition Examination Survey II. USPHS Division of Health Statistics, U.S. Govt. Printing Office, Washington, D.C.

DUCHEATEU, J., DELESPESSE, G., VRIJEN, R. and COOLET, H. 1981. Beneficial effects of oral zinc supplementation on the immune response of old people. Am. J. Med. *70*, 1001–1004.

EBADI, M. and SWANSON, S. 1988. The status of zinc, copper, and metallothionein in cancer patients. *In* Nutrition, Growth, and Cancer, Alan R. Liss, New York.

FABRIS, M. *et al.* 1984. Thymic hormone deficiency in normal aging and Down's syndrome: Is there a primary failure of the thymus? Lancet *1*, 983–986.

FABRIS, N. *et al.* 1986. Thyroid function modulates thymus endocrine activity. J. Clin. Endocrinol. Metab. *62*, 474–478.

FABRIS, N. *et al.*. 1988a. AIDS, zinc deficiency, and thymic hormone failure. JAMA *259* (6), 839–840.

FABRIS, N., MOCCHEGIANI, E. and PALLONI, R. 1988b. Zinc-dependent failure of thymic hormone in human pathologies, *In* Trace Elements in Man and Animals. L. S. Hurtley (ed.). Plenum Publishing Corp., New York.

FABRIS, N. and MOCCHEGIANI, E. 1985. Endocrine control of thymic serum factor production in young-adult and old mice. Cell Immunol. *91*, 325–385.

FABRIS, N., MOCCHEGIANI, E., MUZZIOLI, M. and PROVINCIALI, M. 1990. Zinc, immunity and aging. *In* Biochemical Advances in Aging. A. L. Goldstein (ed.). Plenum Publishing Corp., New York (In press).

Food and Nutrition Board. 1980. Recommended Dietary Allowances, 9th Ed. National Academy of Sciences, Washington, D.C.

FRAKER, P. J., HAAS, S. and LUECKE, R. W. 1977. Effect of zinc deficiency on the immune response of the young adult A/Jax mouse. J. Nutr. *107*, 1889–1895.

GASTINEL, L. N., DARDENNE, M., PLEAU. J. M. and BACH, J. F. 1984. Studies on the zinc binding site to the serum thymic factor. Biochem. Biophys. Acta *797*, 147–155.

GIBSON, R. A., ANDERSON, B. M., and SABRY, J. H. 1983. The trace metal status of a group of post-menopausal vegetarians. J. Am. Dietet. Assoc. *82*, 246–251.

IWATA, T. *et al.* 1979. Circulating thymic hormone levels in zinc deficiency. Cell. Immunol. *47*, 100–105.

JOYNSON, D. H. M., JACOBS, A., MURRAY, W. D. and DOLBY, A. E. 1972. Defect of cell-mediated immunity in patients with iron-deficiency anaemia. Lancet *2*, 1058–1062.

KULAPONGS, P., VITHAYASAI, V., SUSKIND, R. and OLSON, R. E. 1974. Cell-mediated immunity and phagocytosis and killing function in children with severe iron-deficiency anaemia. Lancet *2*, 689–694.

LEVINE, R. A., STREETEN, D. H. P. and DOISY, R. J. 1968. Effects of oral chromium supplementation on the glucose tolerance of elderly human subjects. Metabolism *17*, 114–120.

LIGHTMAN, *et al.* 1986. Use of the serum copper/zinc ratio in the differential diagnosis of ovarian malignancy. Clin. Chem. *32* (1), 101–103.

McCLAIN, C. S. 1985. Zinc metabolism in malabsorption syndromes. J. Am. Coll. Nutr. *4*, 49–64.

MOCCHEGIANI, E. and FABRIS, N. 1990a. Neuroendocrine-thymus interactions. I. *In vitro* modulation of thymic factor secretion by thyroid hormones. J. Endocrinol. Invest. *13*, 139–147.

MOCCHEGIANI, E., PAOLUCCI, P. and FABRIS, N. 1990b. Zinc deficiency and low thymic hormone activity in young cancer patients. Abst. Cong. Int. ISNIM, Florence, Italy, May 1990, p. 23–26.

NADLER, B. N., MAHONEY, A. W., RAMAKRISHNAN, R. and HENDRICKS, D. G. 1972. Sensitivity of the immunological response to the nutritional status of rats. J. Nutr. *102*, 535–545.

PRASAD, A. S. 1982. History of zinc in human nutrition in clinical applications of recent advances in zinc metabolism. Alan R. Liss, New York.

PRASAD, A. S. 1985. Clinical, endocrinological and biochemical effects of zinc-deficiency. Clin. Endocrinol. Metab. *14* (3), 567–589.

SOLOMONS, N. W. 1985. Biochemical, metabolic, and clinical role of copper in human nutrition. J. Am. Coll. Nutr. *4*, 83–105.

SUSKIND, R. M., KULAPONGS, P., VITHAYASAI, C. and OLSON, R. E. 1977. Iron deficiency anaemia and the immune response. *In* Malnutrition and the Immune Response. R. M. Suskind (ed.). Raven Press, New York.

TRAVAGLINI, P. *et al.* 1989. Effect of oral zinc administration on prolactin and thymulin circulating levels in uremic patients. J. Clin. Endocrinol. Metab. *68* (1), 186–190.

TURNLUND, J. R., DURVIN, N., COSTA, F. and MARGEN, S. 1986. Stable isotope studies of zinc absorption and retention in young and elderly men. J. Nutr. *116* (7), 1239–1247.

UNDERWOOD, E. J. 1977. Trace Elements in Human and Animal Nutrition, 4th Ed. Academic Press, New York.

USDA. 1980. Science and Education Administration, Food and Nutrient Intakes of Individuals in One Day in the United States, Spring 1977. Prelim. Rep. No. 2. U.S. Department of Agriculture, Washington, DC.

WAGER, P. A. *et al.* 1983. Zinc nutriture and cell mediated immunity in the aged. Int. J. Vitam. Nutr. Res. *53*, 94–101.

CHAPTER 15

NUTRITION AND THE AGING HEMATOLOGICAL SYSTEM

DAVID A. LIPSCHITZ, M.D., Ph.D.
Geriatric Research, Education and Clinical Center
John L. McClellan Memorial Veterans Hospital
and
Division on Aging
University of Arkansas for Medical Sciences
Little Rock, Arkansas

INTRODUCTION

The aging process is characterized by a diminished reserve capacity. Thus while function may be normal in the basal state, response to maximal stimulation is frequently compromised. A classic example is the diminished ability of elderly humans to clear an intravenous glucose load. This review will present evidence that the aging hematopoietic system has a decreased reserve capacity. This reduction results in pathologic abnormalities with relatively minor stress that would be unlikely to cause problems in the young. In this regard we believe that subtle alterations in nutritional status may play a critical role in hematopoietic alterations that are erroneously attributed to the aging process.

THE AGING HEMATOPOIETIC SYSTEM

A finite replicative capacity of normal cells is one of the major theories of cellular aging (Hayflick 1965). When this replicative capacity has been reached, the cell's ability to divide is lost and death occurs. The evidence that the pluripotential hematopoietic stem cell has a limited self-renewal capacity is controversial. Results from *in vivo* serial transplantation studies suggest a limited life span and proliferative capacity of these cells (Ogden and Micklem 1974). However, there is evidence that the pluripotent stem cell compartment can maintain hematopoiesis for a period that far exceeds the maximum life expectancy of the animal being studied (Harrison 1975b). Further support for a finite replicative capacity for pluripotent stem cells comes from studies employing long-term bone marrow cultures. These studies have demonstrated an inverse correlation between hematopoietic cell production and the age of the donor from which the long-term bone marrow culture was initiated (Lipschitz *et al.* 1983; Mauch *et al.* 1982).

Of particular relevance to this review is the fact that many variables affect hematopoietic function. Thus, the interpretation of the effect of age on hematopoiesis is made difficult by the fact that even healthy elderly persons frequently have co-existing diseases or nutritional deficiencies or have been exposed to drugs and toxicants that have profound effects on the bone marrow. Because of this fact, information obtained from the studies of animal models is important. Numerous reports have shown anemia to be universal in the aged mouse. A closer evaluation of hematopoiesis in this animal model, however, demonstrates that the anemia primarily reflects an expansion of plasma volume, as red cell mass is unchanged with aging (Boggs 1983; Williams *et al.* 1986). A careful evaluation of the effect of age on hematopoiesis in the mouse has failed to demonstrate any age-related alteration in the number of formed elements in the peripheral blood, or in the number of differentiated precursors in the marrow of these animals. Furthermore, measurement of the committed myeloid progenitor cell (colony-forming unit-culture, [CFU-C]) or erythroid progenitor cells (burst-forming unit-erythroid [BFU-E] or colony-forming unit-erythroid [CFU-E]) have shown no age-related reduction as healthy aged animals approach their maximum life expectancy. Evaluation of the kinetics of erythropoiesis have demonstrated that plasma iron turnover and erythron iron turnover are unchanged with aging, and red cell survival is not altered. It is apparent from the study of animal models that minimal if any change in basal hematopoiesis occurs with aging.

There is, however, good evidence that hematopoietic reserve capacity is compromised. The rate of return of hematocrit values to normal following phlebotomy is decreased in aged mice (Harrison 1975a), and *in vivo* and *in vitro* studies have shown that the erythropoietic cells from animals respond less well to increased stimulation than do erythroid cells from young animals (Udupa and Lipschitz 1974). Similarly, a compromise in granulocyte production following increased stimulation has been demonstrated in the aged mouse (Rothstein *et al.* 1987).

Biologically, the effect of age on hematopoiesis in man should be similar to that found in animals. Thus, basal hematopoiesis should be unchanged with aging. There is good evidence that a reduction in cellularity of the bone marrow occurs in the elderly, but the functional significance of this observation is unknown (Hartsock *et al.* 1965). Although a reduction in hematocrit is common even in healthy elderly subjects, the cause is usually not obvious. Thus, in a survey of very carefully selected healthy elderly subjects living in the Little Rock, Arkansas, area we found a high prevalence of modest reductions in hematocrit (Lipschitz *et al.* 1981). However, a careful evaluation to reveal the cause showed that iron deficiency, the anemia of chronic disease, folate deficiency, hemolysis, and other, rarer causes of anemia were uncommon. The elderly males and females with this unexplained anemia had significantly lower leukocyte and neutrophil counts than nonanemic subjects suggesting mild failure of the marrow. In a further study careful assessment of hematopoiesis in these individuals revealed significant decreases in differentiated bone marrow hematopoietic cells of the myeloid, erythroid, and megakaryocytic lines (Lipschitz *et al.* 1984). When the committed hematopoietic progenitor cells were measured, a significant reduction in the myeloid (CFU-C) and late erythroid (CFU-E) precursors was found. In contrast, the most primitive hematopoietic precursors that were measured, namely the BFU-E, were not decreased. This finding suggests that rather than an absolute decrease in stem cell numbers, an abnormality in cellular proliferation existed in elderly subjects with anemia. A major unanswered question is whether these alterations result from the aging process or some other related abnormalities. Since aging does not by itself alter basal hematopoiesis, suspicion is increased that the unexplained anemia we describe is not exclusively due to aging. As will be discussed below, nutritional factors may well exert an influence on these age-related changes in hematopoietic function.

PREVALENCE OF ANEMIA

A series of epidemiologic studies from the United States, Canada and Europe (Hill 1967; McLennan *et al.* 1973; Myers *et al.* 1968; Information Canada 1973; Parson *et al.* 1965), demonstrated a high prevalence of anemia in the elderly. In women older than age 59, anemia occurs as frequently as that noted in women of child bearing age. In men a definite increase in the prevalence of anemia is found in older age groups. Studies from Great Britain are important since they have determined the incidence of anemia in large number of subjects older than 60 years. In both men and women, the prevalence of anemia increased significantly with each successive age decade. A recent analysis of the second National Health and Nutrition Education Survey (NHANES II) demonstrated a significant reduction in hemoglobin levels with advancing age in apparently healthy males and a minimal, statistically significant decrease in elderly females (Yip *et al.* 1984). Based upon a lower normal limit of 14 g/dL, a very large percentage of elderly males would be found to be anemic. This study proposed that the reduction for males was a consequence of aging and suggested that age-specific reference standards for hemoglobin concentration for the elderly be adopted.

A major unanswered question is whether or not this decline in hemoglobin with advancing age is a consequence of the normal aging process or reflects some yet to be defined abnormality. Of particular importance in this regard is the recent finding that anemia is extremely rare in an affluent, healthy elderly population examined in New Mexico (Garry *et al.* 1983). None of the elderly males and females in this group were anemic. Furthermore, longitudinal monitoring of these subjects over a five year period failed to demonstrate an increased prevalence of anemia. Based upon this observation it seems highly likely that the decrease in hemoglobin seen commonly with advancing age is not a consequence of the normal aging process and is related to some extrinsic variable that remains to be determined.

Recent studies have implicated inflammation or chronic disease as the likely etiology of the anemia (Dallman *et al.* 1984). A second possibility is that the anemia has a nutritional basis. This is suggested by a closer examination of data obtained in epidemiologic surveys in which anemia has been shown to be most prevalent in low socioeconomic populations. This population also has a high prevalence of other nutritional deficiencies. We have performed a comprehensive nutritional and hematologic evaluation on a group of 73 elderly veterans living in a domiciliary facility. A high prevalence of anemia was present in this population. A close evaluation demonstrated that iron deficiency, folate deficiency, or other usually described causes of anemia were rare. We then performed a multivariate analysis of the data using age, hematopoietic and nutritional factors as covariants. We demonstrated that while age appeared to be the major variable accounting for the decline in immunologic measurements observed in this elderly population, age did not appear to be an important factor in the prevalence of anemia. In contrast, serum albumin, transferrin and prealbumin, which assess nutritional status, appeared to be excellent predictors of anemia. This information provides indirect evidence that a nutritional variable may contribute to the anemia seen in these elderly populations.

THE EFFECT OF GROUP HOUSING ON HEMATOPOIESIS IN THE AGED MOUSE

The most universal finding of anemia prevalence in population studies is its relationship to poverty. The poorer the population group, the higher the prevalence of anemia; the abnormality becomes most apparent in the elderly. It is this population group that also has a high incidence of nutritional deficiencies. It is highly likely that the major hematopoietic change with age is a diminished reserve capacity and an increased susceptibility to stress resulting in pathology not observed in the young. The study of the effect of group housing on hematopoiesis in the aged mice provides a good example of the fragility of the hematopoietic system in mice approaching their maximum life expectancy (Williams *et al.* 1986).

The median life span of C57BL/6 mice is 24 months, but the maximum reported life expectancy is 48 months. Provided 42-month-old mice are housed in individual cages (one animal per cage), no change in hematopoiesis is seen. If, however, they are housed in groups of 5 animals per cage, a significant alteration of bone marrow function occurs (Table 15.1). The animals become more anemic and the number of progenitor cells in their bone marrow decreases. Significant decreases also occur in the morphologically recognizable erythroid precursors. These findings are identical to hematopoietic changes described with overcrowding. The effects of overcrowding, however, are only seen when young, or even 24-month-old animals are

TABLE 15.1
HEMATOLOGIC PARAMETERS IN YOUNG (6-MONTH) AND OLD (42-MONTH) MICE CAGED IN SINGLE OR GROUP HOUSING

	Single Housed				Group Housed			
Parameter	Young (n)[1]		Old (n)[2]		Young (n)[1]		Old (n)[2]	
Body weight (g)	28.4 ± 0.3*	(27)	33.1 ± 0.3	(10)	27.7 ± 1.0	(12)	32.9 ± 0.6	(14)
Hematocrit (%)	49.4 ± 0.4	(23)	46.1 ± 0.7	(10)	50.0 ± 0.5	(12)	4.9 ± 0.7***	(14)
WBC (μL)	8710 ± 689	(23)	10,679 ± 1003	(10)	9915 ± 1003	(12)	9850 ± 774	(18)
Marrow cells/kg (× 10^9)	23.9 ± 1.4	(20)	24.2 ± 1.6	(10)	22.7 ± 0.8	(12)	19.8 ± 0.9**	(20)
Myeloid, total/kg (× 10^9)	12.2 ± 0.6	(23)	12.6 ± 0.9	(10)	11.9 ± 0.7	(12)	12.1 ± 0.7	(20)
Myeloid, mitotic/kg (× 10^9)	8.2 ± 0.3	(23)	8.6 ± 0.6	(10)	8.0 ± 0.4	(12)	9.2 ± 0.5	(20)
Erythroid, total/kg (× 10^9)	7.6 ± 0.5	(23)	6.5 ± 0.6	(10)	7.1 ± 0.3	(12)	4.7 ± .0.3**	(20)
BFU-E/kg (× 10^6)	5.5 ± 0.5	(23)	4.9 ± 0.4	(10)	4.8 ± 0.4	(10)	3.4 ± 0.2**	(13)
CFU-E/kg (× 10^6)	131 ± 10	(26)	139 ± 8	(10)	112 ± 8	(12)	61 ± 2**	(14)
CFU-C/kg (× 10^6)	48.1 ± 3.0	(23)	46.1 ± 2.9	(10)	42.0 ± 3.1	(10)	24.2 ± 1.1**	(13)

Source: Adapted from Williams *et al.* (1986).
[1]Results combined from 5 separate studies.
[2]Results combined from 3 separate studies.
*Mean ± SEM.
**Group-housed very old significantly lower than single-housed very old or young animals ($P < 0.01$).
***Group-housed very old significantly lower than single-housed very old or young animals ($P < 0.02$).

housed in groups of 10 mice per cage. This finding indicates that a minor stress, which does not effect hematopoiesis in young animals, causes significant abnormalities in aged animals.

The mechanism accounting for these age-related changes are unknown. Possibilities include minor infection, increased activity when strange animals are housed in groups or increased competition for nutrients. The overcrowding animal model has many similarities to the environmental variables likely to exist in low socioeconomic population groups. If the etiology is nutritional the mechanism is clearly more complex than those currently proposed for nutritional anemia in the young.

PROTEIN CALORIE MALNUTRITION IN THE ELDERLY

Further evidence suggesting that a nutritional factor may contribute to the anemia seen in older persons comes from the observation that there is a marked similarity between the alterations in immunologic and hematopoietic function that occur with aging and those that occur with protein deprivation (Table 15.2). A high incidence of protein energy malnutrition has been demonstrated in hospitalized subjects and in the elderly with a wide array of medical disorders. This raises the possibility that protein deprivation in some form may contribute to alterations in host defense normally ascribed to aging. To examine this possibility, we have recently performed an evaluation of immune and hematopoietic status in hospitalized elderly subjects with protein energy malnutrition (Lipschitz and Mitchell 1982). We confirmed previous reports that nutritional rehabilitation can improve delayed cutaneous hypersensitivity and increase the lymphocyte count. A close evaluation of the hematopoietic system also revealed dramatic improvements following correction of the nutritional deficits. A highly significant increase in hemoglobin values occurred that was accompanied by elevations in serum iron levels and in the total iron-binding capacity. Simultaneously the serum ferritin fell, presumably owing to a redistribution of iron from stores to circulating red cells. In selected individuals we demonstrated that correction of nutritional deficiencies results in significant increases in the number of bone-marrow differentiated cells, as well as marked increases in bone marrow stem cell numbers (Lipschitz and Mitchell 1982). The improved immune and hematopoietic function following rehabilitation in the elderly supports the possibility that nutritional factors contribute to age-related changes in these organ systems.

The interpretation of improved immune and hematopoietic status in malnourished aged subjects, however, is extremely difficult. Any hospitalized elderly individual has coexisting diseases (including infection, dehydration, and psychoneurological changes) that markedly affect immune and hematopoietic function. Thus, the overall improvement seen with nutritional rehabilitation may reflect an overall improvement in the health status of the patient. To evaluate this possibility more closely, we next examined the effect of increased feeding on the immune and hematopoietic status of elderly persons who lived at home and were ambulatory, but were

TABLE 15.2
SIMILARITIES BETWEEN CHANGES IN IMMUNE AND HEMATOPOIETIC FUNCTION CAUSED BY AGING OR PROTEIN ENERGY MALNUTRITION

	Aging	Protein Energy Malnutrition
Cell Mediated Immunity		
Delayed cutaneous hypersensitivity	decreased	decreased
T-cell number	decreased	decreased
% T-suppressor cell	increased	increased
Blastogenic response to mitogen	decreased	decreased
Humoral Immunity		
B-cell number	unchanged	unchanced
Antibody production	moderately decreased	moderately decreased
Erythropoiesis		
Hemoglobin	decreased	decreased
Marrow erythroid cells	decreased	decreased
CFU-E number	decreased	decreased
BFU-E number	normal	normal
Myelopoiesis		
Granulocyte number	reduced	reduced
Granulocytosis after endotoxin administration	decreased	decreased
CFU-C number	decreased	decreased

underweight and had marginal evidence of protein energy deprivation (Lipschitz *et al.* 1985). By providing polymeric dietary supplements to these subjects between meals, it was possible (for a 16-week period) to maintain a 50% increase in total protein and caloric intake. Weight gain and significant increases in nutritional parameters indicated that the nutritional status of these subjects could be substantially improved. Thus, incremental increases in serum albumin and total iron-binding capacity occurred and highly significant elevations in selected vitamin measurements were seen. Despite improved nutritional status, the immune function and hemoglobin levels, which prior to the study were abnormal to the extent usually seen in healthy elderly persons, failed to show any increase over the 16 weeks. Thus no anergic subject showed improved delayed hypersensitivity, and measurement of T- and B-cell function failed to show an improvement (Table 15.3). In addition, no increase in hemoglobin levels was seen. Conclusions from this study, and that on the severely malnourished elderly, suggest that nutritional deficiencies aggravate immune and hematopoietic function in the elderly. Correction of coexisting disease and nutritional rehabilitation in the severely malnourished are associated with dramatic im-

TABLE 15.3
EVALUATION OF HEMATOLOGIC AND LYMPHOCYTE FUNCTION IN MILDLY MALNOURISHED ELDERLY PERSONS PRIOR TO AND FOLLOWING 16 WEEKS OF NUTRITIONAL SUPPLEMENTATION

	Week 0	Week 16
Hemoglobin (g/dL)	12.5± 0.4[1]	12.9± 0.9
Granulocyte count (× $10^3/\mu L$)	3.2± 0.1	3.4± 0.4
Mean absolute lymphocyte count (× $10^3/\mu L$)	1.4± 0.2	1.6± 0.2
Mean absolute T-lymphocytes (× $10^3/\mu L$)	0.9± 0.5	1.1± 0.4
Mean absolute T-helper lymphocytes (× $10^3/\mu L$)	0.5 ±0.3	0.3± 0.3
Mean absolute T-suppressor lymphocytes (× $10^3/\mu L$)	0.4± 0.3	0.4± 0.2

Source: Adapted from Lipschitz *et al.* (1985).
[1]Mean (± SE)

provements in host defense parameters. Mildly malnourished elderly individuals who have changes in immune and hematopoietic function, not unlike those seen in healthy elderly, do not show an improvement in their function despite obvious improved nutritional status. A reasonable conclusion from these studies is that neither protein nor calorie deprivation is the major cause of host defense changes seen in the elderly.

THE EFFECT OF AGE ON NEUTROPHIL FUNCTION

The most important function of neutrophils is to phagocytose and kill bacteria. For this to occur the neutrophil must be able to adhere to endothelial surfaces, migrate to the site of inflammation (chemotaxis), engulf and then kill the ingested bacteria. Killing is achieved by the generation of a series of toxic radicals and microbicidal halogens and by the release of a series of enzymes located in neutrophil granules. The process of bacterial killing is associated with a hundred-fold increase in neutrophil metabolism and oxygen uptake. This reaction is referred to as the respiratory burst (Babior and Cohen 1981; Babior *et al.* 1973). The neutrophil also plays an important role in the inflammatory response.

Neutrophil function can be assessed by measuring the ability of the neutrophils to phagocytose and kill bacteria. Alternatively, they can be exposed to a series of chemotactic peptides or other reagents which stimulate the respiratory burst and cause the secretion of enzymes from neutrophil granules. The burst can be evaluated by assessing oxygen metabolism in the cells, or the end products of the burst, namely the production of superoxide which is the first step in the generation of toxic radicals.

Utilizing these approaches a series of studies have examined the effects of aging on neutrophil function. In response to a wide variety of stimuli, respiratory burst activity of neutrophils from elderly individuals is decreased, and the level of various neutrophil enzymes secreted during degranulation is reduced (McLaughlin *et al.* 1986; Nagel *et al.* 1982; Suzuki *et al.* 1982; Lipschitz *et al.* 1988). The key question is whether or not the decline in neutrophil function, described as a consequence of aging, has any clinical relevance. Although neutrophil function is diminished with aging, the defect is not large enough to interfere with the ability of neutrophils from the elderly to phagocytose or to kill bacteria. However, the diminished neutrophil reserve capacity does have relevance. We have recently shown that when mice are made protein deficient, a modest reduction occurs in neutrophil function which is very similar to that seen with aging (Lipschitz and Udupa 1986). In old mice the effect of protein deficiency and aging are additive, so that in this circumstance neutrophil function decreases to a level where the ability of the cell to undertake its most critically important role of phagocytosis, and bacterial killing is severely compromised (Fig. 15.1). This finding is of particular importance as it may help explain the high prevalence of serious bacterial infection in hospitalized and older individuals who are frequently malnourished. It also demonstrates the relevance of diminished reserve capacity resulting in increased susceptibility of disease.

CONCLUSIONS

The studies described here indicate that nutritional factors play an important role in alterations in hematopoiesis seen in the elderly. There is strong evidence that nutrition may be important in the anemia seen in low socioeconomic older persons. If nutritional factors do account for the anemia, then mechanisms other than a simple nutrient deficiency must be postulated. It is possible that nutrient deficiencies not felt to be severe enough to cause pathology in a younger individual may result in abnormalities in the elderly. It is also possible that marginal deficiencies of one or more nutrients acting alone or in combination over a prolonged period of time may modulate or cause the hematopoietic changes usually ascribed to aging. Alternatively, nutrient delivery to the target organ may be altered with aging and, finally, nutrient-target interactions may change with aging.

The importance of diminished hematopoietic reserve capacity must be emphasized. Thus, a relatively minor stress, not affecting hematopoietic function in the young, clearly causes abnormalities in the old. Furthermore declines in function as a consequence of aging and nutritional deprivation appear to be additive resulting in much more significant abnormalities. The importance of these observations lies in the fact that nutritional variables can be corrected or improved, with positive effects on hematopoietic function that could contribute to diminished morbidity and mortality in the elderly.

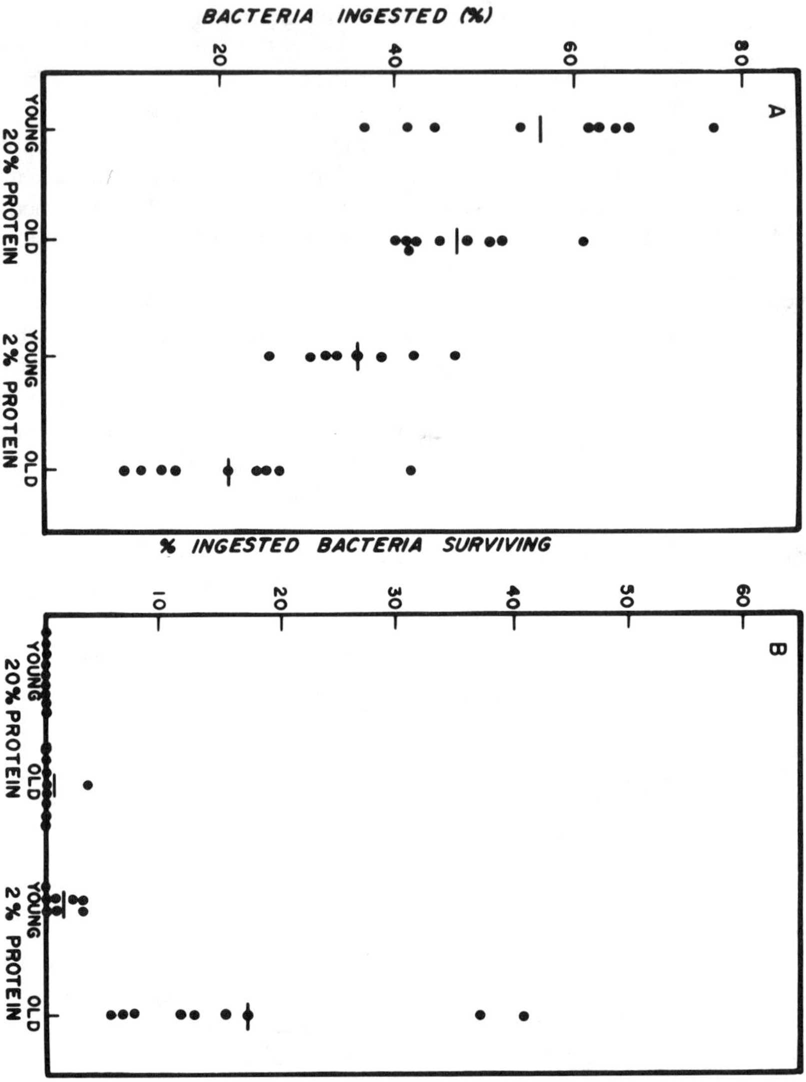

From Lipschitz and Udupa (1986)

FIG. 15.1. PHAGOCYTOSIS (PANEL A) AND BACTERIAL CELL KILL (PANEL B) IN NEUTROPHILS OBTAINED FROM THE PERITONEAL CAVITY OF YOUNG AND OLD MICE FED A 20% OR 2% PROTEIN DIET FOR 3 WEEKS

Phagocytosis is significantly lower in old animals fed a 2% protein diet. In addition a significant fraction of ingested bacteria are not killed in old animals fed the low protein diet.

REFERENCES

BABIOR, B. M. and COHEN, H. J. 1981. Measurement of neutrophil function: Phagocytosis, degranulation, the respiratory burst and bacterial killing. *In* Leukocyte Function, M. J. Cline (ed.). Churchill Livingstone, New York.

BABIOR, B. M., KIPNES, R. S. and CURNUTTE, J. T. 1973. Biological defense mechanisms. The production by leukocytes of superoxide, a potential bactericidal agent. J. Clin. Invest. *52*, 741–744.

BOGGS, D. R. 1985. Hematopoiesis and aging. III. Anemia and a blunted erythropoietic response to hemorrhage in aged mice. Am. J. Hematol. *19*, 327–339.

DALLMAN, P. R., YIP, R. and JOHNSON, C. 1984. Prevalence and causes of anemia in the United States, 1976 to 1980. Am. J. Clin. Nutr. *39*, 437–445.

GARRY, P. J., GOODWIN, J. S. and HUNT, W. C. 1983. Iron status and anemia in the elderly. J. Am. Geriatr. Soc. *31*, 389–399.

HARRISON, D. E. 1975a. Defective erythropoietic response of aged mice not improved by young marrow. J. Gerontol. *30*, 286–291.

HARRISON, D. E. 1975b. Normal function of transplanted marrow cell lines from aged mice. J. Gerontol. *30*, 279–285.

HARTSOCK, R. J., SMITH, E. B. and KETTAN, C. S. 1965. Normal variation with aging of the amount of hematopoietic tissue in bone marrow form the anterior iliac crest. Am. J. Clin. Pathol. *43*, 325–331.

HAYFLICK, L. 1965. The limited in vitro lifetime of human diploid cell strains. Exp. Cell. Res. *37*, 614–636.

HILL, R. D. 1967. The prevalence of anemia in the over-65s in a rural practice. Practitioner *217*, 963–967.

Information Canada. 1973. Nutrition Canada: National Survey. Information Canada, Ottawa.

LIPSCHITZ, D. A., MITCHELL, C. O. and THOMPSON, C. 1981. The anemia of senescence. Am. J. Hematol. *11*, 47–54.

LIPSCHITZ, D. A., McGINNIS, S. K. and UDUPA, K. B. 1983. The use of long-term bone marrow culture as a model of the aging process. Age *6*, 122–127.

LIPSCHITZ, D. A. and MITCHELL, C. O. 1982. The correctability of the nutritional, immune and hematopoietic manifestations of protein calorie malnutrition in the elderly. J. Am. Coll. Nutr. *1*, 17–25.

LIPSCHITZ, D. A., MITCHELL, C. O. and MILTON, K. Y. 1982. Nutritional evaluation and supplementation of elderly participants in a Meals on Wheels program. J.P.E.N. *9*, 343–347.

LIPSCHITZ, D. A. and UDUPA, K. B. 1986. Influence of aging and protein deficiency on neutrophil function. J. Gerontol. *41*, 690–694.

LIPSCHITZ, D. A., UDUPA, K. B. and BOXER, L. A. 1987. Evidence that microenvironmental factors account for the age-related decline in neutrophil function. Blood *70*, 1131–1135.

LIPSCHITZ, D. A., UDUPA, K. B. and BOXER, L. S. 1988. The role of calcium in the age-related decline of neutrophil function. Blood *71*, 659–665.

LIPSCHITZ, D. A., UDUPA, K. B., MILTON, K. Y. and THOMPSON, C. 1984. Effect of age on hematopoiesis in man. Blood *63*, 502–509.

McLAUGHLIN, B., O'MALLEY, K. and COTTEN, T. G. 1986. Age-related differences in granulocyte chemotaxis and degranulation. Clin. Sci. *70*, 59–62.

McLENNAN, W. J., ANDREWS, G. R., MACLEOD, C. and CAIRD, F. I. 1973. Anaemia in the elderly. Q. J. Med. *52*, 1–13.

MAUCH, P. *et al.* 1982. Decline in bone marrow proliferative capacity as a function of age. Blood *60*, 245–252.

MYERS, M. A., SAUNDERS, C. R. G. and CHALMERS, D. G. 1968. The hemoglobin level of fit elderly people. Lancet *2*, 261–263.

NAGEL, J. E., PYLE, R. S., CHREST, F. J. and ADLER, W. H. 1982. Oxidative metabolism and bactericidal capacity of polymorphonuclear leukocyte from young and aged adults. J. Gerontol. *37*, 529–534.

OGDEN, D. A. and MICKLEM, H. S. 1974. The fate of serially transplanted bone marrow cell populations from young and old donors. Transplantation *22*, 287–293.

PARSON, P. L., WHITHEY, J. L. and KILPATRICK, G. S. 1965. The prevalence of anemia in the elderly. Practitioner *195*, 656–660.

ROTHSTEIN G., CHRISTENSEN, R. D. and NIELSON, B. R. 1987. Kinetic evaluation of pool sizes and proliferative response of neutrophils in bacterially challenged aging mice. Blood *70*, 1836–1841.

SUZUKI, K. *et al.* 1982. Age-related decline in lysosomal enzyme release from polymorphonuclear leukocytes after N-Formyl-Methionylleucyl-Phenylalanine stimulation. Exp. Hematol. *11*, 1005–1013.

UDUPA, K. B. and LIPSCHITZ, D. A. 1974. Erythropoiesis in the aged mouse: I. Response to stimulation in vivo. J. Lab. Clin. Med. *103*, 574–580.

WILLIAMS, L. H., UDUPA, K. B. and LIPSCHITZ, D. A. 1986. An evaluation of the effect of age on hematopoiesis in C57BL/6 mouse. Exp. Hematol. *14*, 827–832.

YIP, R., JOHNSON, C. and DALLMAN, P. R. 1984. Age-related changes in laboratory values used in the diagnosis of anemia and iron deficiency. Am. J. Clin. Nutr. *93*, 427–436.

CHAPTER 16

ENDOGENOUS DNA DAMAGE AS RELATED TO NUTRITION AND AGING

BRUCE N. AMES, Ph.D.
Division of Biochemistry and Microbiology
University of California
Berkeley, California

INTRODUCTION

Progress in identifying the important endogenous processes damaging DNA and developing methods to assay this damage in individuals is presented. This approach may aid studies on nutritional modulation of the aging process.

The endogenous background level of oxidant-induced DNA damage *in vivo* has been assayed by measuring 8-hydroxydeoxyguanosine (oh^8dG), thymine glycol and thymidine glycol in urine and oh^8dG in DNA. oh^8dG is one of about 20 adducts found on oxidizing DNA, e.g., by radiation. The level of oxidative DNA damage as measured by oh^8dG in normal rat liver is shown to be extensive especially in mtDNA (1/130,000 bases in nuclear DNA and 1/8,000 bases in mitochondrial DNA). We also discuss three hitherto unrecognized antioxidants in man.

AGING, CANCER, AND ENDOGENOUS SOURCES OF DNA DAMAGE

The marked increase in life span that has occurred in 60 million years of primate evolution has been accompanied by a marked decrease in age-specific cancer rates. Cumulative cancer risk increases with approximately the fourth power of age (Fig. 16.1), both in short-lived species such as rats and mice (about 30% have cancer

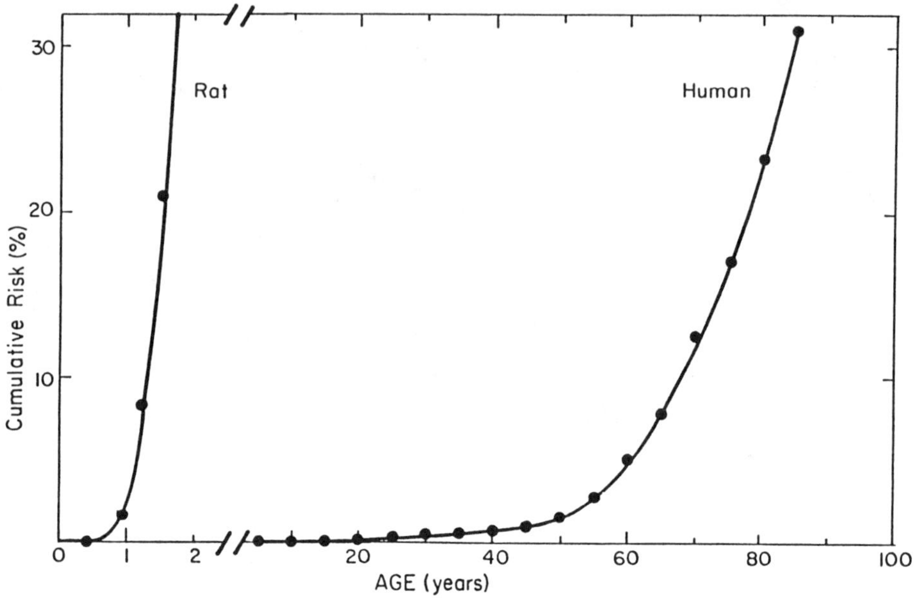

From Ames et al. 1985

FIG. 16.1. CUMULATIVE NET RISK OF DEATH FROM CANCER FOR RATS AND HUMANS

by the end of their 2- to 3-year life span) and in long-lived species such as humans (about 30% have cancer by the end of their 85-year life span). Thus, cancer is fundamentally a degenerative disease of old age, though it can be increased (e.g., cigarette smoking in humans) or decreased (e.g., calorie restriction in rodents) by exogenous factors.

One important factor in longevity appears to be basal metabolic rate (Cutler 1984), which is much lower in man than in rodents and could markedly affect the level of endogenous mutagens produces by normal metabolism. We assume that DNA damage is likely to be critical for both cancer and aging. One view of the somatic damage theory of aging is that the amount of maintenance and repair of somatic tissues is always less than that required for indefinite survival. Thus, some DNA damage in somatic cells induced by endogenous mutagens will accumulate with time.

Four important endogenous processes leading to significant DNA damage are likely to be oxidation (Totter 1980; Ames 1983; Cutler 1984), methylation, deamination, and depurination (Saul and Ames 1986). In support of this are the existence of specific DNA repair glycosylases for oxidative, methylated and deaminated adducts, and a repair system for apurinic sites produced by spontaneous depurination (Lindahl 1982). The measurement of DNA adducts by new methods shows that oxidation is a major type of DNA damage.

MEASUREMENT OF OXIDATIVE DNA DAMAGE

Oxidants are produced as byproducts of normal metabolism and of lipid peroxidation (Fig. 16.2 and 16.3). Oxidative damage of cellular DNA has been detected by chemical, physical, enzymatic, and immunochemical methods. The methods have been sensitive enough to detect DNA damage induced by severe stresses such as kilorad doses of radiation, but have not generally been useful for examining the background levels of damage products formed from normal aerobic metabolism.

$$O_2 \xrightarrow{e^-} O_2^{\overline{\cdot}} \xrightarrow{e^-} H_2O_2 \xrightarrow{e^-} \cdot OH \xrightarrow{e^-} H_2O$$

$$O_2 \xrightarrow[\text{LIGHT}]{\text{DYE}} {}^1O_2$$

From Ames et al. 1985

FIG. 16.2. THE FORMATION OF SUPEROXIDE, HYDROGEN PEROXIDE, AND HYDROXYL RADICALS BY SUCCESSIVE ADDITIONS OF ELECTRONS TO OXYGEN
Cytochrome oxidase adds 4 electrons fairly efficiently during energy generation in mitochondria, but some of these toxic intermediates leak out. Singlet oxygen is generated from oxygen by the absorption of energy from a dye activated by light.

Our laboratory has overcome this problem by using an approach based on the pathways shown in Fig. 16.4. Nonspecific DNA repair enzymes excise DNA adducts to release deoxynucleotides, or specific DNA repair glycosylases release free bases. Deoxynucleotides are enzymatically hydrolyzed to the deoxynucleosides which are not usually further metabolized, and both these and the free bases may be recovered in the urine. Two products of oxidative damage to DNA are thymine glycol and 5-hydroxymethyluracil. We have described a specific DNA repair enzyme, a DNA glycosylase from mouse cells, which repairs 5-hydroxymethyluracil and differs from the specific DNA glycosylase repair enzyme for thymine glycol in mouse cells (Hollstein *et al.* 1984). The existence of these specific repair enzymes points to the importance of this type of DNA damage *in vivo*.

Our method suffers from being an indirect measurement of what was in the DNA and being potentially subject to artifacts. Nevertheless, it has two very powerful advantages. It can be made extremely sensitive, in part because DNA lesions from all the cells in the body are concentrated in a relatively small volume of urine, and it is noninvasive.

In order to quantify the daily removal of these lesions from DNA, we developed a high performance liquid chromatography (HPLC) assay for the known radiation

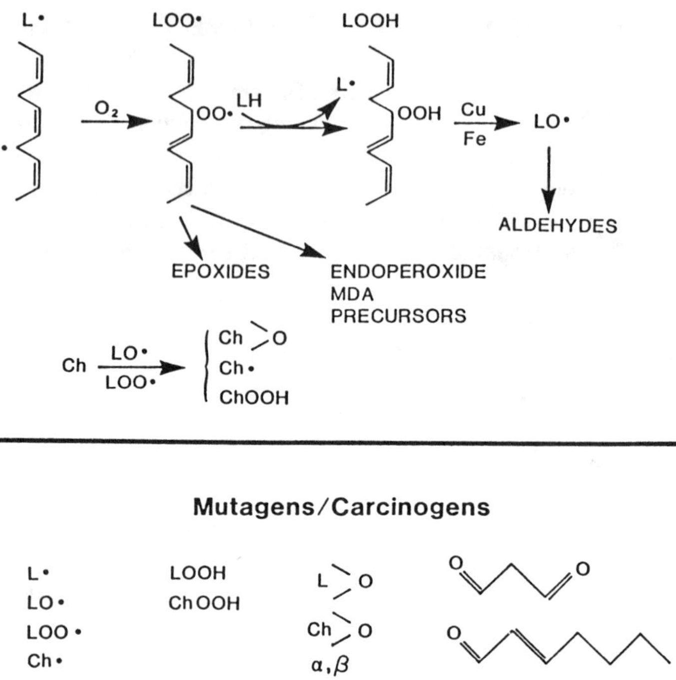

From Ames 1988

FIG. 16.3. LIPID PEROXIDATION

L = lipid radical; L• = alkoxy lipid radical; LOO• = hydroperoxy lipid radical; LOOH = lipid hydroperoxide; Ch = cholesterol; Ch O = cholesterol epoxide; L O = lipid epoxide; MDA = malondialdehyde.

damage products thymine glycol, thymidine glycol, hydroxymethyluracil, and hydroxymethyldeoxyuridine in urine (Cathcart *et al.* 1984; Saul *et al.* 1987; B. N. Ames and R. L. Saul, unpublished observations). Our results indicate that normal humans excrete a total of about 100 nmol/day of the first 3 compounds. We have considerable evidence that most of this total is derived from repair of oxidized DNA, rather than from alternative sources, e. g., diet or bacterial flora (Cathcart *et al.* 1984; Saul *et al.* 1987; Ames and Saul 1988). This total may therefore represent an average of about 10^3 oxidized thymine residues per day for each of the body's 6×10^{13} cells. Because these products are only 3 of about 20 products of oxidative damage of DNA (Cadet and Berger 1985; von Sonntag 1987), the total number of all types of oxidative hits of DNA per cell per day in man may be more than 10^4.

Metabolic Rate and Oxidant-induced DNA Damage

Although considerable speculation about the relationships among oxidants, cancer, and aging abounds, the experimental evidence is still weak. The impressive interspecies correlation between the specific metabolic rate and the rate of aging, i.e., species with high metabolic rates also have a high age-specific cancer incidence (Fig. 16.1), is circumstantial evidence implicating oxidants in aging. The faster rate of aging and the faster accumulation of carcinogenic events for mammals with higher specific metabolic rates may be explained by assuming that these species have higher rates of production of oxidants per cell, leading to faster accumulation of somatic damage, carcinogenic events, and aging. We now have data on four species that provide additional circumstantial evidence for this theory and are consistent with the possibility that DNA is a critical target in aging. Rats, which have a higher specific metabolic rate and a shorter life span than humans, excrete about 15 times more thymine glycol and thymidine glycol per kilogram of body weight than do humans (Fig. 16.5) (Cathcart *et al.* 1984; Adelman *et al.* 1988). Mice have an even higher metabolic rate and a shorter life span, and they have higher levels of thymine glycol and thymidine glycol than rats. Data obtained with monkeys are consistent with this relationship (Adelman *et al.* 1988).

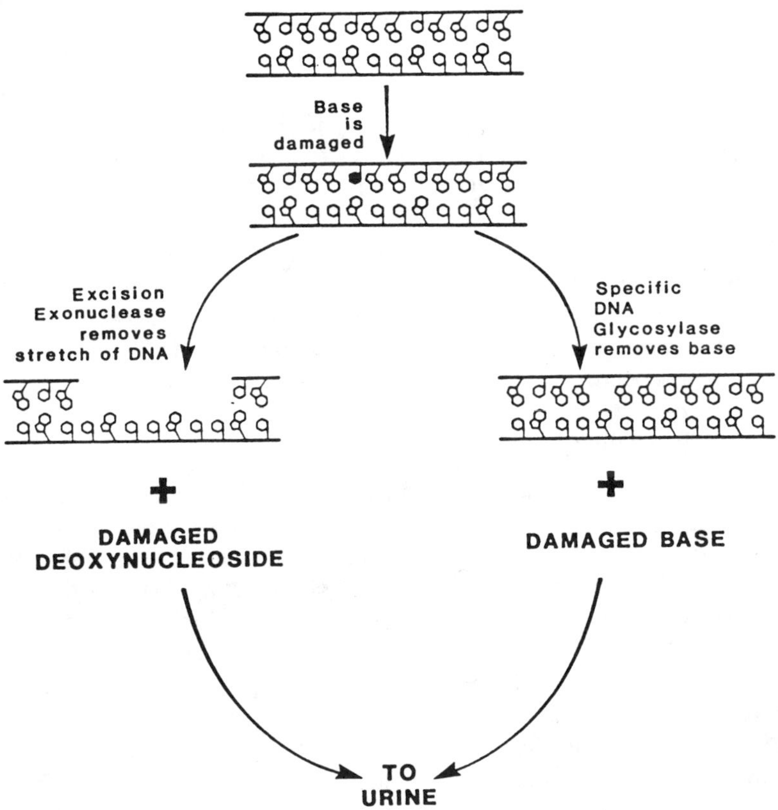

From Ames et al. 1985

FIG. 16.4. REPAIR OF A DAMAGED DNA BASE BY EXCISION REPAIR OR A SPECIFIC GLYCOSYLASE

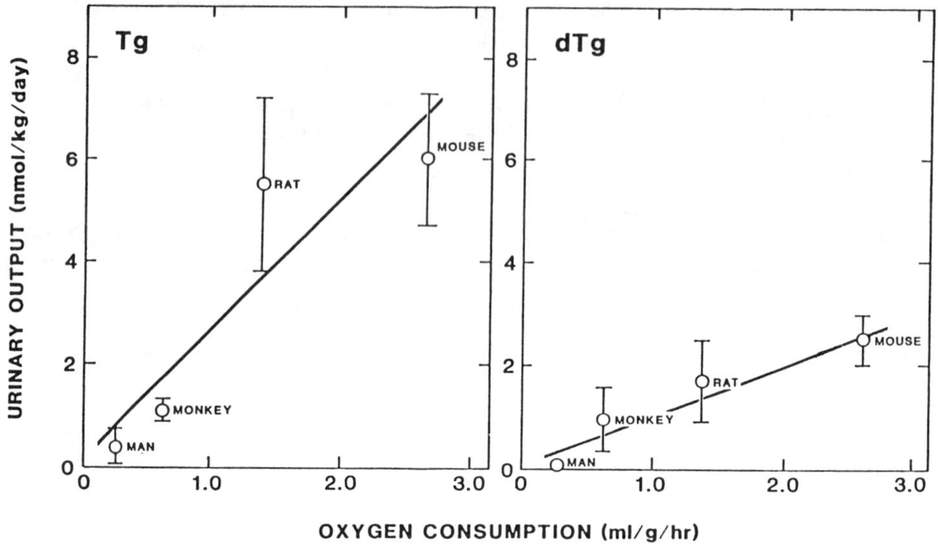

From Adelman et al. 1988

FIG. 16.5. AVERAGE URINARY OUTPUT OF THYMINE GLYCOL (Tg) AND THYMIDINE GLYCOL (dTg) FOR FOUR DIFFERENT SPECIES, EXPRESSED AS A FUNCTION OF THE SPECIFIC METABOLIC RATE

We have now tested urines for thymine glycol and thymidine glycol from normal human volunteers aged 22–84 years (Saul *et al.* 1987). The preliminary evidence is that their urinary outputs are age-independent, which suggests that the rate of oxidative DNA damage in man does not change substantially with age. This is consistent with age-independent somatic damage theories of aging (Peto *et al.* 1985).

Urinary 8-Hydroxydeoxyguanosine

Our urinary thymine glycol assay is difficult and takes about 3 weeks. We are thus developing a simpler urinary assay for 8-hydroxydeoxyguanosine (oh^{8}dG), which has been measured in DNA by electrochemical detection at about 1000 times the sensitivity of UV detection (Floyd *et al.* 1986; Kasai *et al.* 1986; Kuchino *et al.* 1987). This new assay (Cundy *et al.* 1988; Shigenaga *et al.* 1989) can be done quickly and thus will enable a much more rapid and simpler assay of urine for oxidized DNA. The level in human urine is of the same order as dTg and is much lower than the level in rodents. We also have evidence for the presence of 8-hydroxyguanosine, a measure of oxidative damage to RNA. We have used this assay to measure oh^{8}dG in urine of humans with chronic granulomatous disease (Cundy *et al.* 1988). These people lack the respiratory burst from phagocytic cells, yet they still produce oh^{8}dG in their urine. This is evidence that the presence of oxidized DNA bases in urine is not a consequence of normal cell turnover.

8-Hydroxydeoxyguanosine in DNA

Since our work on urinary excretion of oxidized bases did not distinguish between damage to nuclear and mitochondrial DNA, we have examined the level of 8-hydroxydeoxyguanosine, one of about 20 known radiation damage products, in both mitochondrial and nuclear DNA of normal rat liver (Richter *et al.* 1988). It is present at a level of 1/130,000 bases in nuclear DNA and 1/8,000 bases in mitochondrial DNA. Our preliminary evidence suggests that the level of oh^8dG does not increase with age. The extremely high level in mitochondrial DNA may be caused by the immense oxygen metabolism, relatively inefficient DNA repair and the absence of histones in mitochondria. Thus, mitochondria may be accumulating mutations with age which could compromise energy supplies to the cell. Mitochondria are likely to be a major source of the oxidants damaging nuclear DNA.

7-Methylguanine in DNA

The 7-methylguanine (m^7G) adduct in the DNA of rat liver has been determined as an indicator of exposure to exogenous and endogenous methylating agents (Park and Ames 1988). A new method for the analysis of m^7G adducts has been developed by combining the selectivity of separation of reversed-phase high-performance liquid chromatography with the specificity and high sensitivity of electrochemical detection (Park and Ames 1988). The sensitivity of the method is about 10,000-fold that of optical methods and is sufficient to determine the endogenous background of DNA methylation.

DEFENSES AGAINST OXIDANTS

Many defense mechanisms within the organism have evolved to limit the levels of reactive O_2 species and the damage they induce. Among the defenses are SOD, catalase, and GSH peroxidase as well as the antioxidants β-carotene, tocopherols, and vitamin C. We have discussed several previously unappreciated antioxidants that have appeared in evolution.

Uric Acid

Uric acid is a powerful antioxidant that appeared in primate evolution concomitant with the development of a long life span and large, metabolically active brain (Ames *et al.* 1981). Uric acid is the main antioxidant in saliva and is 300 μM in human blood. It is present in much lower amounts in animals before the primates. Uric acid levels increased in primate evolution at about the same time as we lost the ability to synthesize ascorbic acid, so that these events may be related.

Bilirubin

Heme is degraded to biliverdin, and in mammals biliverdin is converted to bilirubin, both of which are shown to be powerful antioxidants (Stocker *et al.* 1987a, 1987b; Stocker and Ames 1987). The bilirubin in human blood is bound at a specific site on albumin at a concentration of 20 μM (Stocker *et al.* 1987a, 1987b; Stocker and Ames 1987). This is a much higher level than in rat blood. Conjugated bilirubin also appears to be the most important antioxidant in bile, and with the copper ions present in bile forms a powerful redox system for oxidizing xenobiotics and destroying hydroperoxides (Stocker and Ames 1987).

Carnosine

Carnosine, which is present in high concentrations in human muscle and brain, has been shown to have antioxidant properties and to chelate copper and iron ions so as to inhibit oxidative reactions. We have postulated that it is a physiologically significant antioxidant (Kohen *et al.* 1988).

Other Defenses

Because of the finite time between generation of oxidants and their destruction by a defense mechanism, low levels can exist for sufficient time to produce damage to cellular macromolecules (Chance *et al.* 1979). For nuclear DNA, however, the mammalian cell has three more levels of defense. First, nuclear DNA is compartmentalized away from mitochondria and peroxisomes where most oxidants are probably generated. Second, most nonreplicating nuclear DNA is surrounded by histones and polyamines which may protect against oxidants. Finally, most of the types of DNA damage produced can be repaired by efficient enzyme systems. The net result of this multilevel defense is that nuclear DNA is very well, but not completely, protected from oxidants.

ENDOGENOUS DNA DAMAGE COULD CAUSE AGING BY VARIOUS MECHANISMS

Several models relate endogenous DNA damage, cancer, and aging. One possibility is that mutagens react with nuclear DNA to produce somatic mutations, both point mutations and clastogenic events such as deletions. The sources of mutagenic oxidants could include: long-lived oxidants generated outside the nucleus in the mitochondria and cytoplasm and capable of crossing the nuclear membrane, lipid-soluble oxidants generated in the nuclear membrane itself, and oxidants generated within the nucleus. Methylation of DNA could cause both point mutations and apurinic sites which lead to breaks and clastogenic events. Somatic mutation could disrupt the cell by altering gene products or by altering their regulation.

Another model for mutagenic damage is that the high rate of oxidative damage to mitochondria causes an accumulation of mutations with age in mitochondrial DNA that results in energy deficiencies in old cells. This would, in turn, lead to deficiencies in repair enzymes, or to cell death.

In addition to mutation, DNA damage can prevent DNA replication and lead to cell death. This can cause neighboring cells to proliferate, a promotional stimulus for carcinogenesis in cells that do not normally undergo DNA replication.

Oxidation or methylation could also cause loss of 5-methylcytosine, an epigenetic change. 5-methylcytosine is important in turning off genes in differentiation so that its loss by DNA damage could cause de-differentiation and contribute to cancer and aging (Wilson *et al.* 1987; Holliday 1987). By analogy with 5-hydroxymethyluracil, 5-hydroxymethylcytosine could be formed by oxidative damage (Cannon *et al.* 1988). This could lead to lack of methylation after DNA replication as the DNA maintenance methylase is not likely to recognize 5-hydroxymethylcytosine as 5-methylcytosine. Similarly, 8-hydroxyguanine and 7-methylguanine are likely to interfere with maintenance methylation at neighboring or base-paired cytosines and cause loss of 5-methylcytosine.

ACKNOWLEDGMENTS

This work was supported by National Cancer Institute Outstanding Investigator Grant CA39910 and by National Institute of Environmental Health Sciences Center Grant ES01896. This paper was adapted in part from Ames (1989).

REFERENCES

ADELMAN, R., SAUL, R. L. and AMES, B. N. 1988. Oxidative damage to DNA: Relation to species metabolic rate and life span. Proc. Natl. Acad. Sci. USA *86*, 2706–2708.

AMES, B. N. 1983. Dietary carcinogens and anticarcinogens. Oxygen radicals and degenerative diseases. Science *221*, 1256–1264.

AMES, B. N. 1988. Measuring oxidative damage in humans: Relation to cancer and aging. *In* Methods for Detecting DNA Damaging Agents in Humans: Applications in Cancer Epidemiology and Prevention, H. Bartsch, K. Hemminki and I. K. O'Neill (eds.). IARC Scientific Publications No. 89. International Agency for Research on Cancer, Lyon, France.

AMES, B. N. 1989. Endogenous DNA damage as related to cancer and aging. Mutation Res. *214*, 41–46.

AMES, B. N. CATHCART, R., SCHWIERS, E. and HOCHSTEIN, P. 1981. Uric acid provides an antioxidant defense in humans against oxidant- and radical-caused aging and cancer: A hypothesis. Proc. Natl. Acad. Sci. USA *78*, 6858–6862.

AMES, B. N. and SAUL, R. L. 1988. Cancer, aging, and oxidative DNA damage. *In* Theories of Carcinogenesis, O. H. Iversen (ed.). Hemisphere Publishing Corp., Washington, D. C.

AMES, B. N. *et al.* 1985. Oxidative DNA damage as related to cancer and aging: The assay of thymine glycol, thymidine glycol, and hydroxymethyluracil in human and rat urine.

In Molecular Biology of Aging: Gene Stability and Gene Expression, R. S. Sohal, L. S. Birnbaum and R. G. Cutler (eds.). Raven Press, New York.

BARROW, L. R. and MAGEE, P. N. 1982. Nonenzymatic methylation of DNA by S-adenosylmethionine *in vitro*. Carcinogenesis *3*, 349–351.

CADET, J. and BERGER, M. 1985. Radiation-induced decomposition of the purine bases within DNA and related model compounds. Int. J. Radiat. Biol. *47*, 127–143.

CANNON, S. V., CUMMINGS, A. and TEEBOR, G. W. 1988. 5-Hydroxymethylcytosine DNA glycosylase activity in mammalian tissue. Biochem. Biophys. Res. Commun. *151*, 1173–1179.

CATHCART, R., SCHWIERS, E., SAUL, R. L. and AMES, B. N. 1984. Thymine glycol and thymidine glycol in human and rat urine: A possible assay for oxidative DNA damage. Proc. Natl. Acad. Sci. USA *81*, 5633–5637.

CHANCE, B., SIES, H. and BOVERIS, A. 1979. Hydroperoxide metabolism in mammalian organs. Phys. Rev. *59*, 527–605.

CUNDY, K., KOHEN, R. and AMES, B. N. 1988. Determination of 8-hydroxydeoxyguanosine in human urine: A possible assay for *in vivo* oxidative DNA damage. *In* Oxygen Radicals in Biology and Medicine, M. G. Simic, K. A. Taylor, J. F. Ward and C. von Sonntag (eds.). Plenum Publishing Corp., New York.

CUTLER, R. G. 1984. Antioxidants, aging, and longevity. *In* Free Radicals in Biology, Vol. 6, W. A. Pryor (ed.). Academic Press, New York.

FLOYD, R. A. *et al.* 1986. Hydroxyl free radical adduct of deoxyguanosine: Sensitive detection and mechanisms of formation. Free Rad. Res. Comm. *1*, 163–172.

HOLLIDAY, R. 1987. The inheritance of epigenetic defects. Science *238*, 163–169.

HOLLSTEIN, M. C., BROOKS, P., LINN, S. and AMES, B. N. 1984. Hydroxymethyluracil DNA glycosylase in mammalian cells. Proc. Natl. Acad. Sci. USA *81*, 4003–4007.

KASAI, H. *et al.* 1986. Formation of 8-hydroxyguanine moiety in cellular DNA by agents producing oxygen radicals and evidence for its repair. Carcinogenesis *7*, 1849–1851.

KOHEN, R., YAMAMOTO, Y., CUNDY, K. and AMES, B. N. 1988. Antioxidant activity of carnosine, homocarnosine, and anserine present in muscle and brain. Proc. Natl. Acad. Sci. USA *85*, 3175–3179.

KUCHINO, Y. *et al.* 1987. Misreading of DNA templates containing 8-hydroxydeoxyguanosine at the modified base and at adjacent residues. Nature *327*, 77–79.

LINDAHL, T. 1982. DNA repair enzymes. Annu. Rev. Biochem. *51*, 61–87.

PARK, J.-W. and AMES, B. N. 1988. 7-Methylguanine adducts in DNA are normally present at high levels and increase on aging: Analysis by HPLC with electrochemical detection. Proc. Natl. Acad. Sci. USA *85*, 7467–7470, 9508.

PETO, R., PARISH, S. E. and GRAY, R. G. 1985. There is no such thing as ageing, and cancer is not related to it. *In* Age-Related Factors in Carcinogenesis, A. Likhachev, V. Anismov and R. Montesano (eds.). IARC Scientific Publications No. 58, International Agency for Research on Cancer, Lyon, France.

RICHTER, C., PARK, J.-W. and AMES, B. N. 1988. Normal oxidative damage to mitochondrial and nuclear DNA is extensive. Proc. Natl. Acad. Sci. USA *85*, 6465–6467.

SAUL, R. L. and AMES, B. N. 1986. Background levels of DNA damage in the population. *In* Mechanisms of DNA Damage and Repair: Implications for Carcinogenesis and Risk Assessment, M. G. Simic, L. Grossman and A. C. Upton (eds.). Plenum Publishing Corp., New York.

SAUL, R. L., GEE, P. and AMES, B. N. 1987. Free radicals, DNA damage, and aging. *In* Modern Biological Theories of Aging, H. R. Warner, R. N. Butler, R. L. Sprott and E. L. Schneider (eds.). Raven Press, New York.

SHIGENAGA, M. K., GIMENO, C. J. and AMES, B. N. 1989. Urinary 8-hydroxy-2′-deoxyguanosine as a biological marker of *in vivo* oxidative DNA damage. Proc. Nat. Acad. Sci USA *86*, 9697–9701.

STOCKER, R. and AMES, B. N. 1987. Potential role of conjugated bilirubin and copper in the metabolism of lipid peroxides in bile. Proc. Natl. Acad. Sci. USA *84*, 8130–8134.

STOCKER, R., GLAZER, A. N. and AMES, B. N. 1987a. Antioxidant activity of albumin-bound bilirubin. Proc. Natl. Acad. Sci. USA *84*, 5918–5922.

STOCKER, R. *et al.* 1987b. Bilirubin is an antioxidant of possible physiological importance. Science *235*, 1043–1045.

TOTTER, J. R. 1980. Spontaneous cancer and its possible relationship to oxygen metabolism. Proc. Natl. Acad. Sci. USA *77*, 1763–1767.

VON SONNTAG, C. 1987. The Chemical Basis of Radiation Biology. Taylor and Francis, London.

WILSON, V. L., SMITH, R. A., MA, S. and CUTLER, R. G. 1987. Genomic 5-methyldeoxycytidine decreases with age. J. Biol. Chem. *21*, 9948–9951.

CHAPTER 17

MODULATION OF IMMUNE FUNCTIONS AND AGING BY OMEGA-3 FATTY ACIDS AND/OR CALORIE RESTRICTION

GABRIEL FERNANDES, Ph.D.
Departments of Medicine, Microbiology and Physiology
The University of Texas Health Science Center at San Antonio
San Antonio, Texas

INTRODUCTION

For several years, food restriction has been known to increase life span by inhibiting the rise in several age-associated diseases in both mice and rats. Although several observations carried out recently by many investigators have offered some clue in understanding the mechanism of how food restriction acts in the prolongation of life span, the precise mechanism for modulating the immune system has not been discovered. Our results indicate food restriction alters various lymphocyte subsets minimally in Fischer-344 male rats, and yet enhancement in functional activity of T-cells has been observed during aging in food-restricted rats. Food restriction prevented changes in membrane fluidity and loss of high-affinity interleukin-2 (IL-2) receptor molecules, facilitated production of higher IL-2, maintained increased natural killer cell (NK) activity and inhibited oncogene expression during aging.

Recently, besides utilization of calorie restriction for understanding the aging process and/or the development of autoimmune disorders, a significant interest in the utilization of Menhaden fish oil as a dietary lipid supplement, without reducing the caloric intake, to control autoimmune disease processes has been receiving greater attention. The lifelong feeding results showed either food restriction or fish oil diet alone can inhibit autoimmune disease, whereas diets containing lard or corn oil accelerated the disease and caused early deaths. The beneficial effects of both food restriction and/or fish oil diet with adequate antioxidants appear to be due to the following major physiological changes: (1) decrease in plasma prolactin levels; (2) prevention of loss of Lyt-2 cells; (3) prevention of rise in la^+, lg^+ and $Ly1/B^+$ cells; and (4) decrease in anti-DNA antibodies levels. Further, decreased arachidonic acid (20:4), increased n-3 fatty acids (20:5 and 22:6), higher fluidity, and decreased oncogene mRNA expression in spleen cells of fish-oil fed and food-restricted mice was also noted.

Our current data demonstrate that food restriction may have a marked effect on lengthening the life span of both long-lived Fischer-344 rats and short-lived B/W mice; however, our ongoing studies reveal that Omega-3 fatty acids may serve as an alternative approach to inhibit autoimmune disease and to lengthen the life span of short-lived strains of mice without reducing their calorie intake. However, further studies are required to compare the effect of Omega-3 fatty acids on Fischer-344 rats without reducing the lifelong calorie intake to prolong their life span.

Excessive nutritional intake has been implicated as an influence on the development of many chronic diseases, including arteriosclerosis, cardiovascular disease, several forms of cancer, and autoimmune disorders (Levy and Moskowitz 1982). Involution of thymus and the consequent loss of several T-cell effectors and immunoregulatory functions linked to the genetic background may underlie the development of many of these age-related diseases and early deaths (Fernandes 1984). The maintenance of active immunological function during aging may be a likely basis for the prevention of at least some of these diseases during aging. On the other hand, long-term chronic diet and nutrition deficiency, particularly of essential vitamins and trace elements, in humans has been associated with an increase susceptibility to infectious diseases (Chandra and Newberne 1977). However, carefully controlled animal studies have shown that moderate total calorie restriction and/or lowering dietary fat intake can enhance immune function, prolong life and lower the incidence of or delay the onset of autoimmune disease, particularly renal disease and malignancy.

Autoimmune diseases, particularly rheumatoid arthritis (RA), affect over 7,000,000 adults, and systemic lupus erythematosus (SLE) strikes approximately 1 in 1,000 individuals of the general population. Patients with these disorders are mostly females and both diseases are multisystem autoimmune phenomena characterized by the production of a variety of autoantibodies with resulting immune-mediated inflammation (Am. Rheumatism Assoc. 1973; Smith and Steinberg 1983). The inflammatory process in autoimmune diseases may spare the major organs of the body or may involve vital organs such as brain and kidney. There is no known cure for either SLE or RA, but several treatments are directed at relieving symptoms as well as preventing progression of the disease (Balow 1986; Steinberg and Decker 1974). However, many of the drugs (corticosteroid, azathioprine, cyclophosphamide, gold salts, etc.) used for this purpose have substantial toxicities and, therefore, studies are urgently needed to balance the potential risks of therapy with the potential benefits. Patients with these diseases regularly seek dietary cures as therapies that have no toxicity, but scientific evidence is lacking and so far does not support any particular food or vitamin as having a dramatic effect on arthritis or lupus disease (Balow 1986). On the other hand, experimental studies have shown that either calorie or dietary fat restriction has a profound effect on autoimmune SLE in mice (Homsy *et al.* 1986). Nonetheless, patients with arthritis are encouraged to follow nutritionally well-balanced diets. Although stringent caloric restriction may have a profound value as a preventive measure in reducing age-related disease, it may not have practical therapeutic value in many chronic diseases. Although weight reduction in obesity seems to alleviate RA symptoms in many of these patients, no specific dietary factor yet described either improves autoimmune disease or reduced drug dosage and toxicities.

ANIMAL MODELS

MRL/*lpr*/*lpr* and NZB×NZW F_1 mice spontaneously develop an autoimmune disease manifested clinically by arthritis, vasculitis and immune complex glomerulonephritis. As such, these mice also represent a murine model for RA and SLE (Andrews *et al.* 1978; Theofilopoulos and Dixon 1985). Because strains homozygous for the *lpr* gene exhibit profound T-cell lymphadenopathy associated with polyclonal B-cell activation, autoantibody production, and specific T-cell unresponsiveness, such mice have served as a useful model for studying the mechanisms underlying B-cell hyperactivity, and its relationship to increased la antigen expression, which may be influenced by dietary and endocrine systems, particularly to the excess production of various lymphokines (Theofilopoulos *et al.* 1980). On the other hand, Fischer-344 rats, which are known to develop chronic renal disease in 100% of the animals, has been extensively utilized to study the mechanism of prolonged life span by food restriction (Masoro *et al.* 1982; Yu 1985). We and others have observed food restriction indeed maintains higher T-cell function, retards malignancy and chronic renal disease, and extends life span significantly (Weindruch *et al.* 1979; Fernandes *et al.* 1976).

AGE-RELATED CHANGES IN IMMUNE CELLS

A progressive decline in T-cell immune function, particularly cellular immunity as a function of age, is well established (Walford *et al.* 1981; Makinodan and Kay 1980). Further, loss of the T-cell surface antigen recognition system occurs earlier than loss of B-cell function. Evidence has also been presented that T-cells, after acquiring self/nonself discriminatory ability in the thymus, conduct immune surveillance by seeking changes in major histocompatibility-coded surface antigens in normal and transformed cells (Dorf and Benacerraf 1984). Many studies show that T-cells from aging animals and humans respond to various stimuli less vigorously than those from young animals, and that the defects are intrinsic to aged T-cells (Tam and Walford 1978). Further alteration in T-cell proliferative response is also related to increased suppressor cell populations of both T-cell and macrophage lineage. In addition to a possible increase in number of nonspecific suppressor cells during aging, a significant decrease in cytotoxic T-cell function and NK function in aging animals is implicated by many in the increased incidence of malignancy in aged animals (Weksler and Siskind 1983).

CLASS II ANTIGEN EXPRESSION

In the context of an association between major histocompatibility complex class II (la) antigen expression and disease, both B/W and *lpr* mice are particularly interesting because they have been shown to exhibit an age-related increase in both the proportion and absolute number of la$^+$ macrophages and B-cells that parallel lymphoid hyperplasia and symptoms of lupus (Kelley and Roths 1982; Kofler *et al.* 1984). Further, T-cell involvement in autoimmunity has been demonstrated in several ways. For example, B-cells of lupus mice, as with normal B cells, require the presence of T-cell derived, accessory signals to proliferate and differentiate in response to exogenous antigen and *lpr* and B/W disease is prevented or inhibited by *in vivo* treatment with anti-la and T-cell monoclonal antibodies (Wofsy *et al.* 1986), as well as by neonatal thymectomy (Steinberg *et al.* 1980). Food restriction also normalizes several immune functions, particularly T-cell functions both in short-lived autoimmune-prone mice as well as in long-lived strains of mice and rats.

INTERLEUKIN-2 AND IL-2 RECEPTOR FUNCTIONS

Considerable progress has been made in characterizing T-cell and NK-cell functions, particularly membrane properties, in relation to their abilities to respond to various lymphokines with maximum cytolytic activity. IL-2 binding to its receptor has been found to drive cells into proliferation. Because IL-2 is a key immunomodulator, changes in its expression could be an important factor in age-related alterations in other immune cells, e.g., NK and Mϕ functions. In recent years, it has been shown that IL-2 produced by T cells in response to antigen and lectin stimulation causes expression of IL-2 receptors in other T-cells. Both IL-2 production and IL-2 receptor expression play a crucial role in both the etiologies and potential therapies of several diseases. In addition to its requirement in the culturing and cloning of T-cells, IL-2 potentiates the release of a number of other important lymphokines including γ-interferon, B-cell growth factor and B-cell differentiation factor (Smith 1984). IL-2 deficiency or defects in its production or function not only have been implicated in the aging process, but also in many pathological states such as congenital and acquired immunodeficiency, autoimmunity and cancer (Gillis *et al.* 1982; Dauphinee *et al.* 1981).

Although some studies have shown that cytotoxic/suppressor T-cells as well as helper T-cells can produce IL-2, IL-3, IL-4, IL-5, IL-6, etc., well-defined studies at the single-cell level indicate that helper T-cells are the major source of IL-2 (Miller 1983), whereas responding receptor-positive cells are found to be of the cytotoxic/ suppressor lineage. Several factors may modulate the availability of IL-2 and/or the expression of IL-2 receptors during aging or disease states. For example: (1) action of secreted IL-2 may be limited by an increase in the affinity of cellular receptors: thus, during aging, available IL-2 may be bound by fewer target cells (Robb *et al.* 1981); (2) serum inhibitor may appear during aging that neutralizes the IL-2 as its concentration declines; (3) IL-2 secretion may be down-regulated by an increase in suppressor cells (Gullberg and Larsson 1982) or by a loss in the expression of IL-2 receptor that may be an age-related phenomenon occurring at transcriptional level. We observed that in Fischer-344 rats (Masoro *et al.* 1982, Yu *et al.* 1985 and Chapter 8 in this book for details on feeding, housing and changes in several physiological parameters) *ad libitum* feeding not only causes a rapid reduction in the production of IL-2 during aging (Fig. 17.1) but also leads to a loss in responsiveness to recombinant IL-2. Similarly aged lymphocytes from food-restricted rats produced higher levels of IL-2 and responded more vigorously to IL-2, indicating that food restriction may act at the molecular level to prevent early loss in T-cell function (Fernandes *et al.* 1987a; Fernandes 1988).

We have observed that the ratio of helper to nonhelper T-cells remains constant until at least 18 months of age in Fischer-344 rats (Fig. 17.2–17.4). Our recent results of an increased IL-2 receptor expression in purified T-cells in food-restricted rats

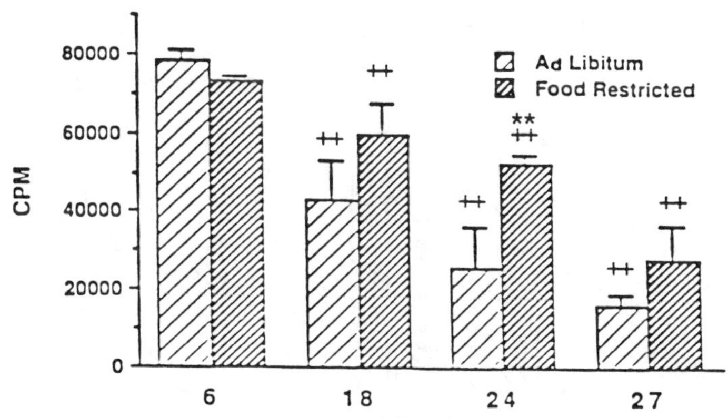

FIG. 17.1. EFFECT OF DIET ON IL-2 PRODUCTION BY SPLEEN CELLS

Spleen cells were cultured for 48 h. in the presence of Con-A and the supernatants were used to measure IL-2 activity against CTLL-1 cells

++ Significantly different from 6-month *ad libitum* fed control rats at < 0.05 level.

**Significantly different from age-matched *ad libitum* fed animals at < 0.05 level.

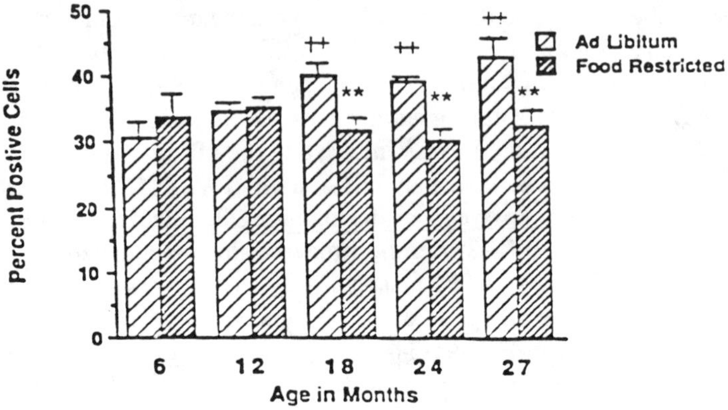

FIG. 17.2. PERCENT OX6 POSITIVE (la) SPLEEN CELLS
Viable spleen cells were analyzed with FACS instrument after staining with fluorescinated OX6 monoclonal antibody. When cells stained for various age groups, 6-month-old cells from *ad libitum* fed groups were used as controls

$^{++}$significantly different from 6-month-old *ad libitum* fed control rats at < 0.05 level.

**significantly different from same age *ad libitum* fed animals at < 0.05 level.

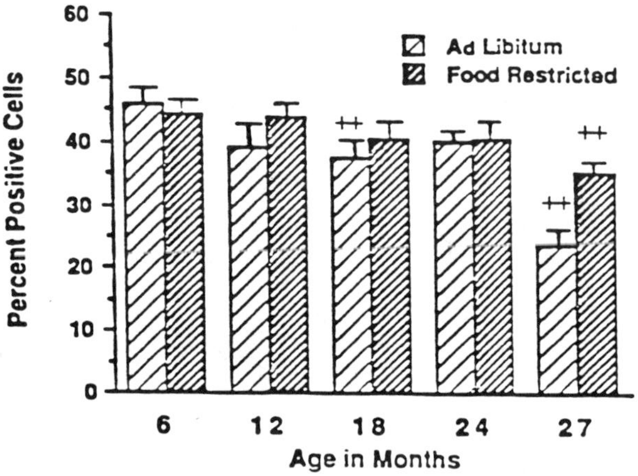

FIG. 17.3 W3/25^{+} HELPER T-CELLS
Spleen cells from Fischer-344 male rats fed *ad libitum* and food-restricted dietary regimens were analyzed with FACS instrument after staining with fluorescinated W3/25 monoclonal antibodies which stain only helper T-cells

$^{++}$significantly different from 6 month *ad libitum* fed control rats at < 0.05 level.

may, therefore, reflect a selective influence of food restriction on helper T-cell activation (Iwai and Fernandes 1989). Elevated T-cell functions were also observed in food-restricted rats in response to alloantigen with a low dose of rIL-2 (2×10^2U/mL) and in response to a high dose of rIL-2 (2×10^3U/mL). It has been reported that HA IL-2 receptor promotes the rapid receptor-mediated internalization of IL-2 receptor complex and that this internalization causes DNA synthesis and activation of several growth factor genes which ultimately induces mitosis in cells (Robb *et al.* 1984; Weissman *et al.* 1986). Our results so far suggest enhanced IL-2 receptor function in food-restricted animals may not allow spontaneous activation of oncogenes and thus could maintain a prolonged T-cell immune function in food-restricted rats (Iwai and Fernandes 1989).

MOLECULAR DEFECTS DURING AGING

Several recent studies have shown that dietary restriction begun at weaning age and continued throughout life extends the life span and maintains better immune function. Several reports indicate that the beneficial effects exerted by dietary manipulations may be due to a direct effect at the molecular level. For example, Leveille *et al.* (1984) reported age-related effects of dietary restriction on preventing the loss of soluble gamma crystallin. In addition, protein restriction showed an

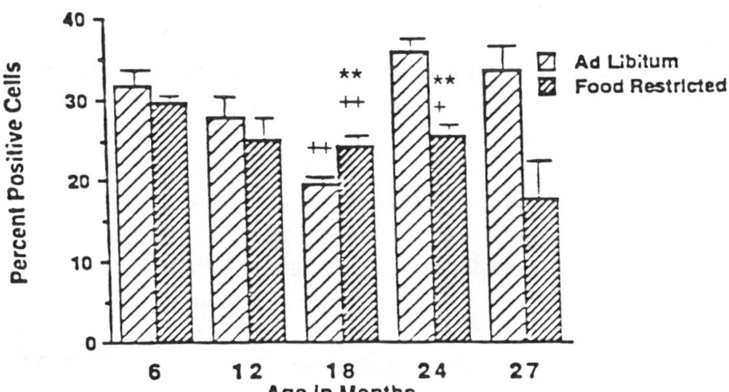

FIG. 17.4. PERCENT OX8 POSITIVE SUPPRESSOR T CELLS

Spleen cells from Fischer-344 male rats fed *ad libitum* and food-restricted dietary regimens were analyzed with FACS instrument after staining with fluorescinated OX8 monoclonal antibody which recognizes only nonhelper T cells.

++ significantly different from 6 month *ad libitum* fed control rats at < 0.05 level.

**significantly different from same age *ad libitum* fed animals at < 0.05 level.

effect on hepatic mRNA in azotemic rats; the effect was equally seen also on pair-fed controls, indicating that food restriction acts at transcriptional levels (Kinlaw *et al.* 1984). However, no effect of caloric restriction on immune function and longevity correlating with relevant mRNA levels has yet been established.

Several recent reports clearly establish the effect of aging on total RNA synthesis in a variety of rodent cells and tissues. Many studies have reported a 30–80% decline in RNA synthesis *in vivo* and *in vitro* for both mice and rats (Richardson 1985). More recent studies have further described both increases and decreases in the rates of synthesis of specific types of RNA (Merry *et al.* 1987). Recently, Richardson (1985) showed that the rate of poly $(A)^+$ RNA (mRNA) synthesis by hepatocytes declines significantly with increasing age. However, the amounts of poly $(A)^+$ RNA in the liver and the cell-free translational efficiency of poly $(A)^+$ RNA from the liver do not change with age. The age-related changes in levels of various mRNA species appeared to parallel changes seen in the levels of the proteins coded for by these mRNAs. For example: (1) the level of albumin mRNA and the synthesis of albumin by hepatocytes were both increased after 24 months of age; (2) the age-related decrease in α_{2u}-globulin protein in the liver; (3) the age-related decrease in IL-2 production in response to Con-A was found to be identical to the decrease in the induction of IL-2 mRNA, thus implying that transcription of mRNA may become defective as a function of age (Wu *et al.* 1986).

In a collaborative study with Richardson *et al.* (1987), we measured α_{2u}-globulin mRNA levels in the liver of 18-month-old *ad libitum* fed and food-restricted Fischer-344 rats. The results indicate that food restriction delays the loss of α_{2u}-globulin mRNA levels in the livers (see also Chapter 10 in this book). Furthermore, we completed a detailed molecular study with Chatterjee *et al.* (1989) which not only confirmed the loss of mRNAs for α_{2u}-globulin with age in *ad libitum* fed Fischer-344 rats and lesser loss in food-restricted rats, but also revealed changes in senescence marker protein (SMP-2) that was maintained at a much lower level in food-restricted rats. *Ad libitum* fed rats showed an age-associated rise for the SMP-2 protein confirming food restriction could have profound influence on modulating crucial mRNA levels in various tissues during aging. Although food restriction does not alter the ratio of T-cells, B-cells and macrophages, IL-1 production by macrophages in the spleen initially appears to be reduced, and IL-2 production by T-cells increased in food-restricted rats (unpublished data). Wu *et al.* (1986) reported that no age-related changes occurred in the size or rate of degradation or in the post-transcriptional processing of IL-2 mRNA in rats. The induction of IL-2 mRNA was, however, decreased by 85% at 28 months of age in rats. Our studies using phytohemagglutinins (PHA) and Con-A have shown an increased proliferative response to these two mitogens, as well as active IL-2 receptor activity, up to 27 months of age in food-restricted rats. It will be important to compare the effect of food restriction at various ages on IL-2 and for various oncogene mRNA levels in purified T-cells and IL-1 mRNA levels in aging macrophages.

The maintenance of competent cellular immune activity of T-cells (Table 17.1) and NK-cells in food-restricted rats parallels the survival rate of these rats (Fig.

TABLE 17.1
EFFECT OF AGING AND FOOD RESTRICTION IN FISCHER-344 RATS ON PROLIFERATIVE RESPONSE OF SPLEEN CELLS TO MITOGENS

Age	[^{3}H]-Thymidine Incorporation (CPM)							
	Media		PHA		Con A		BCM	
(Months)	AL	FR	AL	FR	AL	FR	AL	FR
6	7331	6330	54,745	78,121	101,179	113,746	17,101	27,243
12	2284	7960	35,752	60,899	77,021	96,480	12,439	19,845
18	4112	7041	33,034	98,850	126,731	208,442	14,412	41,526
24	735	920	35,367	85,532	53,985	143,713	6,454	14,092
27	573	1323	12,003	34,395	22,460	77,227	704	5,658

AL = *ad libitum*; FR = food restriction. PHA = phytohemagglutinin, Con A = concanavalin A, and BCM = B-cell mitogen. Values ± SEM (n = 6–8) are cpm ^{3}H-methyl-thymidine incorporated/5 × 10^5 cells/48 h culture. The stimulatory effects of food restriction reached significance ($P < 0.05$) with 18, 24, and 27-month-old rats.

17.5). The overall incidence of tumors is unchanged by food restriction (Maeda *et al.* 1985). However, *ad libitum* fed rats die with a chronic renal disease and with a variety of tumors between 18–30 months, and their immune function shows a rapid decline between 12–24 months of age. Similar tumor incidence appears in food-restricted rats between 30–43 months of age. We described briefly in a series of studies a dramatic reduction in immune function after 24 months of age in food-restricted rats (Fernandes *et al.* 1987a; Fernandes 1988). Thus, it can be implied that appearance of tumors and death are directly correlated with loss of T-cell and NK-cell activities in both groups of rats (Fig. 17.1 and 17.5).

AGING AND ONCOGENES

A few years ago, oncogenes were exclusively relegated to causing various types of tumors in both rodents and humans. This concept has changed dramatically after the realization that oncogene-coded protein products are involved in the functioning of normal cells from species as diverse as fruit flies and man (Weinberg 1985; Leder *et al.* 1986). This suggests that oncogenes are also involved in the control of cell division and metabolism. Some oncogenes are now known to code for enzymes with tyrosine kinase activity and others for growth factors, plasma-membrane receptors and/or nuclear DNA-binding substances. It is possible that oncogenes may become mutated and rearranged under the influence of an inappropriate environment, and cause abnormal immune function, eventually resulting in life-shortening diseases such as autoimmunity and cancer. It will, therefore, be useful to compare several oncogene mRNA levels between *ad libitum* fed and food-restricted rats. Our initial findings suggest that mRNA levels in the spleen of food-restricted rats is inversely correlated with immunity and extended life span. A recent report suggests increased NK activity against oncogene-activated target cells. In that study, transfection of

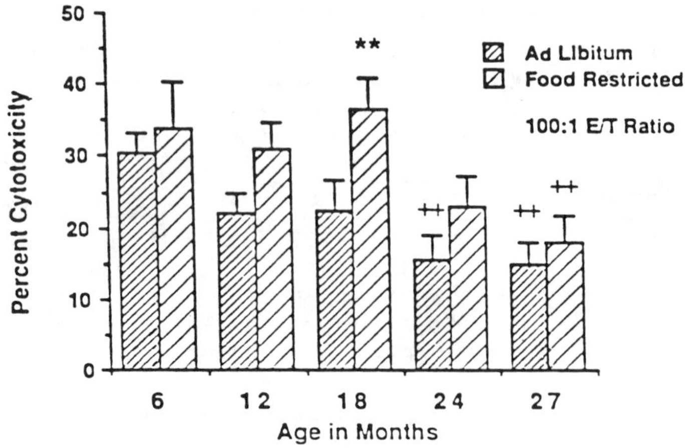

FIG. 17.5. NATURAL KILLER CELL ACTIVITY IN FISCHER RATS
Spleen cells were incubated with ^{51}Cr labelled YAC-1 tumor cells as targets (1:100 ratio) for 4 h and the supernatants were counted in a gamma counter to measure ^{51}Cr release

$^{++}$Significantly different from 6 month *ad libitum* fed control rats at < 0.05 level.

**significantly different from same age *ad libitum* fed animals at < 0.05 level.

the V-Ki-ras oncogene into rat fibroblasts yielded a cell line that was malignant, yet highly sensitive to lysis by NK cells (Johnson *et al.* 1985).

A more compelling reason to look for activation of oncogenes in lymphoid cells in aging rats is based on the findings of Maeda *et al.* (1985), that a significant proportion of tumors (20%) in aged food-restricted rats occurred in the lymphoreticular and hematopoietic systems, as compared to only 3% of the tumors in *ad libitum,* fed rats. *Ad libitum* feeding, on the other hand, showed an increased incidence of tumors in endocrine and other systems much earlier. It is generally known that food restriction lowers the incidence of several tumors, particularly hormone-dependent tumors. It may be of greater interest to follow the changes, if any, in a battery of oncogenes in lymphoid tissues of both dietary groups to identify any trend in mRNA levels occurring prior to the appearance of frank tumor growth. Our pilot studies have revealed changes in oncogene mRNA levels in spleen and liver of *ad libitum* fed rats. Spleen cells of food-restricted older rats show reduced oncogene mRNA expression compared to *ad libitum* fed rats. Reduced mRNA levels are not caused by decreased cell numbers, because lymphoid cell concentration does not vary with age. It is important, therefore, to compare changes in gene expression specifically to see if food restriction modulates activation of any specific oncogenes (viral or cellular) as a function of age, and/or preferentially inhibits oncogenes in a subpopulation of aging lymphoid cells (Ferrari *et al.* 1985; Boumpas *et al.* 1986; Reed *et al.* 1985; Heldin and Westermark 1984).

DIET AND AUTOIMMUNITY

Variations in the intake of specific dietary factors, including vitamins and trace metals, are known to influence the immune response (Fernandes *et al.* 1979; Chandra 1982; Biegel 1982), but only relatively recently has much attention been directed to the role of dietary fat. We reported back in 1972 the role of dietary fat on autoimmune disease in NZB mice (Fernandes *et al.* 1972). Since then several studies have described both protective and adverse effects of dietary lipids in autoimmune-prone animal systems. In the past, most studies were concerned with the regulation of immunocompetence by dietary modification of amounts on n-6 fatty acids, especially linoleic acid, which is present in high quantity in vegetable oil (safflower oil, corn oil, etc.). Diets enriched with these oils increase the level of linoleic acid in tissue phosphoglycerides and usually tend to elevate arachidonic acid levels (Johnson and Marshall 1984; Meade and Mertin 1978). Arachidonate is metabolized to other mediators including prostaglandins (PG), thromboxanes and leukotrienes which may all adversely affect immune function if chronically elevated. Elevated arachidonic acid metabolites levels may in turn alter binding and activity of hormones, peptide growth factors, neurotransmitters, and even those of food antigens to specific target tissues. Occupancy of such receptors is known to inhibit the production of active messengers including cAMP and cGMP; also, current interest is directed at messenger molecules derived from phosphoinositides such as arachidonate, inositol 1,4,5-triphosphate [Ins(1,4,5)P_3] and 1-2-diacylglycerol.

In contrast, feeding oils rich in n-3 fatty acids, such as fish oil or linseed oil, lowers the level of arachidonic acid in phosphoglycerides of tissue membranes, including those of macrophages (Johnson and Marshall 1984; Meade and Mertin 1978; Marshall and Johnson 1982). This would be expected to reduce PG production, not only by reducing the availability of substrate but also because activation of phospholipase will release n-3 polyunsaturated fatty acids. These acids will compete with the arachidonic acid cyclo-oxygenase pathway to reduce levels of the 2-series PG or even to lead to the formation of 3-series PG's with different biological activities. Nonetheless, due to higher risk of cardiovascular disease caused by saturated dietary fat intake, there has been a shift toward greater intake of dietary vegetable fats, thus promoting increased production of PGE_2 *in vivo*; this alone is most likely to decrease IL-2 production as well as to inhibit the response of T-cells to IL-2 (Goodwin and Ceuppens 1983). In addition, PGE_2 may enhance immunoglobulin production and appears to inhibit T-cell suppression of B-cell functions (Staite and Panayi 1986). Such adverse hormonal effects of polyunsaturated fats on normal lymphocytes and on autoimmune-prone mice have also been noted (Marshall 1987; Morrow *et al.* 1985; Levy *et al.* 1982; Leslie *et al.* 1985).

Years of study have indicated genetic, viral and various immunologic abnormalities in autoimmune animals (Talal and Steinberg 1974; Theofilopoulos and Dixon 1985). In humans, the concordance of lupus disease expression in identical twins is about 67% (Arnett and Schulman 1967). This implies that external factors must also influence the expression of this disease. Dietary effects on autoimmunity, therefore, require close scrutiny. In the case of RA and SLE in humans, however, the role of diet has not yet received great attention; nonetheless, in recent years both clinical and experimental studies have focused on the role of food antigens, lipids, and caloric content in modifying immune function (Panush *et al.* 1983; Gershwin *et al.* 1985; Fernandes *et al.* 1978; Fernandes 1984; Morrow and Levy 1983; Kelly and Izui 1983). Recently, intake of fish and/or fish oil supplemented diets have been found to protect against not only cardiovascular diseases but also autoimmune disease in humans and also animals (Dyerberg and Bang 1979; Thorngren and Gustafson 1981; Sanders *et al.* 1981; Prickett *et al.* 1981; Robinson *et al.* 1985; Leslie *et al.* 1985; Fernandes *et al.* 1987b; Fernandes 1987; Morrow *et al.* 1985; Fernandes *et al.* 1983; Hurd *et al.* 1981; Enig *et al.* 1978; Johnston 1985).

Our recent studies are directed toward identifying dietary fats which are less detrimental to the immune system and ameliorate renal and vascular disease. Several studies by others in autoimmune mice using either essential-fatty-acid-deficient (EFAD) saturated fat (coconut oil) or polyunsaturated fatty acids (PUFA) with an n-3 (n = Omega) double bond, such as fish oil, have demonstrated protective effects not seen with either vegetable PUFA fats (n-6), corn oil or safflower oil, or saturated animal fats (beef or lard) (Morrow *et al.* 1985; Fernandes *et al.* 1983; Hurd *et al.* 1981). Because PUFA lower cholesterol levels and protect against cardiovascular disease, considerably higher levels (8–10 times) of vegetable fat intake have been noted in recent years in the United States (Enig *et al.* 1978). As these fats do not protect against experimental autoimmune disease, the mechanism of protection seen with fish oil or coconut oil is considered to be mostly due to decreased production of immunosuppressive prostaglandins (PG) of the E series (Johnston 1985).

Changes in dietary fat intake can lead to profound alterations in physiological functions, including changes in cell membrane structure, fluidity and signal transduction. The exact mechanism by which dietary fatty acids become incorporated into cellular membranes is not known. Fatty acid components of ingested lipids are absorbed in the intestines as monoglycerides. Fatty acids become incorporated into lipoproteins after reesterification, and then enter the circulation. It is known that high intake of 18:2 n-6 leads to higher synthesis of PG (via cyclo-oxygenase) in stimulated tissues, whereas the effect of dietary 18:3 n-3 is primarily on the lipoxygenase pathway that results in increased leukotriene production (Johnston 1985).

DIETARY LIPIDS AND CALORIE RESTRICTION—EXPERIMENTAL EVIDENCE

During the past few years we have intensified our efforts to study the effect of the following high (20%) dietary fats on mice prone to develop autoimmune lupus disease: (1) saturated (lard); (2) polyunsaturated (corn oil); and (3) fish oil (Menhaden) with additional vitamin E (instead of 30 IU/kg of food we supplemented 250 IU/kg). Fatty acid composition of oils used in the present studies is given in Table 17.2.

TABLE 17.2
FATTY ACID COMPOSITION OF DIETARY FATS
USED IN OUR PRESENT STUDIES

Fatty Acid	No. Carbon Double Bond	Corn Oil	Fish Oil	Lard
Lauric	12:0	0.304	—	—
Myristic	14:0	0.240	8.090	1.302
Palmitic	16:0	10.972	18.835	24.741
Palmitoleic	16:1	—	12.372	3.001
Stearic	18:0	2.063	5.065	18.592
Oleic	18:1	26.776	15.148	40.333
Linoleic	18:2	58.270	5.062	9.693
Linolenic	18:3	1.304	1.672	0.794
Arachidonic	20:4	—	0.301	—
Eicosapentaenoic	20:5	—	15.208	—
Docosahexaenoic	22:6	—	11.038	—
Other		0.071	7.239	1.544

Source: Fernandes (1989).
Fatty Acid Analysis: Lipids from oils were extracted in 2:1 chloroform/methanol and fatty acids derivatized with methanolic-HC1. Fatty esters were determined by gas-liquid chromatography (Hewlett-Packard) using a fused silica capillary column.

These diets were compared to a control diet containing 5% corn oil (CO), as well as to a diet utilizing calorie restriction with supplemented vitamin E. Extensive studies were carried out using large groups of NZB×NZW F_1 mice (Fernandes *et al.* 1987; Fernandes *et al.* 1986). Only food-restricted mice showed significantly lower body weight. However, in the case of fish-oil fed mice, their body weight was closer to the other three groups, e.g., 5% CO, 20% CO and 20% lard-fed mice; yet the fish-oil fed mice lived as long as food restricted mice, whereas mice fed diets containing lard or corn oil 20% and 5% (normal caloric intake) or laboratory chow all died significantly earlier, indicating either food restriction or a diet containing fish oil is most effective in prolonging the life span of both female and male B/W mice (Fernandes 1989).

DIETARY LIPIDS AND IMMUNOLOGICAL MECHANISMS

While summarizing our immunological studies in B/W mice, we noticed a few striking findings that led us to establish and follow closely several new approaches toward understanding the immune mechanism by which dietary saturated and polyunsaturated fats can influence autoimmune disease and also the mechanism by which fish oil and/or food restriction are able to retard the disease. First, extensive fluorescence activated cell sorter (FACS) data analysis gathered for spleen cells revealed that loss of T-cells, particularly Lyt-2$^+$ or CD-8$^+$ cells, and increase in

B-cells (lg$^+$ or la$^+$) was significantly greater in mice fed high levels of corn oil and lard, whereas high levels of fish oil and/or food restricted mice showed fewer changes (Fernandes 1989). Secondly, the Ly1/B$^+$ cell population, which is linked to the production of autoantibodies in the sera of autoimmune-prone mice, was also much lower in fish-oil fed and food-restricted B/W mice, and the level of circulating anti-DNA antibodies was less in these mice (Fig. 17.6) (Fernandes 1989).

DIET AND SERUM HORMONE LEVELS

Because T-cells, particularly Lyt-2$^+$ (CD8$^+$) cells, are extremely sensitive to estrogen treatment (Ansar Ahmed *et al.* 1985), and B/W disease is known to be hormone-dependent, we measured serum hormone levels in B/W mice. The data showed increased prolactin levels ($P < 0.01$) and higher uterus weight (< 0.01) in B/W female mice, decreased testosterone levels ($P < 0.05$) in male mice in both 20% corn-oil and lard fed mice, whereas weight-matched, fish-oil fed mice showed lower prolactin and higher testosterone levels (Fernandes *et al.* 1987b). Since it was recently shown that prolactin significantly increases la antigen expression (Bernard *et al.* 1986) and our FACS data demonstrated increased la$^+$ cells in corn-oil and lard fed mice, we hypothesize that diet-induced prolactin elevation in 20% fat fed mice may be indirectly responsible for modulating la antigen expression in macro-

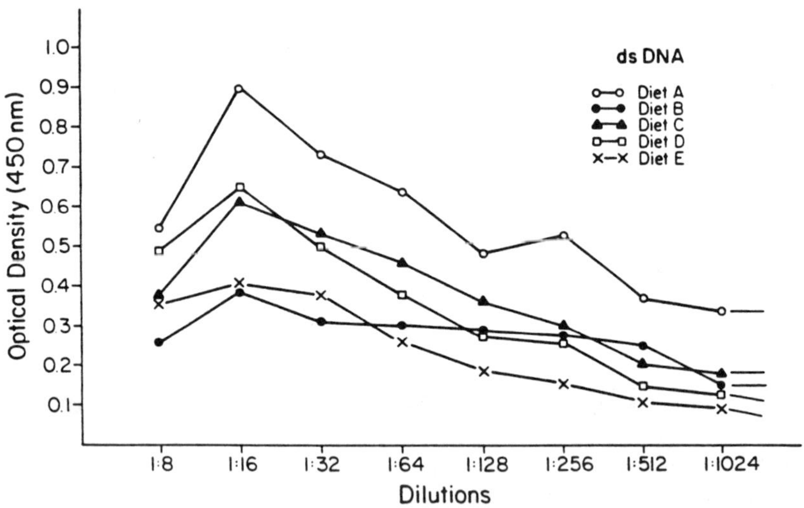

From Fernandes 1989

FIG. 17.6. EFFECT OF VARIOUS DIETS ON THE ANTI-ds DNA LEVELS IN THE SERUM OF B/W FEMALE MICE

Diet A (corn oil 5%, 20 cal.); Diet B (corn oil 5%, food restriction); Diet C (corn oil 20%); Diet D (lard 20%); Diet E (fish oil 20%). Please note less anti-ds DNA levels at 1:16 and 1:32 dilutions in Diet B and E groups.

phages and in B-cells. In addition, prolactin is an immunostimulatory polypeptide for T-lymphocytes (Spangelo *et al.* 1985). Furthermore, it is known that cyclosporin A can inhibit autoimmune disease in B/W mice (Israel-Biet 1983). Recently, not only the existence of prolactin receptor on T- and B-lymphocytes has been described, but cyclosporin has also been found to dramatically affect prolactin receptors (Russell *et al.* 1985). Thus, it is quite possible that fish oil may act similarly to cyclosporin treatment, thereby inhibiting prolactin action on lymphocytes in B/W mice. We have proposed that certain dietary fats appear to operate adversely, particularly on endocrine systems of genetically susceptible strains of mice. A similar mechanism could influence acceleration of various autoimmune diseases in humans as well. Indeed, carefully planned clinical studies are urgently required to clarify these issues further.

HISTOPATHOLOGICAL FINDINGS

It is a well-established fact that females in general have increased immune function compared to males. SLE is common in women during their active reproductive age. Indeed, SLE patients have higher estrogen and lower androgen levels, in addition to abnormal sex steroid metabolism (Lahita *et al.* 1982). Further, other factors, such as oral contraceptive and exogenous estrogens, have been implicated in increased risk of vascular diseases such as venous thromboembolism, stroke and myocardial infarcts (Wahl *et al.* 1983). One mechanism resulting in increased risk for myocardial infarction in RA and SLE may be increased serum triglyceride and cholesterol concentrations. We have observed high cholesterol levels in both female and male mice fed lard, as well as higher levels in mice fed corn oil. In contrast, both fish-oil

TABLE 17.3
EFFECT OF DIETARY FAT ON SERUM CHOLESTEROL LEVELS IN NZB×NZW F_1 MICE (AGE 5–10 MONTHS)

Diet	Sex	n	Cholesterol (mg/dL)
Corn oil 5%	F	23	160±19
	M	24	201±17
Corn oil 5% (R)	F	14	134±17
	M	21	140±7
Corn oil 20%	F	12	163±14
	M	10	221±26
Fish oil 20%	F	10	105±4
	M	12	115±6
Lard 20%	F	10	245±26
	M	11	357±36

Source: Fernandes (1989).
Cholesterol: Serum was analyzed for total cholesterol using Sigma diagnostic kits, measuring hydrogen peroxide produced from cholesterol and O_2 by the action of cholesterol oxidase.

fed and food-restricted mice showed significantly lower proteinuria and cholesterol levels (Fernandes *et al.* 1989) (Table 17.3). Histological studies clearly show severe glomerulosclerosis and periarteritis in kidneys of animals fed lard, and less so in fish-oil fed animals (Fig. 17.7 and 17.8). Thus, high prolactin and/or estrogen levels may be very important determinants leading to deleterious effects caused by diet in B/W mice. The oils which we used are similar to those consumed in human diets and contained no measurable estrogens.

OMEGA-3 FATTY ACIDS AND ANTIOXIDANTS

Although we noted significant protection of B/W disease afforded by fish oil, nonetheless our present experimental diets demonstrate marked variations in survival among different strains of animals. For example, B/W mice tolerated fish oil much better than C3H/*lpr* mice. However, C57BL/6 or C57BL/*lpr* mice were highly sensitive to fish oil, and the fish oil diet even caused premature deaths in some instances. Indeed, variable effects of food restriction and/or protein restriction on genetically different strains of mice on their survival was originally noted by us (Fernandes *et al.* 1976). This observation is recently confirmed by Harrison (see Chapter 9) and extended further for changes in immune and other physiological parameters. Our recent studies are directed to analyze fatty acid content in different tissues and

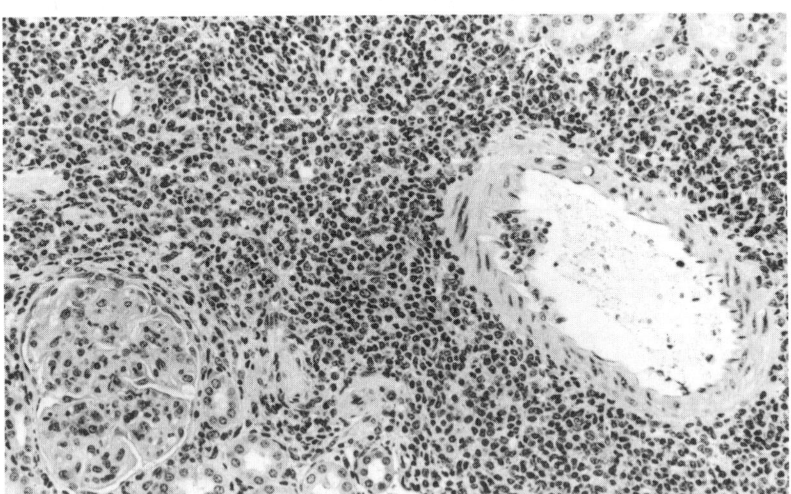

FIG. 17.7. HISTOPATHOLOGICAL PHOTOMICROGRAPH SHOWING MARKED INCREASE IN MESANGIAL CELLULARITY AND INCREASE IN MESANGIAL MATRIX OF GLOMERULUS AS WELL AS THE VESSEL SHOWING PERIVASCULAR INFILTRATE IN LARD-FED (20%) MICE (×50)

changes in the composition of lymphoid cells in plasma membranes in both rats and mice. Both a fish-oil diet and food restriction caused loss of 18:2, 20:4, increase in 20:5, 22:6 fatty acids (not only in spleen tissues [Table 17.4] but also in mitochondrial and microsomal membranes of liver cells), and increased malondialdehyde (MAD) metabolism (Laganiere and Fernandes 1987). The latter observations suggest a possible antioxidant deficiency in fish oil diets. Furthermore, measurement of vitamin E content in mitochondrial and microsomal membrane fractions confirmed that fish oil depletes vitamin E levels in the membranes. Finally, measurement of vitamin E in the serum further confirmed that fish oil causes a severe vitamin E deficiency, which may be the primary reason that we saw variations among strains in the past in the absence of additional vitamin E.

We also noted that, although mitogen-induced T- and B-cell responses were greatly increased in food-restricted mice, the fish-oil fed B/W mice showed less mitogen response and their natural killer cell (NK) activity was generally lower. This led us to test the effect of dietary lipids on resistance to viral infection, e.g., coxsackie B3. Experiments carried out with this virus indicated more deaths and increased myocarditis in fish-oil fed mice in the absence of additional vitamin E supplementation. Since low NK activity is correlated with elevated viral-induced lesions (Godeny and Gauntt 1986), it appears fish-oil containing diets can increase viral infections (Goodnight *et al.* 1982; Willis 1981). Thus, it is very important to supplement fish oil with adequate antioxidants to prevent viral infection induced by reduced NK.

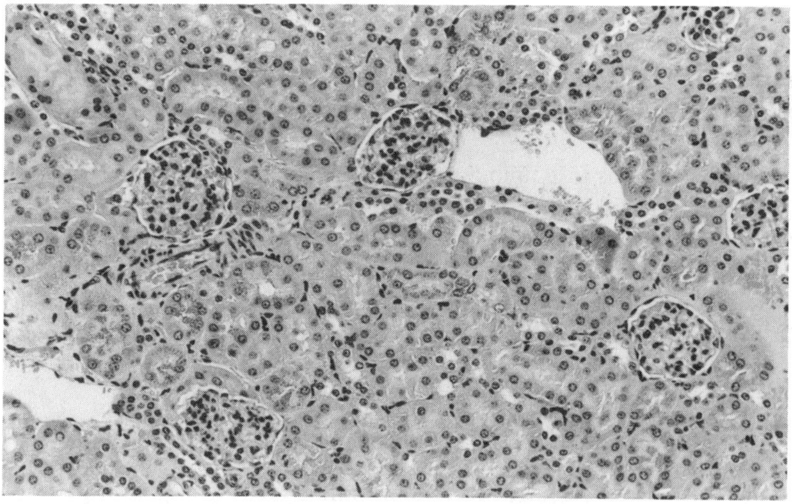

FIG. 17.8. PHOTOMICROGRAPH OF A KIDNEY SHOWING MINIMAL CHANGES IN CELLULARITY AND MESANGIAL MATRIX IN FISH OIL FED MICE (×50)

TABLE 17.4
FATTY ACID ANALYSIS OF SPLEENS FROM 11 MONTH B/W MALE MICE ON VARIOUS DIETS

Fatty Acid	No. Carbons Double Bond	CO 5%	CO 5%(R)	CO 20%	Lard 20%	Fish 20%
Lauric	12:0	—	—	—	—	—
Myristic	14:0	2.600	4.571	2.781	4.178	7.549
Palmitic	16:0	21.678	24.335	18.664	24.423	26.462
Palmitoleic	16:1	3.558	8.132	3.408	3.807	5.675
Stearic	18:0	11.823	7.290	5.443	10.858	8.475
Oleic	18:1	24.330	32.106	24.625	29.857	20.788
Linoleic	18:2	17.122	15.319	27.389	10.438	13.166
Linolenic	18:3	4.017	1.993	1.167	1.603	6.552
Arachidonic	20:4	14.807	6.215	16.542	14.835	3.346
Eicosapentaenoic	20:5	—	—	—	—	5.615
Docosahexaenoic	22:6	—	—	—	—	2.361

Source: Fernandes (1989).
Fatty Acid Analysis: Lipids for spleen tissue were extracted in 2:1 chloroform/methanol and fatty acids derivatized with methanolic-HC1. Fatty esters were determined by gas-liquid chromatography (Hewlett-Packard) using a fused silica capillary column.

DIETARY LIPIDS AND ONCOGENES

Recent studies show abnormal expression of several proto-oncogenes in autoimmune mice (Mountz *et al.* 1984). For example, increased c-myb expression was seen in T-cells of *lpr* mice, whereas significantly elevated c-myc, c-abl, and c-bas was noted in B-cells of most autoimmune mice. In contrast, B-cells with xid gene did not show elevated oncogene expression indicating that modulating a single gene may reduce interactions between oncogenes. We, therefore, compared oncogene expression in the spleens of autoimmune mice. Our data indicate changes in mRNA levels for different oncogenes in both fish-oil and corn-oil fed female B/W mice (Fig. 17.9). We have now expanded these studies in both female and male B/W mice on different diets, particularly fish-oil supplemented diets, with and without calorie restriction, to determine whether protection exerted by lipids is through their action on the expression of various oncogenes which encode growth factors.

PROSTAGLANDINS AND IL-2 RECEPTORS

Our ongoing studies clearly show that both food restriction and fish-oil supplemented diets have a profound influence on fatty acid composition of lymphoid cells, which indeed is known to influence prostaglandin E_2 levels. PG-E_2 is known to influence T-cell function. Our recent data shows that fish-oil supplemented diet

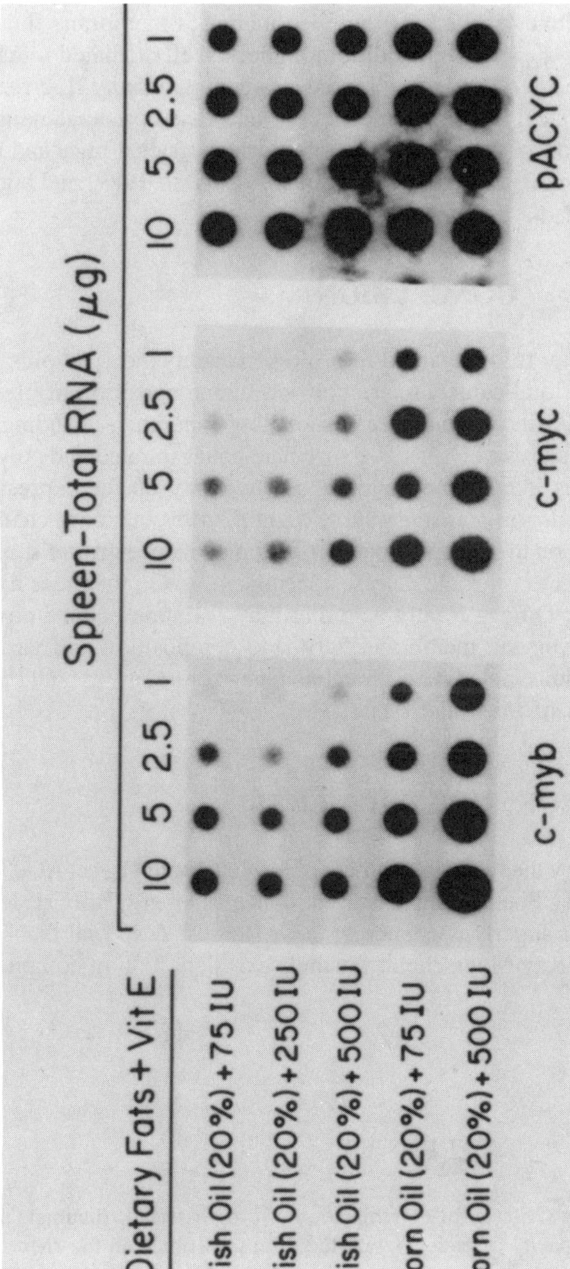

FIG. 17.9. DOT BLOT ANALYSIS OF mRNA LEVELS IN THE SPLEENS OF 8-MONTH-OLD B/W AUTOIMMUNE LUPUS-PRONE FEMALE MICE FED FISH OIL OR CORN OIL DIETS

mRNAS were hybridized with c-myb, c-myc and pACYC probes.

not only decreases serum cholesterol levels, but also increases membrane fluidity in spleen cells (Fernandes *et al.* 1989). In addition, higher T-cell mediated immune functions in fish oil-fed mice are related to decreased loss in high-affinity IL-2 receptors in spleen cells (unpublished data). It appears both decreased prostaglandin E_2 and increased IL-2 production in fish-oil fed and/or calorie-restricted mice and rats are related to the higher high-affinity IL-2 R functions (Iwai *et al.* 1989) and higher membrane fluidity (Gray *et al.* 1989).

CONCLUSION

Studies are now under way to understand the role of various dietary lipids and their restrictions, including total calorie restriction, on the composition of plasma membranes as well as changes in transmembrane signalling apparatus, including the mobilization of intracellular stores of Ca^{2+}. We speculate both saturated and polyunsaturated (n-6) dietary lipids induce abnormalities (1) not only on the expression of membrane antigens but also in transmembrane signalling by inducing changes in membrane fluidity and (2) on membrane proteins which may induce greater susceptibility in developing age-related chronic diseases during aging. On the other hand, both food restriction and/or Omega-3 fatty acid diet may maintain better immune response primarily by altering the membrane fatty acid composition and various growth factor receptor functions including differential gene expression in both short-lived and long-lived strains of mice and rats.

ACKNOWLEDGMENTS

This work was supported by the National Institute of Public Health Grants AG03417 and AG01188 and the Kleberg Foundation. Thanks to Lance Sandberg, Bill Friedricks and Vikram Tomar for their superb assistance in these studies. A special thanks to Dr. Jaya Venkatraman and Kay Meerscheidt for their excellent help in completing the manuscript.

REFERENCES

Am. Rheumatism Assoc. 1973. Criteria for determination of progression of rheumatoid arthritis and of functional capacity of patients with the disease: Primer on the rheumatic disease. JAMA *224*(Suppl.), 140.

ANDREWS, B. *et al.* 1978. Spontaneous murine lupus-like syndromes. Clinical and immunopathological manifestations in several strains. J. Exp. Med. *148*, 1198.

ANSAR AHMED, S., DAUPHINEE, M. J. and TALAL, N. 1985. Effects of short-term administration of sex hormones on normal and autoimmune mice. J. Immunol. *134*, 204.

ARNETT, F. C. and SHULMAN, L. E. 1976. Studies in familial systemic lupus erythematosus. Medicine *55*, 313.

BALOW, J. E. 1986. Lupus nephritis: natural history, prognosis and treatment. Clin. Immunol. Allergy *6*, 353.

BERNARD, D. J. *et al.* 1986. Effect of prolactin on Class II HLA antigen expression by MCF_7 cell line. Anticancer Res. *6*, 79.

BIEGEL, W. R. 1982. Single nutrients and immunity. Am. J. Clin. Nutr. *35*, 417.

BOUMPAS, D. T., MARK, G. E. and TSOKOS, G. C. 1986. Oncogenes and autoimmunity. Anticancer Res. *6*, 491.

CHANDRA, R. K. and NEWBERNE, P. M. 1977. Nutrition, Immunity and Infection. Plenum Press, New York.

CHANDRA, R. K. 1982. Trace elements and immune response. Immunol. Today *4*, 322.

CHATTERJEE, B. *et al.* 1989. Calorie restriction delays age-dependent loss in androgen responsiveness of the rat liver. FASEB J. *3*, 6799.

DAUPHINEE, M. J., KIPPER, S. B., WOFSY, D. and TALAL, N. 1981. Interleukin 2 deficiency is a common feature of autoimmune mice. J. Immunol. *127*, 2483.

DORF, M. E. and BENACERRAF, B. 1984. Suppressor cells and immunoregulation. Ann. Rev. Immunol. *2*, 127.

DYERBERG, J. and BANG, H. O. 1979. Haemostatic function and platelet polyunsaturated fatty acids in Eskimos. Lancet *2*, 433.

ENIG, M. G., MUNN, R. J. and KEENEY, M. 1978. Dietary fat and cancer trends—a critique. Fed. Proc. Fed. Am. Soc. Exp. Biol. *37*, 2215.

FERNANDES, G. 1984. Nutritional factors: modulating effects on immune function and aging. Pharm. Rev. *36*, 123S.

FERNANDES, G. 1987. Influence of nutrition on autoimmune disease. *In* Aging and the Immune Response: Cellular and Humoral Aspects, E. A. Goidl (ed.). Marcel Dekker, New York.

FERNANDES, G. 1988. A possible link between prolactin and immune function or prolongation of life span of SPF Fischer-344 male rats by food restriction. FASEB J. *2*, 5305.

FERNANDES, G. 1989. Effect of dietary fish oil supplement on autoimmune disease: Changes in lymphoid cell subsets, oncogene mRNA expression and neuroendocrine hormones. *In* Health Effects of Fish and Fish Oils, R. Chandra (ed.). ARTS Biomedical Publishers, St. John's, Newfoundland.

FERNANDES, G. *et al.* 1972. Dietary influence on breeding behavior, hemolytic anemia and longevity in NZB mice. Proc. Soc. Exp. Biol. Med. *139*, 1189.

FERNANDES, G. *et al.* 1979. Impairment of cell-mediated immunity functions by dietary zinc deficiency in mice. Proc. Natl. Acad. Sci. *76*, 457.

FERNANDES, G. *et al.* 1983. Influence of diet on vascular lesions in autoimmune-prone B/W mice. Proc. Nat. Acad. Sci. *80*, 876.

FERNANDES, G. *et al.* 1987a. Effect of food restriction and aging on immune cell fatty acids, functions and oncogene expression in SPF Fischer-344 rats. Fed. Proc. *46*, 567a.

FERNANDES, G. *et al.* 1987b. A possible link between dietary fats, hormonal changes and immunological dysfunction in lupus-prone B/W mice. Arthritis Rheum. *30*, S123.

FERNANDES, A. *et al.* 1989. Effect of animal, vegetable and fish oil on serum cholesterol and vitamin-E levels and survival ratio (NZB$\times$NZW) F_1 mice. Fed. Proc. *3*, 4217a.

FERNANDES, G., FRIEND, P. Y., UNIS, E. J. and GOOD, R. A. 1978. Influence of dietary restriction on immunologic function and renal disease in B/W mice. Proc. Nat. Acad. Sci. *75*, 1500.

FERNANDES, G. and SANDBERG, L. E. 1986. Age-related changes in the immune function in SPF Fischer-344 male rats fed six different diets designed to analyze the various effects of food restriction in delaying the aging process. Fed. Proc. *45*, 830 (Abstr. 3929).

FERNANDES, G., SANDBERG, L., KHARE, A. and TROYER, D. 1986. Comparison of calorie restriction against high dietary fats of animal and fish origin on murine lupus disease. Arthritis Rheum. *30*, 172.

FERNANDES, G., YUNIS, E. J. and GOOD, R. A. 1976. Influence of diet on survival of mice. Proc. Natl. Acad. Sci. *73*, 1279.

FERRARI, A. *et al.* 1985. Study of the levels of expression of two oncogenes c-myc and c-myb in acute and chronic leukemia of both lymphoid and myeloid lineage. Leukemia Res. *9*, 833.

GERSHWIN, M. E., BEACH, R. S. and HURLEY, L. S. 1985. Lipids, Nutrition and Immunity. Academic Press, Orlando.

GILLIS, S., KOZAK, R., DURANTE, M. and WEKSLER, M. E. 1982. Immunologic studies of aging: Decreased production of and response to T-cell growth levels from aged humans. J. Clin. Invest. *67*, 937.

GODENY, E. K. and GAUNTT, C. J. 1986. Involvement of natural killer cells in coxsackievirus B3-induced murine myocarditis. J. Immunol. *137*, 1695.

GOODNIGHT, S. H. *et al.* 1982. Polyunsaturated fatty acids, hyperlipidemia and thrombosis. Arteriosclerosis *2*, 87.

GOODWIN, J. S. and CEUPPENS, J. 1983. Regulation of the immune response by prostaglandins. J. Clin. Immunol. *3*, 295.

GULLBERG, M. and LARSSON, E. L. 1982. Studies on induction and effector functions of concanavalin A-induced suppressor cells that limit TCGF production. J. Immunol. *128*, 746.

GRAY, P., IWAI, H., TOMAR, V. and FERNANDES, G. 1989. Modulation of membrane fluidity of spleen cells by food restriction. FASEB J. *3*, 1370a.

HATMAN, L. J. and KAYDEN, H. J. 1979. A high performance liquid chromatography for the determination of tocopherol in plasma and cellular elements of the blood. J. Lipid Res. *20*, 639.

HELDIN, C. H. and WESTERMARK, B. 1984. Growth factors. Mechanism of action and relation on oncogenes. Cell *37*, 9.

HOMSY, J., MORROW, W. J. W. and LEVY, J. A. 1986. Nutrition and autoimmunity: A review. Clin. Exp. Immunol. *65*, 473.

HURD, E. R. *et al.* 1981. Prevention of glomerulonephritis and prolonged survival in New Zealand Black/New Zealand White F_1 hybrid mice fed an essential fatty acid-deficient diet. J. Clin. Invest. *67*, 476.

ISRAEL-BIET, D. *et al.* 1983. Marked reduction of DNA antibody production and glomerulopathy in thymulin (FTS-Zn) or cyclosporin A treated (NZB×NZW) F_1 mice. Clin. Exp. Immunol. *54*, 359.

IWAI, H. and FERNANDES, G. 1989. Immunological functions in food-restricted rats: Enhanced expression of high-affinity interleukin-2 receptors on splenic T-cells. Immunol. Lett. *23*, 125.

JOHNSON, P. W., BAUBOCK, C. and RODER, J. C. 1985. Transfection of a rat cell line with the V-Ki-ras oncogene is associated with enhanced susceptibility to natural killer cell lysis. J. Exp. Med. *162*, 1732.

JOHNSON, P. V. and MARSHALL, L. A. 1984. Dietary fat, prostaglandins and the immune response. Prog. Food Nutr. Sci. *8*, 3.

JOHNSON, P. V. 1985. Dietary fat, eicosanoids, and immunity. Adv. Lipid Res. *21*, 103.

KELLEY, V. E. and IZUI, S. 1983. Enriched lipid diet accelerates lupus nephritis in NZB×W mice. Synergistic action of immune complexes and lipid in glomerular injury. Am. J. Pathol. *111*, 288.

KELLEY, V. E. and ROTHS, J. B. 1982. Increase in macrophage la expression in autoimmune mice. Role of *lpr* gene. J. Immunol. *129*, 923.

KINLAW, W. B. *et al.* 1984. Hepatic messenger ribonucleic acid activity profiles in experimental azotemia in the rat. Relationship to food intake and thyroid function. J. Clin. Invest. *74*, 1936.

KOFLER, R., SCHREIBER, R. D., DIXON, F. J. and THEOFILOPOULOS, A. N. 1984. Macrophage la expression production of and response to macrophage stimulation lymphokines in murine lupus strains. Cell Immunol. *87*, 92.

LAGANIERE, S. and FERNANDES, G. 1987. High peroxidizability of subcellular membrane induced by high fish oil diet is reversed by vitamin E. Clin. Res. *35*, 565a.

LAHITA, R. G., BRADLOW, L., FISHMAN, J. and KUNKEL, H. G. 1982. Estrogen metabolism in systemic lupus erythematosus: patients and family members. Arthritis Rheum. *25*, 843.

LEDER, A. *et al.* 1986. Consequence of widespread deregulation of the c-myc gene intransgenic mice: Multiple neoplasms and normal development. Cell *45*, 485.

LESLIE, C. A. *et al.* 1985. Dietary fish oil modulates macrophage fatty acids and decreases arthritis susceptibility in mice. J. Exp. Med. *162*, 1336.

LEVEILLE, P. J. *et al.* 1984. Dietary restriction retards age-related loss of gamma crystallins in the mouse lens. Science *224*, 1247.

LEVY, J. A. *et al.* 1982. Dietary fat affects immune response, production of antiviral factors and immune complex disease in (NZB×NZW) F_1 mice. Proc. Natl. Acad. Sci. USA *79*, 1974.

LEVY, R. I. and MOSKOWITZ, J. 1982. Cardiovascular research: decades of progress, a decade of promise. Science *217*, 121.

MAEDA, H. *et al.* 1985. Nutritional influences on aging of Fischer-344 rats: II pathology. J. Gerontol. *40*, 671.

MAKINODAN, T. and KAY, M. M. B. 1980. Age influence on the immune system. Adv. Immunol. *29*, 287.

MARSHALL, L. A. and JOHNSON, P. V. 1982. Modulation of tissue prostaglandins synthesizing capacity by increased ratios of dietary alpha-linolenic acid to linoleic acid. Lipids *17*, 905.

MARSHALL, P. 1987. Lymphocyte hormone receptors. Ann. Rev. Immunol. *5*, 621.

MASORO, E. J., YU, B. P. and BERTRAND, H. A. 1982. Action of food restriction in delaying the aging process. Proc. Natl. Acad. Sci. *79*, 4239.

MEADE, G. F. J. and MERTIN, J. 1978. Fatty acids and immunity. Adv. Lipid Res. *16*, 127.

MERRY, B. J., HOLEHAN, A. M., LEWIS, S. E. M. and GOLDSPINK, D. F. 1987. The effects of aging and chronic dietary restriction on *in vivo* hepatic protein synthesis in the rat. Mech. Ageing Dev. *39*, 189.

MILLER, R. A. 1983. IL-2 production by mitogen-stimulated T-cell subsets: helper-precursors are predominantly Lyt-2-. J. Immunol. *131*, 2864.

MORROW, W. J. W. and LEVY, J. A. 1983. Dietary regulation of the autoimmune process in murine lupus. Immunol. Today *4*, 249.

MORROW, W. J. W. *et al.* 1985. Dietary fat and immune function. I. Antibody responses, lymphocytes and accessory cell function in (NZB×NZW) F_1 mice. J. Immunol. *135*, 3857.

MOUNTZ, J. D. *et al.* 1984. Autoimmunity and increased c-myb transcription. Science *226*, 1087.

National Research Council (Comm. on Diet, Nutr. and Cancer, Assem. of Life Sci.). 1982. Diet, Nutrition and Cancer. National Academy Press, Washington, D. C.

PANUSH, R. S. *et al.* 1983. Diet therapy for rheumatoid arthritis, Arthritis Rheum. *26*, 462.

PRICKETT, J. D., ROBINSON, D. R. and STEINBERG, A. D. 1984. Dietary enrichment with the polyunsaturated fatty acid eicosapentaenoic acid prevents proteinuria and prolongs survival in NZB×NZW F_1 mice. J. Clin. Invest. *68*, 556.

REED, J. NOWELL, P. C. and HOOVER, R. G. 1985. Regulation of c-myc in RNA levels in normal human lymphocytes by modulators of cell proliferation. Proc. Natl. Acad. Sci. USA *82*, 4221.

RICHARDSON, A. 1985. The effect of age and nutrition on protein synthesis by cells and tissue from mammals. *In* Handbook of Nutrition in the Aged, R. R. Watson (ed.). CRC Press, Boca Raton.

RICHARDSON, A. *et al.* 1987. Effect of age and dietary restriction on the expression of α_{2u}-globulin. J. Biol. Chem. *262*, 12821.

ROBB, R. J., GREENE, W. C. and RUSK, M. C. 1984. Low and high affinity cellular receptors for interleukin-2: Implications for the level of Tac antigen. J. Exp. Med. *160*, 1126.

ROBB, R. J., MUNCK, A. and SMITH, K. A. 1981. T-cell growth factor receptors. Quantitation, specificity, and biological relevance. J. Exp. Med. *154*, 1455.

ROBINSON, D. R. *et al.* 1985. The protective effect of dietary fish oil on murine lupus. Prostaglandins *30*, 51.

RUSSELL, D. H. *et al.* 1985. Prolactin receptors on human T- and B-lymphocytes: antagonism of prolactin binding of cyclosporin. J. Immunol. *134*, 3027.

SANDERS, T. A. B. , VICKERS, M. and HAINES, A. P. 1981. Effect on blood lipids and haemostasis of a supplement of cod-liver oil, rich in eicosapentaenoic acid and docosahexaenoic acids, in healthy young men. Clin. Sci. *61*, 317.

SMITH, H. R. and STEINBERG, A. D. 1983. Autoimmunity—a perspective. Ann. Rev. Immunol. *1*, 175.

SMITH, K. A. 1984. Interleukin-2. Ann. Rev. Immunol. *2*, 319.

SPANGELO, B. L., HALL, N. A. and GOLDSTEIN, A. L. 1985. Evidence that prolactin is an immunomodulatory hormone in prolactin, basic and clinical correlates. Fidia Res. Ser. *1*, 342.

STAITE, N. D. and PANAYI, G. S. 1986. Prostaglandin regulation of B-lymphocyte function. Immunol. Today *5*, 175.

STEINBERG, A. D. and DECKER, J. L. 1974. A double-blind controlled trial containing cyclophosphamide, azathioprine, and placebo in the treatment of lupus glomerulonephritis. Arthritis Rheum. *17*, 923.

STEINBERG, A. D. *et al.* 1980. Effects of thymectomy or androgen administration upon the autoimmune disease of MRL/MP/*lpr*/*lpr* mice. J. Immunol. *125*, 871.

TALAL, N. and STEINBERG, A. D. 1974. The pathogenesis of autoimmunity in NZB mice. Curr. Top. Microbiol. Immunol. *64*, 79.

TAM, C. F. and WALFORD, R. L. 1978. Cyclic nucleotide levels in resting and mitogen-stimulated spleen cell suspensions from young and old mice. Mech. Aging Rev. *7*, 309.

THEOFILOPOULOS, A. N. and DIXON, F. J. 1985. Murine models of systemic lupus erythematosus. Adv. Immunol. *37*, 269.

THEOFILOPOULOS, A. N., SHAWLER, D. L. EISENBERG, R. A. and DIXON, F. J. 1980. Splenic immunoglobulin secreting cells and their regulation in autoimmune mice. J. Exp. Med. *151*, 446.

THORNGREN, M. and GUSTAFSON, A. 1981. Effects of 11-week increases in dietary eicosapentaenoic acid on bleeding time, lipids, and platelet aggregation. Lancet *11*, 1190.

WAHL, P. *et al.* 1983. Effect of estrogen/progestin potency on lipid/lipoprotein cholesterol. N. Engl. J. Med. *308*, 862.

WALFORD, R. L. *et al.* 1981. The immunopathology of aging. *In* Annual Review of Gerontology and Geriatrics, Vol. 2, C. Eisdorfer *et al.* (eds.). Springer Publishing Co., New York.

WEKSLER, M. E. and SISKIND, G. W. 1983. The cellular basis of immune senescence. Monogr. Dev. Biol. *17*, 110.

WEINDRUCH, R. H. *et al.* 1979. Influence of controlled dietary restriction on immunologic function and aging. Fed. Proc. *38*, 2007.

WEINBERG, R. A. 1985. The action of oncogenes in the cytoplasm and nucleus. Science *230*, 770.

WEISSMAN, A. M. *et al.* 1986. Only high-affinity receptors for interleukin-2 mediate internalization of ligand. Proc. Nat. Acad. Sci. USA *83*, 1463.

WILLIS, A. L. 1981. Nutritional and pharmacological factors in eicosanoid biology, Nutr. Rev. *39*, 289.

WOFSY, D., HARDY, R. R. and SEAMAN, W. F. 1986. The proliferating cells in autoimmune MRL/*lpr* mice lack L3T4, an antigen or "helper" T-cells that is involved in the response to class II major histocompatibility antigens. J. Immunol. *132*, 2686.

WU, W., PAHLAVANI, M., CHEUNG, H. T. and RICHARDSON, A. 1986. The effect of aging on the expression of interleukin-2 messenger ribonucleic acid. Cell Immunol. *100*, 224.

YU, B. P., MASORO, E. J. and McMAHAN, C. A. 1985. Nutritional influences in aging Fischer-344 rats: physical, metabolic and longevity characteristics. J. Gerontol. *40*, 657.

SECTION V

Nutritional Influences on Aging of the Central Nervous System

CHAPTER 18

EFFECTS OF DIETARY RESTRICTION ON BRAIN AND BEHAVIORAL FUNCTION IN AGING RODENTS

DONALD K. INGRAM, Ph.D.
Molecular Physiology and Genetics Section
Laboratory of Cellular and Molecular Biology
Nathan W. Shock Laboratories
Gerontology Research Center[1]
National Institute on Aging
Francis Scott Key Medical Center
Baltimore, Maryland

INTRODUCTION

When the caloric intake of postweaning or mature laboratory rodents is reduced up to 50% below *ad libitum* levels for a major portion of their life span, mean and maximum life span can be incremented substantially (Barrows and Kokkonen 1984; Weindruch and Walford 1988). Many different regimens of dietary restriction (DR), including reduced caloric content, increased fiber, or intermittent feeding can be used to reduce caloric intake with similar beneficial results on survival (Weindruch and Walford 1988).

The robust effect of DR on mortality rates is suggested as evidence that the rate of aging can be altered by nutritional means (Sacher 1977; Schneider and Reed 1985; Weindruch and Walford 1988). Additional evidence of this possibility has been provided in a great variety of studies documenting that DR can retard the development of age-related pathology and age-related changes in many genetic, biochemical, endocrinological, and physiological parameters (Weindruch and Walford 1988).

[1]The Gerontology Research Center is fully accredited by the American Association for the Accreditation of Laboratory Animal Care.

When compared to the numerous investigations of the effects of DR on aging in various cell and organ systems, relatively less attention has been paid to the effects of this manipulation on aging in the central nervous system and behavioral consequences (Forbes 1980). Investigation of these effects is important to understanding this phenomenon for several reasons. First, demonstration that age-related decline in specific behavioral and brain function can be retarded would be additional evidence that DR can alter aging rate without having to rely upon collection of mortality data. To this end, much of the behavioral assessment could be accomplished in a noninvasive manner. Second, assessment of brain and behavioral function in animals undergoing DR addresses the issue of *quality* versus *quantity* of life. Some gerontologists have expressed concerns about the potential detrimental effects of DR upon behavioral capacities (Moment 1978). After all, protein-calorie deprivation has been a traditional research subject pertaining to its potentially harmful effects on brain development and behavior (Morgane *et al.* 1978). Therefore, psychobiological analysis of DR in young and aged animals is needed to address these concerns. Finally, recent reviews considering mechanisms of the prolongevity effects of DR in rodents have indicated the possibility for a critical role of centrally mediated neuroendocrine regulation of the phenomenon (Masoro 1988; Weindruch and Walford 1988). Thus, research on mechanisms underlying the effects of DR on aging processes may proceed down neurobiological avenues for answers.

EFFECTS OF DIETARY RESTRICTION ON SURVIVAL

Table 18.1 summarizes data from our laboratory pertaining to the robust effects on longevity observed in rats and mice associated with a regimen of intermittent feeding (Ingram and Reynolds 1987). When the diet (NIH-07; 4.2 kcal/g) is provided every other day (EOD) from weaning, food consumption is reduced (15–30%), and mean life span is incremented, markedly in some cases, compared to counterparts provided the diet *ad libitum* (AL). This effect on survival is also noted in many rodent strains when initiated in adult animals (Ingram and Reynolds 1987). Many of the data to be presented in this review will pertain to the EOD regimen of DR.

EFFECTS OF DIETARY RESTRICTION ON BEHAVIOR

Psychomotor Performance in C57BL/6J Mice

To assess the effects of EOD feeding on behavioral aging, we first examined the performance of male C57BL/6J mice (B6) in a battery of psychomotor tests (Ingram 1983, 1984, 1987). Procedural details have been described previously (Ingram 1983). The correlation of performance in each test with chronological age from a large sample of AL-fed mice is shown in Fig. 18.1 and 18.2. In general, the tests exhibited a relatively high correlation with age (Ingram 1983), demonstrated signifi-

TABLE 18.1
PERCENT CHANGE IN MEAN LIFE SPAN OF GROUPS FED EVERY OTHER DAY OVER *AD LIBITUM* CONTROLS

Rodent Strain[1]	Starting Age (Months)	Change in Mean Life Span (%)
Wistar rats	1.5	82
	10.5	34
	18.0	11
C57BL/6J mice	1.5	27
	6.0	10
	10.0	0
$B6AF_1$ mice	1.5	20
	6.0	19
	10.0	0
A/J mice	1.5	12
	6.0	2
	10.0	−14

[1]All animals were males fed NIH-07 diet.

cant test-retest reliability among aged mice (Ingram 1983), and indicated evidence of predictive validity when future performance or life span were used as criteria (Ingram and Reynolds 1986). However, certain tests were better than others, and considerable variability in test results still existed such that chronological age often cannot account for the majority of variance in performance across the life span (Ingram 1983).

Representative survival curves of B6 mice that had been on the AL diet since weaning or on EOD feeding since 6 months of age are compared in Fig. 18.3 (Talan and Ingram 1985). The EOD regimen significantly increased survival with an 11% increase in mean life span. Thus, this was not a marked prolongevity effect as observed with DR begun at younger ages or in other genotypes or with other regimens. Dietary intake was reduced by about 30% in young (8 month) mice and by about 15% in aged (26 month) animals (Talan and Ingram 1985). The objective of the behavioral assessment was to determine if tests in the psychomotor battery were sensitive enough to detect differences between AL- and EOD-fed groups at older ages near the median life span for these mice but before substantial mortality was manifested (Ingram 1983, 1984).

Comparisons in Fig. 18.4 indicate that every test except grip strength was sensitive to the diet manipulation when assessed relatively late in life. Aged B6 mice that had been fed EOD since 6 months of age exhibited significantly ($P < 0.05$, according to two-tailed t-tests) greater suspension time in the tightrope test, less falls in the rotorod test, and greater locomotor activity in the exploratory and runwheel tests.

Similar results in psychomotor performance have been observed in F-344 rats begun on an EOD regimen at 12 months of age. Campbell and Gaddy (1987) reported

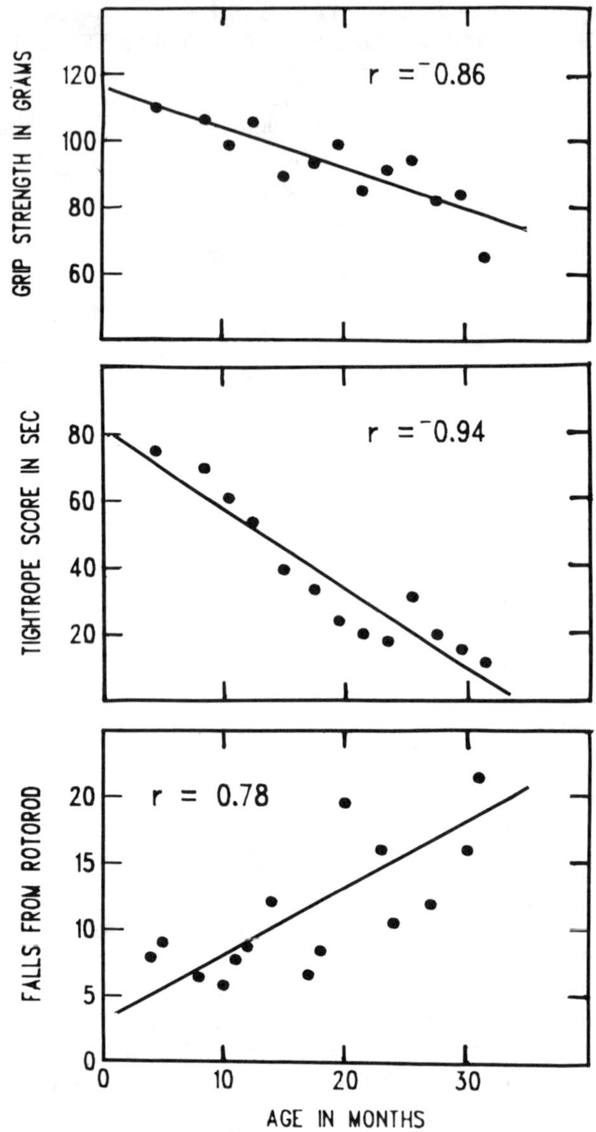

FIG. 18.1. CORRELATION OF AGE WITH PERFORMANCE OF MALE C57BL/6J MICE IN GRIP STRENGTH (MEAN OF 3 TRIALS), TIGHTROPE (MEAN OF 3, 60-S TRIALS), AND ROTOROD (TOTAL NUMBER OF FALLS DURING 3-MIN EXPOSURE TO ROTOROD AT 3 RPM) TESTS

Each point represents mean for 15–20 mice.

superior performance of DR rats compared to AL controls in wire suspension, plank walk, and pole descent tasks. Harrison and Archer (1987) also noted significant effects of DR in open field and tight wire tasks conducted for adult (9–13 months) and aged (25–27 months) C56BL/6J and B6CBAF$_1$/J mice begun on DR (about 33% of control level) at weaning.

Intervening Variables

Do these behavioral effects reflect that aging rate had been altered by DR? The answer to this question is not straightforward. Variables that intervene on such comparisons of psychomotor performance include group differences in body weight, motivational levels, and disease factors. Moreover, Harrison and Archer (1987) noted

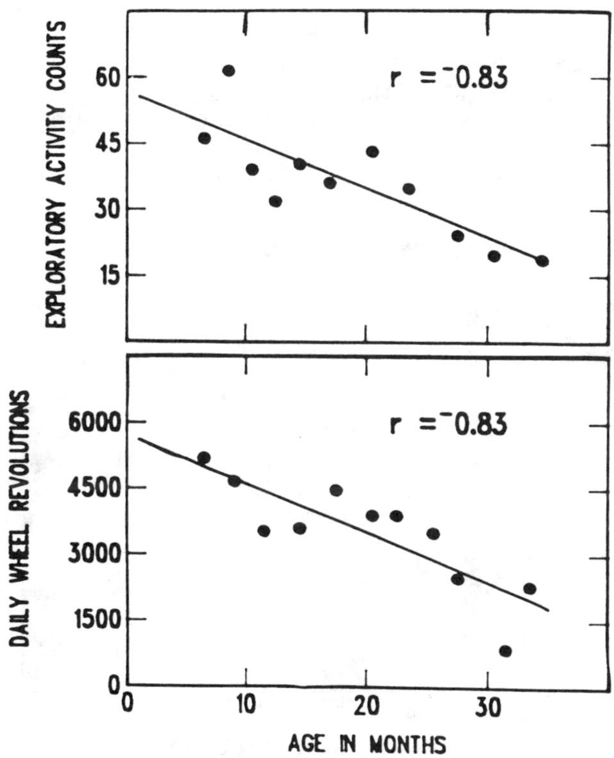

FIG. 18.2. CORRELATION OF AGE WITH PERFORMANCE OF MALE C57BL/6J MICE IN EXPLORATORY ACTIVITY (10 MIN IN OVAL RUNWAY UNDER DIM ILLUMINATION) AND RUNWHEEL (72-H EXPOSURE) TESTS

Each point represents mean for 15–20 mice.

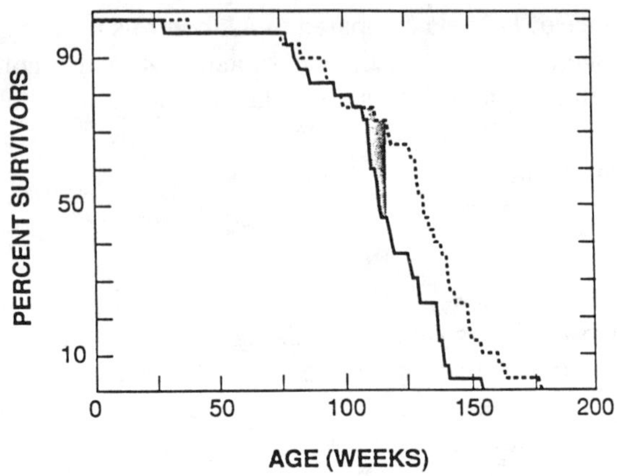

FIG. 18.3. SURVIVAL DISTRIBUTION OF MALE C57BL/6J MICE FED *AD LIBITUM* (SOLID LINE) OR EVERY OTHER DAY (DOTTED LINE) BEGINNING AT 6 MONTHS OF AGE (N = 40 MICE)

Hashed area represents ages at which testing occurred.

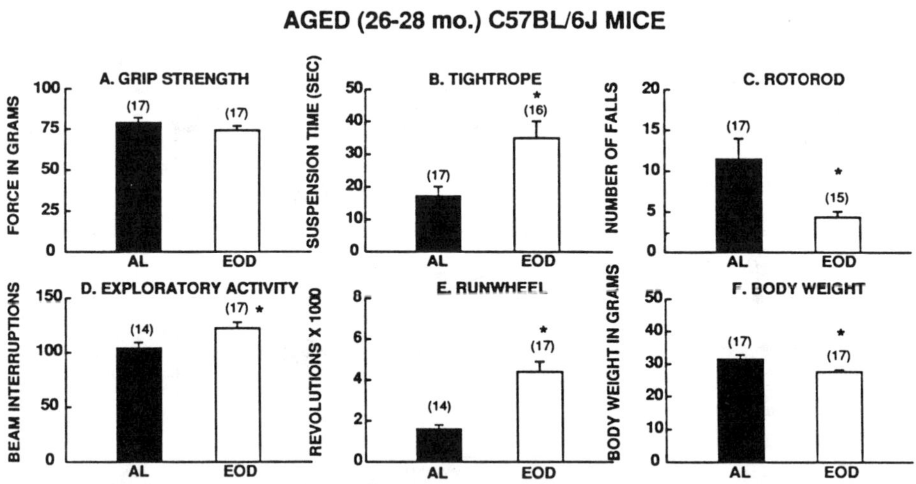

FIG. 18.4. COMPARISON OF MEAN (± SEM) VALUES FOR AGED (26–28 MONTH) MALE C57BL/6J MICE FED *AD LIBITUM* (AL) OR EVERY OTHER DAY (EOD) SINCE 6 MONTHS OF AGE

(A) Grip strength (mean of 3 trials); (B) tightrope (mean of 3, 60-s trials); (C) rotorod (total number of falls during 3-min exposure to rotorod at 3 rpm); (D) exploratory activity (10 min in oval runway under dim illumination); (E) runwheel (72-h exposure) tests; and (F) body weight. Sample sizes are in parentheses. Asterisk indicates significant difference ($P < 0.05$) between AL and EOD groups based on results of two-tailed t-test analysis.

superior performance of C57BL/6J mice on DR in open field and tight wire tasks but shorter survival compared to AL-fed controls.

Body weight is significantly correlated with performance in the tightrope, rotorod, and runwheel tests (Ingram 1983), i.e., heavier mice perform poorly compared to lighter mice of the same age. As usually expected in a DR study, body weight was reduced in EOD-fed mice (about 12%) compared to AL controls (Fig. 18.4F). It stands to reason that lighter mice might have an advantage in a tightrope or rotorod test.

Whether the EOD regimen affects motivational levels is also problematic. To offset this possibility to some degree, the mice were tested only on days after they had 24-h access to food. This was not possible in the runwheel test which extended over 4 days; therefore, EOD mice had 2 feeding days and 2 fasting days. There was a marked reduction in runwheel activity during the feeding days.

Disease factors can also intervene on the behavioral comparisons. Animals that are obviously sick were excluded from analysis, but pathological analysis was not conducted. If DR affects aging rate, then chronic disease processes should be accelerated in the AL-fed groups, and this occurrence appears to be well documented (Weindruch and Walford 1988). If the objective of the behavioral comparison is to confirm this difference in aging rate as reflected in differences in disease incidence, then stringent criteria for exclusion of diseased animals from behavioral testing might not be necessary for DR studies, and disease might not be viewed as an intervening variable. The investigator needs to be aware of these points and decide whether or not control over disease factors is necessary.

Psychomotor Performance in B6AF$_1$/J Mice

The possibility of intervening variation from body weight and motivation factors in DR studies can be addressed by including relevant control groups. One such study was conducted in our laboratory which has not been previously reported. The subjects were male B6AF$_1$/J hybrid mice that had been fed the NIH-07 diet since weaning for all their life or begun on EOD feeding at 6 months of age (Ingram and Reynolds 1987). The effect on survival was very similar to that observed in B6 mice, one of the parental strains. Mortality results indicated about a 19% increase in mean life span of EOD-fed mice when compared to that of AL-fed mice.

Figure 18.5 presents data on performance of these mice in the psychomotor test battery. Comparisons of different groups of AL and EOD mice at young (8–9 month) and aged (26–27 month) intervals were possible. In addition, a control group of aged mice was included. These mice had been on the EOD regimen until about 2 weeks prior to beginning the test battery when they were placed on the AL regimen and maintained that way throughout a 3-week period of testing (EOD-AL). The effect of this treatment was to raise body weight slightly higher than the group maintained on EOD feeding and also to increase motivation ostensively to the same level as that of the AL-fed group. As shown in Fig. 18.5F, the mean body weight of this group was still lower but not significantly so when compared to the aged AL group.

In the grip strength test, the significant age effect of performance of these AL-fed hybrid mice was similar to that observed in B6 mice (Fig. 18.5A). Likewise, no significant diet effect was observed in this psychomotor parameter.

These hybrid mice also exhibited a significant age effect in the tightrope test (Fig. 18.5B). Performance in this test was not affected by diet in the young group but was clearly affected in the EOD groups of aged mice. EOD mice had significantly greater suspension times compared to AL-fed counterparts. However, short-term AL feeding appeared to affect performance as well. Performance declined about 28% in this control group relative to that of aged mice maintained on EOD feeding; however, the level of performance was still significantly greater than that of mice fed AL since weaning.

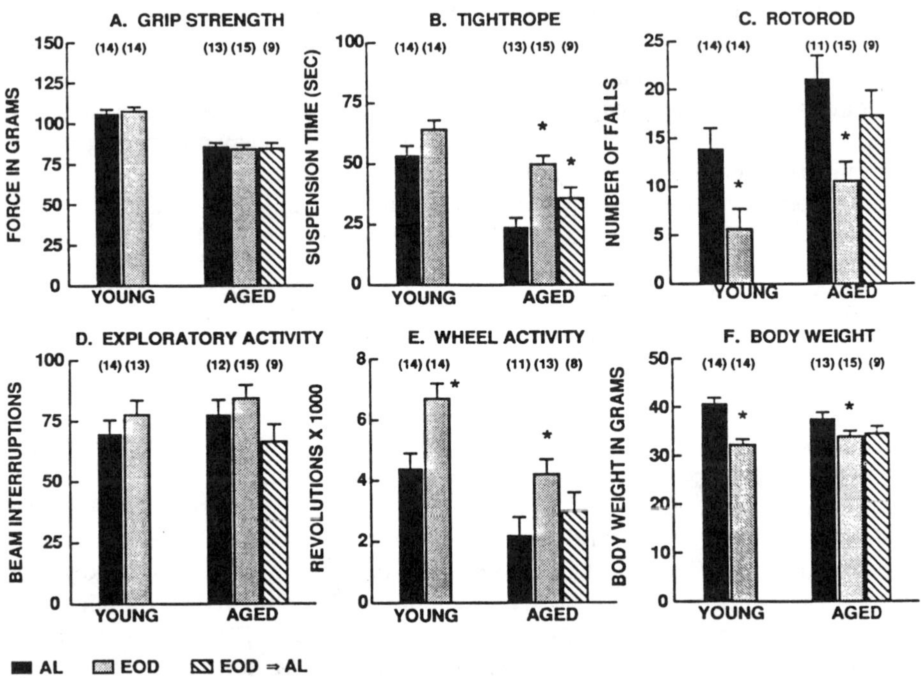

FIG. 18.5. COMPARISONS OF MEAN (± SEM) VALUES FOR AGED (26–28 MONTH) MALE B6AF$_1$/J MICE FED *AD LIBITUM* (AL) OR EVERY OTHER DAY (EOD) SINCE 6 MONTHS OF AGE OR SHIFTED TO AL FEEDING FOR 2 WEEKS PRIOR TO TESTING (EOD → AL)

(A) Grip strength (mean of 3 trials); (B) tightrope (mean of 3, 60-sec trials), (C) rotorod (total number of falls during 3-min exposure to rotorod at 3 rpm); (D) exploratory activity (10-min in oval runway under dim illumination); (E) runwheel (72-h exposure) tests; and (F) body weight. Sample sizes are in parentheses. Asterisk indicates significantly different ($P < 0.05$) from AL group of the same age based on results of two-tailed t-test analysis.

Similar effects were observed in the rotorod test (Fig. 18.5C). A significant age effect was observed among AL-fed groups. However, performance was significantly improved in the young and aged groups by EOD feeding. The marked superiority of performance in young animals on EOD feeding for only a couple of months is indicative of possible body weight/motivational factors. This was confirmed by the performance of the aged EOD-AL group. The mean number of falls increased among these mice relative to the group maintained on EOD feeding to become statistically indistinguishable from that of the aged AL group.

The two tests of locomotor activity yielded different results. No significant age or diet effects were observed in exploratory activity (Fig. 18.5D). A significant age-related decline in runwheel activity was observed in AL-fed mice (Fig. 18.5E). EOD feeding significantly increased activity in both young and aged groups. The aged EOD-AL group showed reduced activity relative to their EOD counterparts; moreover, their mean level of activity, while higher than that of aged AL-fed animals, was not significantly different.

Thus, with the exception of the tightrope test, it could not be concluded with great confidence that the performance differences between aged AL and EOD groups of mice indicated differences in aging rate as reflected at a behavioral level of analysis. This is not to say that inclusion of the EOD-AL group was the best control comparison for drawing these conclusions. Indeed, reintroduction of AL feeding to this group after 20 months of restricted feeding could have had profound effects on neuroendocrine function that negatively impacted upon performance during this short reintroduction. Further investigation could follow this possible outcome. However, this analysis highlighted the difficulty of making careful and controlled behavioral analysis of these dietary treatments.

Psychomotor Performance in $C3B10RF_1$ Mice

With these difficulties in mind, we were able to conduct an additional analysis of psychomotor performance in another mouse strain, $C3B10RF_1$ (Ingram *et al.* 1987). This study was conducted in collaboration with Drs. Richard Weindruch and Roy Walford from the UCLA School of Medicine who had great success in affecting life span parameters in female mice of this strain with a diet restricted about 42% relative to that of controls (Weindruch and Walford *et al.* 1986). Control mice were fed a semipurified diet that was somewhat less than AL levels (~95 kcal/week) on a daily basis; whereas, the restricted mice were fed still on an intermittent basis (Monday, Wednesday, and Friday: ~55 kcal/week). Weindruch *et al.* (1986) reported that the mean life span of control mice on this diet was 33 months versus 42 months for restricted mice.

Before submitting the mice to behavioral testing, all DR animals were returned to the control diet for at least 3 weeks and maintained this way over a 13-week test period. Comparisons are presented in Fig. 18.6 for adults (11–15 months) and aged 31–35 months) groups. Similar to results from the study of $B6AF_1/J$ mice, we observed no age or diet effects on exploratory activity in these hybrid mice (Fig. 18.6A). In the runwheel activity test, no significant age effect was observed: however, DR mice exhibited significantly higher activity at both ages even though they were on the same diet as controls (Fig. 18.6D). Performance in the rotorod test showed a significant age-related decline that was prevented by the restricted diet (Fig. 18.6B).

Body weight differences may have accounted for the rotorod findings since control mice weighed slightly more (about 5%) compared to restricted mice even though both were on the same diet for several weeks. This argument was offset partially by the observation that diet had no significant effect on the performance of the adult group, although their body weights also differed to the same degree. The only other solution to analyzing this possible confound was a statistical one. Analysis of covariance was conducted with body weight as the covariate. The effects of age and diet were still intact with this analysis. Thus, it would appear in these mice that rotorod performance reflected differences in rate of aging and not merely differences in body weight or motivational levels.

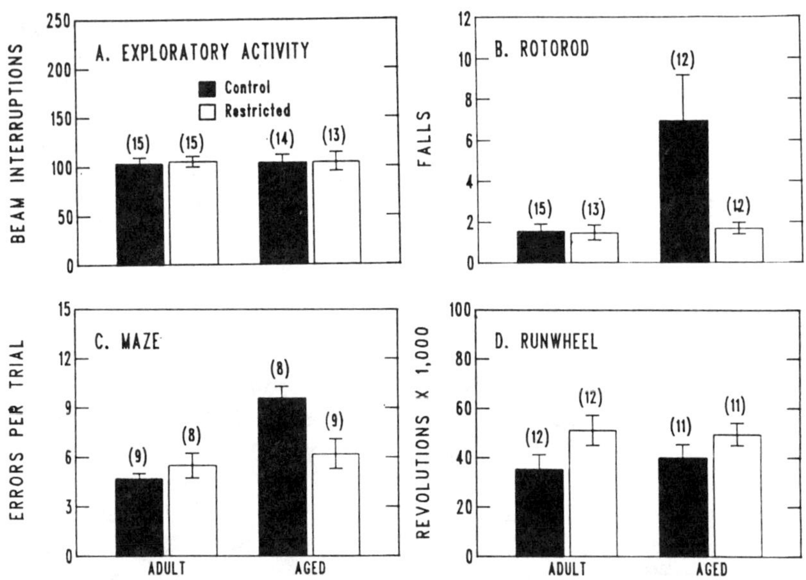

FIG. 18.6. COMPARISONS OF MEAN (± SEM) VALUES FOR ADULTS (11–15 MONTHS) AND AGED (31–35 MONTHS) FEMALE C3B10RF$_1$ FED CONTROL (~95 KCAL/WEEK OR RESTRICTED (~55 KCAL/WEEK) DIETS (A) exploratory activity (10-min in oval runway under dim illumination); (B) rotorod (total number of falls during 3-min exposure to rotorod at 3 rpm); (C) maze learning (errors per trial over 16 trials); and runwheel (72-h exposure) tests. Sample sizes are in parentheses.

Effects of Dietary Restriction on Learning and Memory Performance

The rodent behavioral laboratory at the Gerontology Research Center has a long history regarding the application of a 14-unit T-maze for assessing age-related dysfunction in learning and memory performance (Goodrick 1980; Ingram 1985, 1988). This task provides a robust demonstration of age-related decline in learning ability in several rat and mouse strains under a variety of training and motivational conditions (Ingram 1985, 1988). Thus, this paradigm might also provide a valid assay for assessing the effects of DR on behavioral aging.

Using a food-motivated paradigm, Goodrick (1984) reported that aged (22 month) male Wistar rats fed a life-long AL diet exhibited a higher error rate in learning the 14-unit T-maze compared to the performance of a young (6-month) group undergoing the same diet treatment. In contrast, as observed in Fig. 18.7, the performance of aged (30 month) rats that been fed EOD since weaning was indistinguishable from that of young rats. Thus, the results suggested that DR could preserve the learning abilities of rats into advanced age. However, this interpretation is potentially confounded by the problem of controlling motivational factors in this paradigm in which rats were rewarded with food. In this protocol, the diet

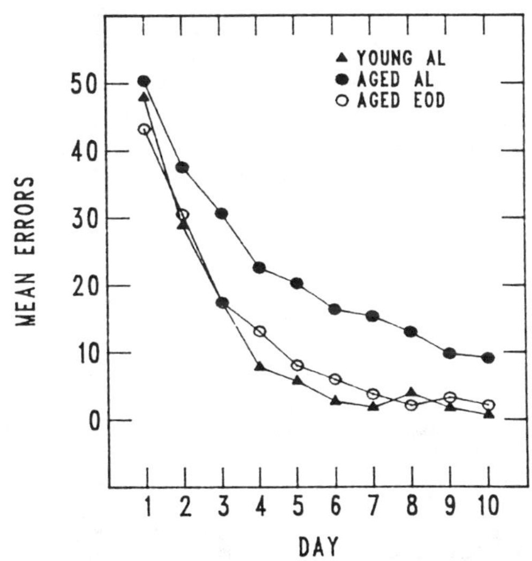

FIG. 18.7. MEAN ERRORS PER TRIAL IN FOOD-MOTIVATED 14-UNIT T-MAZE COMMITTED BY YOUNG (6-MONTH) AND AGED (22-MONTH) MALE WISTAR RATS FED *AD LIBITUM* (AL) AND AGED (30-MONTH) RATS FED EVERY OTHER DAY (EOD) SINCE WEANING

of AL-fed rats had been restricted about 2 weeks before testing to bring their body weights in line with the DR group. The maze testing was conducted on days when food was not available to the EOD group. However, even with this procedure, no other experiments were conducted to determine if the control and experimental groups were equivalently motivated for food rewards. Such experiments might have included latencies to approach food and the amount consumed when provided AL access.

Using a shock-motivated paradigm, Ingram *et al.* (1987) overcame the potential motivational confound to demonstrate that aged DR mice were superior in learning the 14-unit T-maze compared to control counterparts. The subjects were female $C3B10RF_1$ mice from the study mentioned earlier in collaboration with Drs. Weindruch and Walford. Motivational confounding was controlled in two ways. First, food was not used as a reward. All mice were pretrained in footshock avoidance in a straight runway before being tested in the 14-unit T-maze. Only mice meeting a strict performance criterion in this pretraining phase were tested in the complex task; thus, motivation to avoid footshock had been equilibrated in operational terms. Second, as mentioned earlier, all DR mice had been placed on the control diet for several weeks prior to maze testing; thus, both groups were tested under identical nutritional conditions. As observed in Fig. 18.8 the age-related decline in error per-

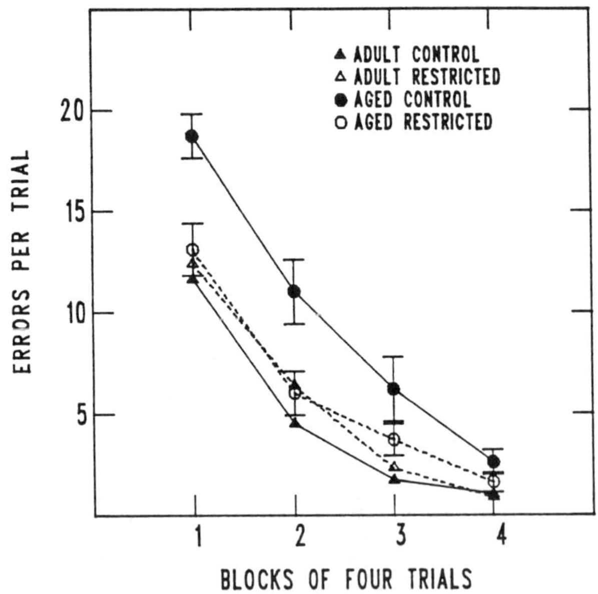

FIG. 18.8. MEAN (± SEM) ERRORS PER TRIAL IN SHOCK-MOTIVATED 14-UNIT T-MAZE COMMITTED BY ADULT (11–15 MONTHS) AND AGED (31–35 MONTHS) FEMALE $C3B10RF_1$ FED CONTROL (~95 KCAL/WEEK) OR RESTRICTED (~55 KCAL/WEEK) DIETS

formance was noted in the control groups, but not in the DR groups. Thus, results generally supported those of Goodrick (1984), but better control over potential motivational confounds rendered the later results easier to interpret.

The observation of superior maze performance among DR mice compared to controls has been reported in at least one other study. Idrobo *et al.* (1987) assessed the performance of 15-month female C57BL/6J mice in a radial arm maze. The task requires the animal to use extramaze cues to remember the location of eight arms radiating from a center arena. The mouse is required to visit each of the arms only once to obtain a water reward. The task is designed as a test of flexible, or *working*, memory since on each trial the animal is required to remember where it has been. Performance in this task has proven to be age-sensitive in rats (Ingram *et al.* 1981; Wallace *et al.* 1980), but not in male C57BL/6J mice (Bernstein *et al.* 1985). No age comparisons were made in the Idrobo *et al.* (1987) study.

In two studies of radial arm maze performance in rats, no differences between DR and control groups have been observed. Beatty *et al.* (1987) reported that aged (21 months) male Sprague-Dawley rats subjected to EOD feeding since 3 months of age did not differ in choice accuracy from controls that had been fed AL. The DR rats were returned to AL feeding for 2 weeks and were then again food restricted in a manner similar to the control rats to motivate maze performance. The paradigm used several delay intervals to assess memory of choices, a procedure that was very sensitive to age differences as determined by the superior performance of young controls (3 month) in this 8-arm maze. However, choice accuracy across delays ranging from 0–5 h did not differ between aged controls and DR groups to indicate that the age-related decline in working memory was not affected by the nutritional manipulation.

Bond *et al.* (1989) examined acquisition performance of male Wistar rats in a 17-arm radial maze without the delay interval. They observed that young rats (5 months) quickly learned choice accuracy, but aged rats (26–28 months) AL-fed exhibited chance performance after 15 trials; also, that the performance of the latter group did not differ significantly from the performance of a group of aged rats (28–30 months) fed a restricted diet (10 g daily) since 6 weeks of age. In addition, these investigators reported an age-related decline in a gustatory neophobia task which measured memory during habituation. Aged control rats took longer to reach an asymptotic level of consumption of a novel saccharin solution compared to young controls; however, there was no significant difference in performance between aged controls and the aged DR group.

What are the reasons for the discrepant findings with respect to the effects of DR on learning and memory performance of aged rodents? Regarding the positive findings in the 14-unit T-maze and the negative findings in the radial maze, a possible explanation is that the tasks involve different memory processes which may be affected differentially by DR. The 14-unit T-maze is a fixed memory task that requires the animal to learn the pathway. The radial maze is a flexible memory task in which the to-be-remembered information changes on every trial. Yet aged rats are impaired in both types of memory events even when tested in the same task (Lowy *et al.* 1985). Moreover, DR mice in the Idrobo *et al.* (1987) study were superior to AL-fed controls. Another explanation for the discrepant results concerns the possibility of sensory confounding in the radial maze task. The inferior performance of aged rats might be due to impaired vision for locating extramaze cues. In the 14-unit T-maze, intact vision is not required for accurate responding (Ingram 1985). Retinal degeneration and cataracts would be two possible impairments in the albino rats used in the radial maze studies. Thus, DR might affect cognitive aging as indicated in the 14-unit T-maze but might not affect aging in the visual system to account for the lack of differences in the radial maze studies. In the mouse radial maze study of Idrobo *et al.*, the pigmented strain of mice might not be as sensitive for age-related visual impairment as were albino strains used in the radial maze studies. The discrepancies will be resolved only by attending to these issues and most directly by comparing aged DR animals in both types of tasks.

EFFECTS OF DIETARY RESTRICTION ON NEUROBIOLOGICAL PARAMETERS

Neurochemical Parameters

A few investigators have attended to possible neurobiological mechanisms underlying the possible beneficial effects of DR on behavioral performance in aged rodents. Most systematic research has involved the nigro-striatal dopamine (DA) system, which has been linked to age-related decline in motor performance (Joseph and Roth 1988; Morgan and Finch 1988).

Levin *et al.* (1981) first reported that the concentration of striatal DA receptors in aged (24 month) male Wistar rats fed on an EOD schedule since weaning was higher than that of age-matched AL-fed controls. Roth *et al.* (1984) confirmed and extended this finding. As observed in Fig. 18.9, the age-related decline in striatal DA receptor concentration was less in DR rats compared to AL-fed controls. Moreover, a short-term DR group (2 weeks) was also examined as a control, and no significant difference between these animals and AL-fed controls was noted, a finding which indicated that the DR effect resulted from chronic treatment.

A behavioral manifestation of these neurochemical findings related to the nigro-striatal system was reported by Joseph *et al.* (1983). Young (6–12 month) and aged (24-month) male rats received unilateral injections of the DA toxin, 6-hydroxydopamine. A week later when injected with the DA agonist, amphetamine, the animals showed a stereotyped turning behavior which is correlated with DA-receptor concentration in the intact striatum (Joseph *et al.* 1981). When comparing AL-fed animals, an age-related decrease in turning behavior was observed. However, the performance of aged rats that had been fed EOD since weaning was indistinguishable from that of young AL-fed rats. When the cholinergic antagonist, atropine, was given to stimulate DA release, young AL-fed rats again showed increased stereotyped behavior compared to aged AL-fed rats. Again the response of aged DR rats was greater than that observed among aged AL rats; however, the response of aged DR rats to this treatment was higher than that of young rats at low doses yet blunted at higher atropine doses to more closely resemble the performance of their aged counterparts than had been observed with amphetamine treatment. These differential responses across neurotransmitter receptors suggested that the cholinergic system may respond differently to DR when compared to the dopaminergic system.

Further evidence of differential effects of DR on neurotransmitter systems was reported by London *et al.* (1985). The subjects were male Wistar rats fed AL or EOD since weaning and compared at 6 and 24 months of age. Total protein content in brain was not affected by age or diet with 1 exception. Hippocampal protein decreased between 6 and 24 months of age but was unaffected by DR. The regional activities of tyrosine hydroxylase (TH), glutamic acid decarboxylase (GAD), and choline acetyltransferase (ChAT) were used as cellular markers for the integrity of the adrenergic, gamma-aminobutyric acid-ergic (GABA), and cholinergic systems, respectively. No diet effects were seen in the adrenergic system except that cortical TH activity was lower among DR rats compared to controls at 6 months of age. Regarding the GABA system, again no significant diet effects were observed except that cortical GAD activity was lower among DR rats compared to controls at 6 months of age. The greatest number of diet effects were observed in cholinergic markers.

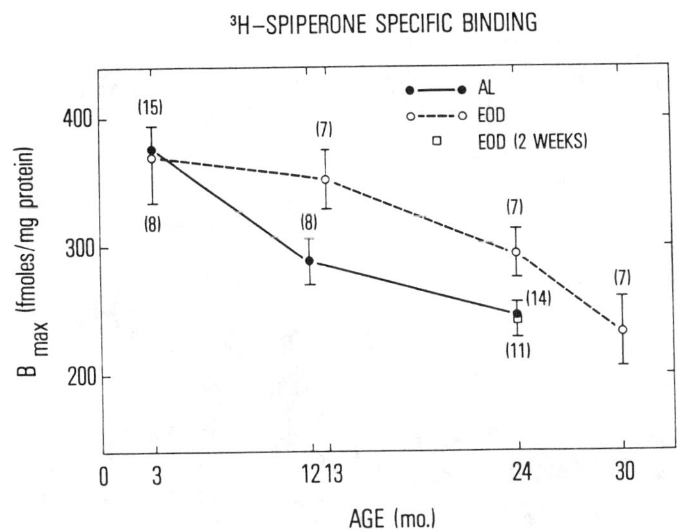

FIG. 18.9. MEAN (± SEM) CONCENTRATIONS OF STRIATAL DOPAMINE RECEPTORS (^{3}H SPIPERONE BINDING) IN MALE WISTAR RATS FED *AD LIBITUM* (AL) OR EVERY OTHER DAY (EOD) SINCE WEANING OR 2 WEEKS PRIOR TO SACRIFICE

Sample sizes are in parentheses.

As observed in Fig. 18.10, ChAT activity was higher in striatum, cerebellum, and hippocampus of 24-month-old DR rats compared to AL control values. Higher hippocampal ChAT activity among EOD animals was also observed at 6 months of age. Concentrations of cholinergic muscarinic receptors were also examined in this study. Diet effects were observed only in the striatum, where receptor concentrations were markedly higher (>40%) among DR rats compared to AL controls.

This higher muscarinic receptor concentration may have accounted for the apparent increased sensitivity to low doses of atropine observed by Joseph *et al.* (1983). Effects on hippocampal cholinergic function are also important to consider with respect to the age-related impairment observed in learning in the 14-unit T-maze (Ingram 1988). Performance in this task can be disrupted by cholinergic antagonists or by lesions to hippocampal cholinergic systems (Ingram 1988). However, London *et al.* (1985) observed no diet effects on the age-related decline in hippocampal muscarinic receptor concentration, although hippocampal ChAT activity was higher among DR rats at 6 and 24 months of age.

Neuromorphological Parameters

Neuromorphological analysis also revealed effects of a chronic regimen of EOD feeding in male Wistar rats. Moroi *et al.* (1989) examined Golgi-stained neurons

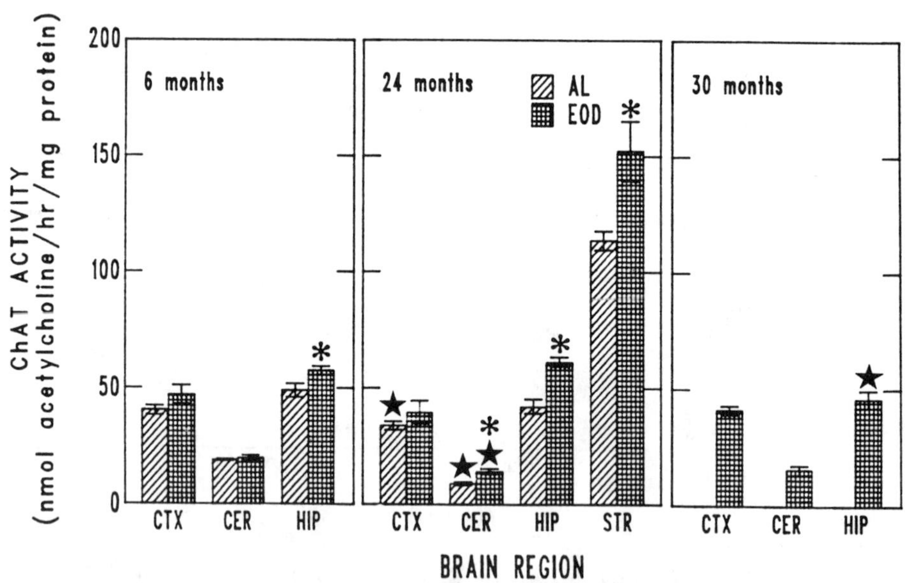

FIG. 18.10. MEAN (± SEM) ACTIVITY OF CHOLINE ACETYLTRANSFERASE (ChAT) IN CEREBRAL CORTEX (CTX), CEREBELLUM (CER), HIPPOCAMPUS (HIP), AND STRIATUM (STR) FROM MALE WISTAR RATS FED *AD LIBITUM* (AL) OR EVERY OTHER DAY (EOD)

Asterisk denotes significant difference from AL group of the same age, $P < 0.05$; star denotes significant difference from previous age on the same diet, $P < 0.05$.

from the parietal cortex of young and aged rats and quantified the morphology of dendritic spines. Among AL-fed groups, spine density decreased (−38%) between 6 and 24 months. When compared to these findings in control groups, spine density exhibited less or no decline in 24- and 30-month-old rats on the EOD regimen since weaning and also in 24-month-old rats undergoing EOD feeding for only 5 months prior to sacrifice. Morphological characterization of L-type (lollipop) and N-type (nubbin) spines also revealed effects of DR. Among AL animals, the proportion of L-type spines exhibits an age-related decline; whereas, all EOD groups exhibited a retention of L-type spines. Thus, these data indicated that DR could prevent some aspects of neuronal aging.

Beneficial effects of DR on other neuromorphological features of the dendritic tree were not confirmed by McNeill *et al.* (1990) in their study of male C57BL/6J mice. The diet manipulation in this study was intermittent feeding (3/7 days/week) since weaning. The analysis focused on the medium spiny neuron of the striatum. No age or diet effects were observed when the number of dendritic arbors, mean total dendritic length per cell, mean total number of segments, and mean segment length were examined. The lack of observable alterations in these neurons was cited as additional evidence of the selective effect of aging and DR on neuronal aging. These neurons are hypothesized to contain either GABA, substance P, or enkephalin as their neurotransmitters. Perhaps striatal cholinergic interneurons would be more affected by aging and thus more responsive to DR.

West *et al.* (1984) also did not observe significant neuromorphological differences between 24-month-old male Sprague-Dawley rats fed AL and counterparts fed a severely restricted diet (body weight maintained at one-third of that for AL controls). Although their analysis was not quantitative and involved small numbers of rats, age-related alterations, including abnormal myelinated axons, intradendritic membranous bodies, and increased lipofuscin, were observed with similar frequency in the auditory cortex of controls and DR groups at 24 months. However, when these investigators examined the brains of 48-month-old DR animals, several phenomena rarely or never observed in younger controls were noted, including thickening of basal lamina of blood vessels, abnormalities in neuroglia, and evidence of neuritic plaques that appeared to have an amyloid core. These latter observations, particularly the report of neuritic plaques, suggested that the extended life span of DR rats permitted the emergence of certain neuropathology not usually manifested in AL rats with shorter life spans.

Lipid Peroxidation

If data are accepted that DR can produce selected retardation of age-associated alterations in brain aging, then a search for mechanisms of this possibility must also be initiated. Retardation of damage produced by normal byproducts of oxidative metabolism has been viewed as a major hypothesis by which DR affects aging processes (Weindruch and Walford 1988). Lipid peroxidation is one possible destructive process that can be retarded by DR. The potential of such damage to cells and to cellular membranes can be measured by several indirect means.

Nandy (1985) assessed one neuronal parameter of lipid peroxidation in female C57BL/6J mice. Production of lipofuscin in neurons can be measured by its autofluorescent quality. The deposition of this pigment is a ubiquitous marker of cytological aging (Nandy 1985). It is considered as an end product of lipid peroxidation and can be manipulated by altering the tissue levels of antioxidants, such as vitamin E (Nandy 1985). When lipofuscin autofluorescence in hippocampus and frontal neocortex was compared between AL-fed controls and mice fed about 50% of the control level since 3 months of age, the DR group exhibited much less evidence of lipofuscin accumulation. No significant effects on brain lipofuscin were observed when the DR regimen was initiated at 24 months of age and assessed up to 6 months later. Chipalkatti *et al.* (1983) confirmed the effects of DR on brain lipofuscin when initiated early in life (at weaning). Examining fluorescence in whole brain preparations from female Swiss albino mice at 4.5 and 12 months of age, these investigators noted that lipofuscin accumulation was higher among AL-fed controls compared to DR mice (about 50% of control intake). Forbes (1980) did not confirm this DR effect when he assessed lipofuscin accumulation in cerebellar Purkinje cells of 7-month-old male Sprague-Dawley rats fed either AL or restricted (2–7.5 g/day) since weaning. There was a trend towards reduced lipofuscin accumulation among DR rats, but perhaps in this study the DR regimen had not been implemented for a sufficient period of time to observe effects on this parameter.

The potential for lipid peroxidation can also be measured with an assay for another end product, malanoaldehyde, with the thiobarbituric assay (TBA). When TBA-reactive material is compared between AL-controls and DR mice at advanced ages, observations of reduced levels in livers of DR mice have been reported (Chipalkatti *et al.* 1983; Koizumi *et al.* 1987), but activity in brain has not been investigated. Chipalkatti *et al.* (1983) did examine the activities of lysosomal enzymes (acid phosphatase and cathepsin) as indices of damage to lysosomes produced by lipid peroxide and found lower enzyme activity in brains of DR mice at 3,6, and 9 months of age. As an index of protection against lipid peroxidation, Chipalkatti *et al.* also examined the activities of superoxide dismutase (SOD), which is an endogenous antioxidant. Brain SOD activity was higher in the DR group at 6 months of age, but lower at 12 months of age.

Immunological Parameters

Neuronal aging may also occur through immunological mechanisms that might be altered by DR (Weindruch and Walford 1988). As one examination of this hypothesis, Nandy (1982) assessed the formation of brain reactive antibodies (BRA) in the frontal cortex and hippocampus of female C57BL/6J mice. At 12 months of age, DR mice (50% of control levels) exhibited virtually no evidence of BRA compared to the high frequency observed among AL-fed controls. When this DR regimen was initiated at 24 months, there was no significant difference between AL control and DR groups in the incidence of BRAs when examined 3 months later (Nandy 1981). Thus, the age-related increase in the potential for autoimmune events appears to be retarded when DR is introduced early but not late in the life of mice.

SUMMARY AND CONCLUSIONS

Results of experiments from several laboratories indicate that DR can retard the age-related decline in motor and cognitive function observed in laboratory rodents. However, in view of some reports of no effects of DR on behavioral function, this conclusion must be qualified. In only a few studies has the issue of adequate control over intervening variables (e.g., body weight, motivation, sensory abilities) been addressed. Further analysis of these behavioral findings that utilize proper tasks and control group is warranted.

Neurochemical analysis of DR effects on brain aging have produced consistent results with respect to the nigro-striatal DA system. The age-associated loss of striatal DA receptors appears to be retarded by DR and to have behavioral consequences. The cholinergic system appears to be especially sensitive to aging and to DR. Several parameters of muscarinic neurotransmission were affected by DR in several brain regions. The GABAergic system appeared less affected by DR, but much less analysis has been conducted of this and other systems.

Neuromorphological analysis of DR effects has produced mixed results. Beneficial effects on dendritic spines in parietal cortex were reported in rats, but aspects of dendritic arborization of striatal medium spiny neurons appeared unaffected by DR in mice. In addition, analysis of many neuromorphological parameters in rats undergoing a severe restriction did not reveal differences between control and DR rats, although the latter developed rare pathology at advanced ages.

Examination of other indices of brain aging, such as the accumulation of lipofuscin and brain reactive antibodies suggested that DR could retard such parameters in mice when initiated shortly after weaning but not when begun during senescence. The importance of these findings is their possible relation to mechanisms of brain aging as manifested in age-related declines in neurochemical and neuromorphological parameters.

In conclusion, this area of research related to the potential for nutritional modulation of aging processes has only begun to be addressed in systematic research. Further, analysis of the behavioral effects of chronic DR regimens is important for assessing the impact of such treatments on function and to indicate possible neurobiological mechanisms. Further analysis of neurobiological effects associated with DR is needed to determine the impact on brain aging and to search for mechanisms of DR at cellular and molecular levels of analysis. This research should focus upon a particular functional system that can be analyzed across behavioral, neurobiological, and molecular levels. Hypothalamic systems would be of considerable interest regarding their regulation and interaction with peripheral neuroendocrine events, yet little systematic research has been conducted to determine effects of DR on this brain region.

ACKNOWLEDGMENTS

This work would not have been possible without the valuable technical assistance of John Freeman, Edward Spangler, Albert Ellis, Kathleen Schrieber, Nancy Cider,

John Whitaker, and Brian Sievers, and the contributions of valued collaborators, including Elaine Bresnahan, Barbara Davis, James Joseph, Edythe London, Thomas McNeill, Ronald Mervis, George Roth, Mark Reynolds, Roy Walford, Steven Waller, and Richard Weindruch. I also wish to thank the American Health Foundation for sponsoring and helping to organize the conference for which this paper was prepared.

REFERENCES

BARROWS, C. H. and KOKKONEN, G. C. 1984. Nutrition and aging: Human and animal laboratory studies. *In* Nutrition in Gerontology, J. M. Ordy, D. Harmon and R. Aflin-Slater (eds.). Raven Press, New York.

BEATTY, W. W., CLOUSE, B. A. and BIERLEY, R. A. 1987. Effects of long-term restricted feeding on radial maze performance by aged rats. Neurobiol. Aging *8*, 325–327.

BERNSTEIN, D. *et al.* 1985. Radial maze performance in young and aged mice: Neurochemical correlates. Pharmacol. Biochem. Behav. *5*, 301–307.

BOND, N. W., EVERITT, A. V. and WALTON, J. 1989. Effects of dietary restriction on radial-arm maze performance and flavor memory in aged rats. Neurobiol. Aging *10*, 27–30.

CAMPBELL, B. A. and GADDY, J. R. 1987. Rate of aging and dietary restriction: Sensory and motor function in the Fischer 344 rat. J. Gerontol. *42*, 154–159.

CHIPALKATTI, S., DE, A. K. and AIYAR, A. S. 1983. Effect of diet restriction on some biochemical parameters related to aging in mice. J. Nutr. *113*, 944–950.

FORBES, W. B. 1980. Dietary restriction, longevity, and CNS aging. *In* The Psychobiology of Aging: Problems and Perspectives, D. Stein (ed.). Elsevier, Amsterdam.

GOODRICK, C. L. 1980. Problem solving and age: A critique of rodent research. *In* Age, Learning Ability, and Intelligence, R. L. Sprott (ed.). Van Nostrand Reinhold, New York.

GOODRICK, C. L. 1984. Effects of lifelong restricted feeding on complex maze performance in rats. Age *7*, 1–2.

HARRISON, D. E. and ARCHER, J. R. 1987. Genetic effects on responses to food restriction in aging micc. J. Nutr. *117*, 376–382.

IDROBO, F. *et al.* 1987. Dietary restriction: Effects on radial maze learning and lipofuscin pigment deposition in the hippocampus and frontal cortex. Arch. Gerontol. Geriat. *6*, 355–362.

INGRAM, D. K. 1983. Toward the behavioral assessment of biological aging in the laboratory mouse: Concepts, terminology, and objectives. Exp. Aging Res. *9*, 225–238.

INGRAM, D. K. 1984. Biological age: A strategy for assessment. *In* Gerontology and Geriatrics Yearbook (U.S.S.R.), F. Cherbotarev, A. V. Tokar and V. P. Viotenko (eds.). Institute for Gerontology, Kiev.

INGRAM, D. K. 1985. Analysis of age-related impairments in learning and memory in rodent models. An. N. Y. Acad. Sci. *444*, 312–331.

INGRAM, D. K. 1987. Motor performance variability during aging in rodents: Assessment of reliability and validity of individual differences. *In* Central Determinants of Age-Related Declines in Motor Function, J. Joseph (ed.). An. N. Y. Acad. Sci. *515*, 70–96.

INGRAM, D. K. 1988. Complex maze learning in rodents as a model of age-related memory impairment. Neurobiol. Aging *9*, 475–485.

INGRAM, D. K. *et al.* 1987. Dietary restriction benefits learning and motor performance of aged mice. J. Gerontol. *42*, 78–81.

INGRAM, D. K., LONDON, E. D. and GOODRICK, C. L. 1981. Age and neurochemical correlates of radial maze performance in rats. Neurobiol. Aging *2*, 41–47.

INGRAM, D. K. and REYNOLDS, M. A. 1986. Assessing the predictive validity of psychomotor tests as measures of biological age in mice. Exp. Aging Res. *12*, 155–162.

INGRAM, D. K. and REYNOLDS, M. A. 1987. The relationship of body weight to longevity within laboratory rodent species. *In* Evolution of Longevity in Animals, A. D. Woodhead and K. H. Thompson (eds.). Plenum Press, New York.

JOSEPH, J. A. and ROTH, G. S. 1988. Upregulation of striatal dopamine receptors and improvement of motor performance in senescence. *In* Central Determinants of Age-Related Declines in Motor Function, J. Joseph (ed.). An. N. Y. Acad. Sci. *515*, 355–362.

JOSEPH, J. A. *et al.* 1983. Lifelong dietary restriction affects striatally mediated behavioral responses in aged rats. Neurobiol. Aging *4*, 191–196.

JOSEPH, J. A., FILBURN, C. R. and ROTH, G. S. 1981. Development of dopamine receptor denervation supersensitivity in the neostriatum of the senescent rat. Life Sci. *29*, 575–584.

KOIZUMI, A., WEINDRUCH, R. and WALFORD, R. L. 1987. Influences of dietary restriction and age on liver enzyme activities and lipid peroxidation in mice. J. Nutr. *117*, 361–367.

LEVIN, P. *et al.* 1981. Dietary restriction retards the age-associated loss of rat striatal dopaminergic receptors. Science *214*, 561–562.

LONDON, E. D., WALLER, S. E., ELLIS, A. T. and INGRAM, D. K. 1985. Effects of intermittent feeding on neurochemical markers in aging rat brain. Neurobiol. Aging *6*, 199–204.

LOWY, A. M. *et al.* 1985. Discrimination learning requiring different memory components in rats: Age and neurochemical comparisons. Behav. Neurosci. *99*, 638–651.

McNEILL, T. H. *et al.* 1991. Assessment of lifelong dietary restriction on neostriatal morphology and peripheral neuroendocrine hormones in aged C57BL/6J mice. *In* The Potential for Nutritional Modulation of Aging Processes, D. K. Ingram, G. T. Baker, III, and N. W. Shock (eds.). Food and Nutrition and Press, Trumbull, CT.

MASORO, E. J. 1988. Food restriction in rodents: An evaluation of its role in the study of aging. J. Gerontol. *43*, B59–B64.

MOMENT, G. 1978. The Ponce de Leon trail today. *In* The Biology of Aging, J. Behnke, C. Finch and G. Moment (eds.). Plenum Press, New York.

MORGAN, D. G. and FINCH, C. E. 1988. Dopaminergic changes in the basal ganglia: A generalized phenomenon of aging in mammals. *In* Central Determinants of Age-Related Declines in Motor Function, J. Joseph (ed.). An. N. Y. Acad. Sci. *515*, 145–160.

MORGANE, P. J. *et al.* 1978. The effects of protein malnutrition on the developing central nervous system in the rat. Neurosci. Biobehav. Rev. *2*, 137–230.

MOROI, S. E., MERVIS, R. F., LONDON, E. D. and INGRAM, D. K. 1989. Dietary restriction suppresses age-related changes in dendritic spines. Neurobiol. Aging, *10*, 317–322.

NANDY, K. 1981. Effects of caloric restriction on brain-reactive antibodies in sera of old mice. Age *4*, 117–121.

NANDY, K. 1982. Effects of controlled dietary restriction of brain-reactive antibodies in sera of aging mice. Mech. Age. Dev. *18*, 97–102.

NANDY, K. 1985. Lipofuscin as a marker of impaired homeostasis in aging organisms. *In* Homeostatic Function and Aging, B. B. Davis and W. G. Wood (eds.). Raven Press, New York.

ROTH, G. S., INGRAM, D. K. and JOSEPH, J. A. 1984. Delayed loss of striatal dopamine receptors during aging of dietarily restricted rats. Brain Res. *300*, 27–32.

SACHER, G. A. 1977. Life table modification and life prolongation. *In* Handbook of the Biology of Aging, C. Finch and L Hayflick (eds.). Van Nostrand Reinhold, New York.

SCHNEIDER, E. L. and REID, JR., J. D. 1985. Life extension. N. Eng. J. Med. 1159–1160.

TALAN, M. I. and INGRAM, D. K. 1985. Effect of intermittent feeding on thermoregulatory abilities of young and aged mice. Arch. Gerontol. Geriat. *4*, 251–259.

WALLACE, J. W., KRAUTER, E. E. and CAMPBELL, B. A. 1980. Animal models of declining memory in the aged: Short-term and spatial memory in the aged rat. J. Gerontol. *35*, 353–363.

WEINDRUCH, R. and WALFORD, R. L. 1988. The Retardation of Aging and Disease by Dietary Restriction. Charles C Thomas, Springfield, IL.

WEINDRUCH, R., WALFORD, R. L., FLIGIEL, S. and GUTHRIE, D. 1986. The retardation of aging in mice by dietary restriction: Longevity, cancer, immunity, and lifetime energy intake. J. Nutr. *116*, 641–654.

WEST, C. D., VOLICER, L. and VAUGHAN, D. W. 1984. Aging in the food-restricted rat: Body temperature, receptor function, and morphologic changes in the brain. *In* Nutritional Intervention in the Aging Process, H. J. Armbrecht, J. M. Pendergast, and R. M. Coe (eds.). Springer-Verlag, New York.

CHAPTER 19

ASSESSMENT OF LIFELONG DIETARY RESTRICTION ON NEOSTRIATAL MORPHOLOGY AND PERIPHERAL NEUROENDOCRINE HORMONES IN AGED C57BL/6J MICE

THOMAS H. McNEILL, Ph.D.
Ethyl Percy Andrus Gerontology Research Center
University of Southern California
Los Angeles, California

BARBARA J. DAVIS, Ph.D. and ROBERT W. HAMILL, M.D.
Departments of Neurology and Neurobiology
University of Rochester School of Medicine
Rochester, New York

and

ELAINE BRESNAHAN, Ph.D. and DONALD K. INGRAM, Ph.D.
Gerontology Research Center
National Institute on Aging
Francis Scott Key Medical Center
Baltimore, Maryland

INTRODUCTION

It is well established that lifelong caloric restriction from weaning can increase mean and maximal life span as well as delay the onset of a variety of age-related pathophysiological conditions in laboratory rodents (Cutler 1981; Weindruch 1984; Barrows and Kokkonen 1984; Masoro 1984a, 1984b; Weindruch and Walford 1982; Walford *et al.* 1974). In addition, previous studies have reported that rats maintained on an alternate day feeding pattern starting one week after weaning prevents normal age-related declines in motor coordination and complex maze performance (Ingram *et al.* 1987; Goodrick 1984; Ingram 1990) as well as rotational behavior and stereotypy induced by intrastriatally administered dopamine-excitatory or cholinergic inhibitory agents (Joseph *et al.* 1983). Although the mechanisms underlying the slowing of these age-related behavioral changes remain unknown, data from previous studies have suggested that caloric restriction may preserve the functional integrity of select neurotransmitter systems of the aged brain as well as retard the loss of dopaminergic receptors in the neostriatum, an essential component of the extrapyramydal motor system (London *et al.* 1985; Levin *et al.* 1981; Roth *et al.* 1984; Joseph *et al.* 1983).

The present study was undertaken to evaluate morphologically the adaptability of the neostriatum to changes within its neurotransmitter environment following a lifetime of caloric restriction (London *et al.* 1985). In addition, we examined the metabolic consequences of lifelong caloric restriction on several neuroendocrine parameters in the periphery which promote both the production and utilization of glucose, the primary source of metabolic energy for the brain. These included plasma glucose, insulin and glucagon, as well as the activity of adrenal tyrosine hydroxylase, the rate limiting enzyme in the synthesis of catecholamines and a marker of sympathoadrenal activity (Cooper *et al.* 1986).

METHODS

Male C57BL/6J mice were obtained from the Jackson laboratories at six weeks of age and were housed in groups of four per cage in the vivarium facility at the National Institute on Aging, Gerontology Research Center, Baltimore, MD. Mice were randomly assigned to one of two experimental groups. Group 1 (*ad libitum*, AD) consisted of mice which were allowed *ad libitum* access to food throughout the experiment while mice in Group 2 (dietary restricted, DR) were calorically restricted and only allowed access to food on Mondays, Wednesdays and Fridays. All mice were fed the standard NIH-07 diet containing 24% protein and 10% fat and all mice had *ad libitum* access to water throughout the experiment. Mice were allowed to survive until they reached either 20 or 27 months of age and were killed between the hours of 1100 and 1400 on the day after having free access to food.

For our study at least five mice per group were examined for each variable measured. Mice were decapitated following cervical dislocation, and trunk blood was collected into chilled heparinized microhematocrit centrifuge tubes. Tubes containing blood were kept on ice until centrifuged (approximately 6 h), and plasma was separated and stored at $-20°C$ until time of assay. At the same time the brain was excised and tissue blocks containing the striatum were dissected and immersed in Golgi Cox solution according to the procedure of Van der Loos (1956). Brains were dehydrated, embedded in Cedukol and cut in a coronal plane at 200 μm.

Slides were coded so that data gathering and analysis were performed blind. Medium spiny I (MSI) neurons of the striatum [classification after DiFiglia (1976)], a principal target population for afferent input, were analyzed from a standardized caudal anatomical level of the striatum based on the topography of both the nigrostriatal (Fallon and Moore 1978; Fallon *et al.* 1978) and corticostriatal projection fields (Gerfen 1984, 1985; Cospito and Kultas-Ilinsky 1981; Ragsdale and Graybiel 1981). In addition, this region of the striatum was selected based on previous biochemical studies which have described dopamine receptor loss (Severson and Finch 1980; Randall *et al.* 1981) as well as reductions of dopamine content (Strong *et al.* 1982; Osterberg *et al.* 1981) and choline acetyltransferase activity, a principal enzyme in the synthesis of acetylcholine (Strong *et al.* 1980) in aged rodent brain. At the time of analysis, cell selection was randomized to avoid clustering and bias based on age-related changes which may be specifically related to MSI neurons that are part of either the "path or matrix" components of the rodent striatum (Graybiel 1983; Gerfen 1984, 1985). Cells were randomized according to the protocol described previously by Coleman *et al.* (1986). A sample of 20 neurons (based on a predetermined 95% confidence interval) was randomly chosen from each mouse from among all well-impregnated MSI neurons. Only cells with their soma in the center one third of the section and whose dendrites which were unobscured by overlying glia, blood vessels, other neurons, or nonspecific deposits of stains were drawn. Based on previous observations, terminal dendritic segments were required to be tapered at their tips and lacking spines indicating the complete impregnation of the dendrite.

Profiles of the cell soma and dendrites were traced using a 40× or 100× objective lens and a camera lucida drawing tube. Cells were entered in an IBM microcomputer system using a digitizing tablet and Dan software (Moyer *et al.* 1985). Analysis of dendritic parameters included total and terminal segment length, as well as the total number of dendritic segments per neuron. In addition, the linear density of dendritic spines on MSI neurons was calculated in 20 μm intervals from the cell body to the tip of the terminal segment. One dendrite from each of 20 cells was used for this analysis, and 5 mice for each age group were examined. Data were expressed as the average total dendritic length of 20 cells per mouse for each age group or as the mean number of dendritic spines for each 20 μm segment per dendrite. Statistical analysis included analysis of variance and nonparametric Mann-Whitney U tests with N equal to the number of mice in each age group.

Plasma glucose was determined using a Beckman Glucose Analyzer (glucose oxidase method). Plasma insulin (Morgan and Lazarow 1963) and glucagon (Hazzard *et al.* 1968) were determined by double antibody radioimmunoassays using commercially prepared RIA kits (Cambridge Medical Diagnostics, Billerica, MA). Adrenal tyrosine hydroxylase (TH) activity was determined on alumina-adsorbed extracts of adrenal medullae using a modification (Melvin and Hamill 1986) of the radiochemical assay of Black (1975). Student t-tests were used to determine significant differences between AD and DR groups for each of the parameters measured.

RESULTS

A summary of the effects of caloric restriction on survival and life span is presented in Fig. 19.1a and 19.1b. Mice maintained on the calorically restricted diet showed a significant increase in life expectancy ($P < 0.0001$) when compared to the *ad libitum* feed group. Caloric restriction also delayed the marked increase in mortality seen at 96 weeks (24 months) of age in AD mice until 132 weeks of age (33.3 months of age) in DR mice. In addition, caloric restriction by intermittent feeding showed a significant increase in both the mean and median life span of C57BL/6J mice with only a small (10%) reduction of food intake. The mean final body weights for AD and DR mice were not significantly different at either 20 or 27 months of age and produced only a 10% reduction of mean body weight through 36 weeks of age.

The average plasma levels of glucose, insulin and glucagon in AD and DR mice are presented in Table 19.1. Plasma glucose levels of DR mice were not significantly different compared to mice fed the *ad libitum* diet. However, we found a significant increase of plasma insulin ($P < 0.01$) and a significant decrease of plasma glucagon ($P < 0.05$) in DR mice when compared with AD mice for the single time point we examined. In addition, there was a significant increase of adrenal TH activity (Table 19.1) in DR mice when compared to the AD group. The increase in plasma insulin levels showed positively correlated with adrenal TH activity in DR mice ($R = 0.85$).

MSI neurons in young AD mice were characterized by a round or oval cell body and represented a majority (greater than 90% over) of all Golgi impregnated neurons of the striatum. Dendritic arbors of MSI neurons had 4–8 primary dendrites that emerged from the cell soma and gave rise to distal segments which branched to form arbors which were usually spherical in shape (Fig. 19.2a). Distal branches were covered by numerous spines of heterogeneous shapes and size while primary dendrites were usually spine free. In addition, there was substantial variation in the size of the dendritic arbor of individual MSI neurons in the striatum (Fig. 19.2a,b). Neurons ranged from having very robust arbors with terminal dendritic arbors of the seventh order and a total dendritic length of greater than 1,200 μm to those that were grossly atrophic and shrunken with only 2–3 segments and a total dendritic arbor of lęss than 500 μm.

Similarly , MSI neurons from 20 month and 27 month AD and DR mice had many of the same general morphological characteristics seen in the young AD mice. Thus, it was impossible to identify either the age or dietary condition of a group based solely on a qualitative morphological assessment of individual Golgi sections. Cell somata from MSI neurons of aged AD and DR mice were either round or oval in shape and gave rise to 3–8 primary dendrites. Secondary and distal segments were covered with numerous spines of heterogeneous size and shape. However, as previously described in aged C57BL/6N mice (McNeill *et al.* 1988b, 1990), many MSI neurons in 27-month-old DR mice had ectopic spines on their cell soma and abnormal dendrites with prominent swellings indicative of ongoing cellular degeneration.

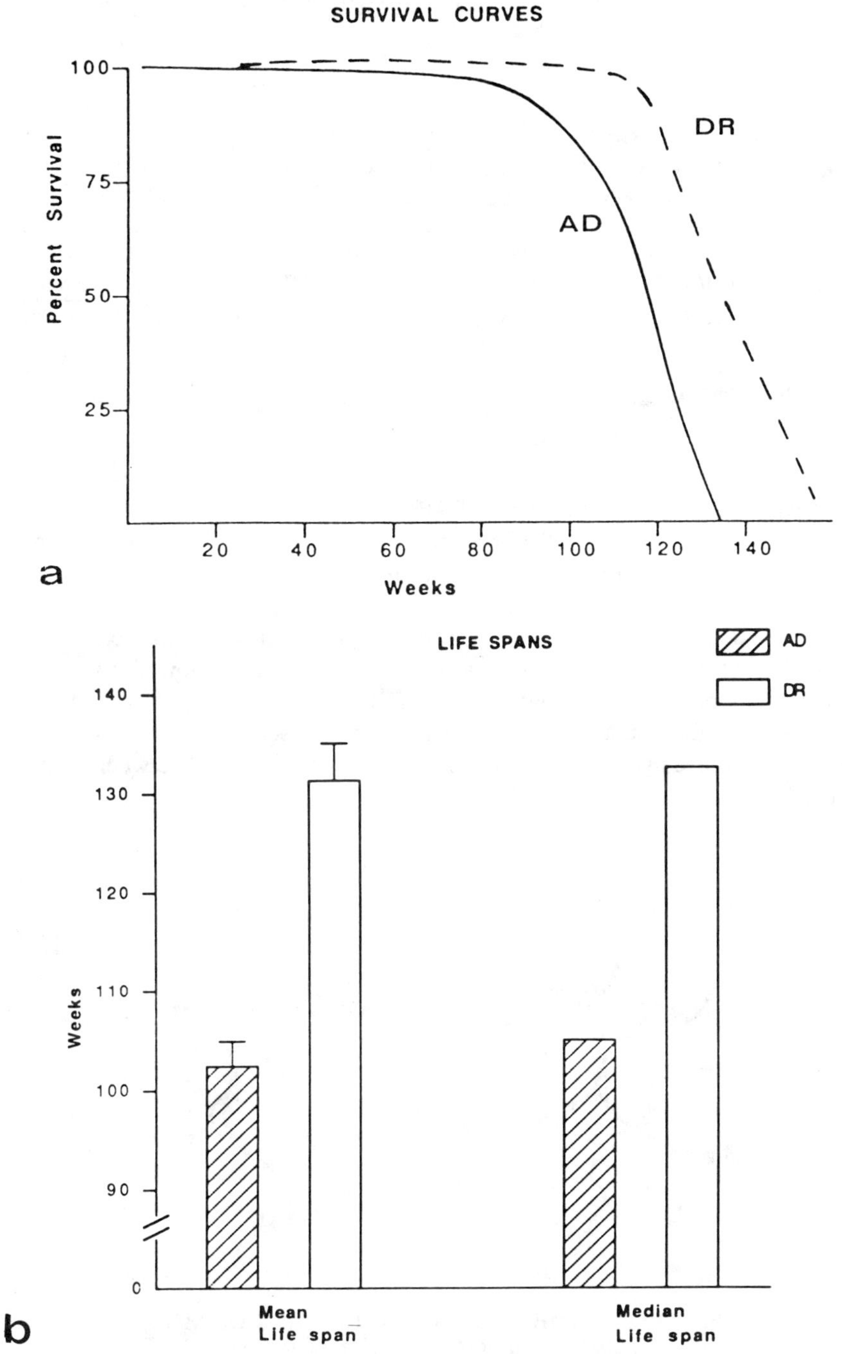

FIG. 19.1. SURVIVAL CURVE (a) AND LIFE SPAN DATA (b) (MEAN ± SEM) OF C57BL/6J MICE FED ACCORDING TO PROTOCOLS DESCRIBED IN THE METHODS SECTION

AD, *ad libitum*; DR, caloric restricted.

TABLE 19.1
EFFECT OF INTERMITTENT FEEDING ON PLASMA LEVELS OF INSULIN (μU/mL), GLUCAGON (pg/mL), GLUCOSE (mg/dL) AND ADRENAL TH ACTIVITY (nM/h/μg PROTEIN) IN 20 MONTH OLD C57BL/6J MICE[1]

Group	Insulin (μU/mL)	Glucagon (pg/mL)	Glucose (mg/dL)	TH Activity (nM/h/μg Protein)
AD	11.3 ± 1.4(12)	2100 ± 733(12)	102.4 ± 5.5(14)	9.24 ± 1.56(10)
DR	31.3 ± 2.1(12)[2]	478 ± 37(12)[3]	106.8 ± 3.8(13)	17.9 ± 2.40(10)

[1]Number of mice shown in parentheses.
[2]$P < 0.01$.
[3]$P < 0.05$.

Quantitative analysis for both AD and DR mice confirmed our qualitative observations (Fig. 19.3). We found that the dendritic arbors of MSI neurons showed no sign of dendritic regression up to 27 months of age with a trend towards an increase in the total dendritic length of MSI neurons in DR mice. However, this increase was not statistically significant. The average total dendritic length per cell, average total number of segments, and average segment length also showed no statistical difference between 27-month-old AD and DR mice. Analysis of MSI dendrites ordered in both the somatopetal and somatofugal directions likewise showed no statistical difference in any of the dendritic parameters examined between 27 month AD and DR mice.

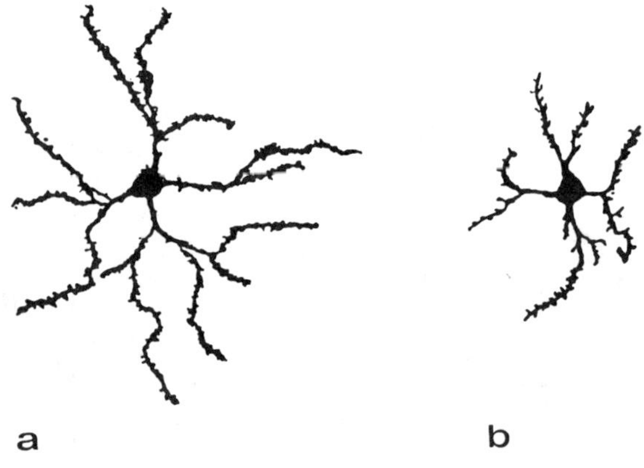

FIG. 19.2. CAMERA LUCIDA DRAWINGS OF MSI NEURONS OF THE STRIATUM FROM 27-MONTH-OLD AD MICE WITH A TOTAL DENDRITIC LENGTH OF (a) 1175 μm OR (b) 415 μm
Neurons with short dendritic branches may be indicative of atrophic changes ultimately leading to cell death.

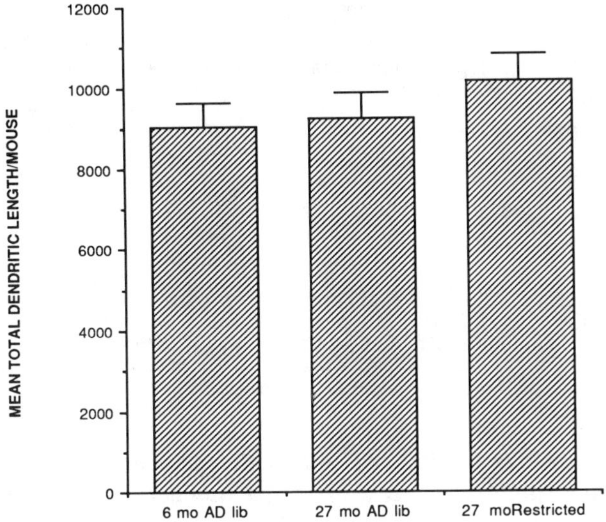

FIG. 19.3. AVERAGE TOTAL DENDRITIC LENGTH OF MSI NEURONS IN 6 MONTH AD, 27 MONTH AD AND 27 MONTH DR MICE
Each mean ± SEM represents the mean total dendritic length for the 20 cells/mouse drawn from 5 mice in each group. There was no significant difference between AD and DR mice.

Because it is known that most synaptic input onto MSI neurons is axospinous, we also examined the effects of caloric restriction on changes in the linear density of dendritic spines in 27-month-old AD and DR mice. As shown in Table 19.2 the linear density of dendritic spines was calculated in 20 μm intervals from the cell body to the tip of the terminal segment. In both young and old AD mice, the linear density of dendritic spines progressively increased from the cell body towards the tip of the dendrite with the highest density of spines found on the 40–60 and 61–80 μm intervals. However, there was no significant changes in dendritic spine density along any interval of the dendrite in old (27 month) AD mice when compared to young (6 month) AD controls. Likewise, there was no significant difference in the linear density of dendritic spines along any interval of the dendrite in 27-month-old DR mice when compared to old AD mice.

DISCUSSION

Data from our study suggests that dietary manipulation imposed by intermittent feeding can extend both mean and maximal life span of C57BL/6J mice and significantly alter the normal pattern of secretion of plasma insulin and glucagon from the endocrine pancreas (Davis *et al.* 1990). These results suggest that when

TABLE 19.2
EFFECTS OF INTERMITTENT FEEDING ON THE LINEAR DENSITY OF DENDRITIC SPINES OF MSI NEURONS

Dendritic Interval (μm)[1]	AD (6 Month)	AD (27 Month)	DR (27 Month)
0–20	6.6 ± 0.97	7.8 ± 0.75	4.7 ± 0.93
21–40	24.6 ± 2.33	22.9 ± 1.42	19.7 ± 0.90
41–60	31.2 ± 1.67	28.9 ± 2.15	26.7 ± 1.62
61–80	30.6 ± 0.60	27.3 ± 3.05	26.5 ± 1.90
81–100	29.7 ± 0.76	27.3 ± 1.57	24.6 ± 0.90
Total	122.9 ± 3.48	114.6 ± 7.65	102.3 ± 4.77

[1]The linear density of dendritic spines was calculated in 20 μm intervals, somatopetally from the cell body to the tip of the terminal segment. Each data point represents the mean number of dendritic spines/20 μm/cell from each of 5 mice.

mice were killed between 1100 and 1400 h after having free access to food for 24 h, they showed a significant increase of plasma insulin, a decrease in plasma glucagon and with no change of plasma glucose. Whether these differences in the hormonal patterns between DR and AD mice are maintained throughout the remainder of the normal dirunal cycle are currently unknown. However, it is important to note that this hormonal profile is similar to what has been reported during the feeding phase for rats trained to consume their total daily allotment of food in a single 2-h meal (Ip *et al.* 1977) and suggests that, metabolically, the intermittent feeding pattern used in our study is similar to a meal-feeding pattern. Similarly, the intermittent feeding pattern used in our study is metabolically similar to the feeding pattern used by Masoro and coworkers in Fischer 344 rats using a protocol of total calorie restriction (Masoro 1984a, 1984b; Yu *et al.* 1984). In those studies rats reportedly consumed their daily allotment of food within 3 h of its presentation (Yu *et al.* 1984), a regimen which has been reported to retard the age-related decline of glucagon and epinephrine-promoted lipolysis in adipose tissue during fasting (Bertrand *et al.* 1987). Together, these data suggest that chronic regimens of intermittent feeding, either by feeding every other day or by meal feeding (feeding restricted amounts of food over 2–3 h period) lead to similar adaptive changes in the liver, adipose tissue and GI tract which enable restricted animals to absorb and store nutrients more rapidly during fasting (Chakrabarty and Leveille 1969; Ip *et al.* 1977). These data also support the concept that chronic intermittent feeding may improve fuel mobilization during fasting and that chronic caloric restriction induced either by intermittent feeding or by restriction of total calories produces a similar alteration of normal age-related patterns of glycogen and fat metabolism found in mice fed an *ad libitum* diet.

Morphological results from our study suggest that caloric restriction does not alter the normal age-related pattern of dendritic remodeling which has been previously reported in this brain region of the C57BL/6N mice (McNeill *et al.* 1988; 1990). Previous studies from our laboratory have found that in the caudal region of the striatum, the dendritic extent of MSI neurons exhibit a significant degree of dendritic proliferation with age while the extent of MSI dendrites in the rostral striatum remain unchanged (McNeill *et al.* 1988, 1990). Changes in the caudal striatum reflect both an increase in the complexity of MSI dendritic branching patterns as well as the elongation of individual dendritic segments. These data support the view that neuronal aging is a dynamic and complex process which summates dendritic changes across individual neurons to accommodate for and respond to age-related changes in both internal and external stimuli (Buell and Coleman 1981; Connor *et al.* 1980; Flood *et al.* 1985; Hinds and McNelly 1977; Coleman *et al.* 1986; Coleman and Flood 1987). In addition, these data support the notion that the effect of caloric restriction does not have a detrimental effect on GABA, Substance P or enkephalin-containing neurons of the striatum. This hypothesis is based on previous immunocytochemical literature which has reported that MSI neurons of the striatum represent separate populations of GABA and Substance P-containing neurons which may co-contain the neurotransmitter, enkephalin in some species (reviewed in Graybiel and Ragsdale 1983). This hypothesis is consistent with the previous biochemical studies of London *et al.* (1985) who reported no change in glutamic acid decarboxylase, an enzyme in the synthetic pathway of GABA in rats maintained on an alternate-day feeding pattern. However, the neurotransmitters Substance P and enkephalin were not measured in their study. To what degree caloric restriction selectively alters that morphology of other neurotransmitter cell types in the striatum is not known. However, the previous studies (London *et al.* 1985; Joseph *et al.* 1983) have suggested the caloric restriction may selectively retard the normal age-related decline in cholinergic markers in the striatum. Thus large aspiny cholinergic neurons are strong candidates for further study.

Our finding that there was no loss in the linear density of dendritic spines on MSI neurons in dietary restricted mice, suggests that the slowing of dopaminergic receptor loss previously reported in dietary restricted rats (Levin *et al.* 1982; Roth *et al.* 1984) is not mediated through selective anatomical changes in the dendritic mantel of at least one population of postsynaptic MSI neurons. Previous studies have shown that the dendritic spines of MSI neurons are a principal target site for afferent dopaminergic fibers of the substantia nigra and the presumed anatomical loci for postsynaptic dopaminergic receptors (Freund *et al.* 1984). Thus, we hypothesized that the loss of dopamine receptors previously described in aged rodents (Severson and Finch 1980; Randall *et al.* 1981), as well as the slowing of age-related dopaminergic receptor loss in calorically restricted rats (Roth *et al.* 1984), may be related to alterations in the linear density of dendritic spines on MSI neurons. However, data from our study suggest that there is no reduction in the overall linear density of dendritic spines in aged mice and that the density of dendritic spines in AD mice is not significantly different from DR mice. Thus, it is unlikely that the slowing of age-related dopaminergic receptor loss in DR mice results from morphological alterations of dendritic spine density on MSI neurons.

Alternatively, we may propose that the loss of dopamine receptors in aged rodents and the subsequent slowing of dopamine receptor loss in DR rodents may be related to an inhibition of age-related cell loss of other dopaminergic receptive neurons in the striatum. One possible candidate to test this hypothesis is the large aspiny cholinergic intraneuron of the striatum. The results from a recent study have shown that with age there is selective loss of transmitter neurons of the striatum with the greatest loss seen in cholinergic cells (McNeill and Koek 1990). In addition, it is known that dopaminergic fibers synapse on cholinergic interneurons of the striatum (Lehman and Langer 1983) and that the loss of cholinergic markers in the striatum in aged rodents (Strong *et al.* 1980) is retarded by caloric restriction (London *et al.* 1985). Thus, we suggest that caloric restriction by some yet undescribed mechanism may slow the loss of cholinergic neurons in this brain region. The previous study by Nadakavukaren and coworkers (1987) has shown that dietary restriction can retard age-related cell loss in the rat corneal endothelium, and studies are currently underway to examine whether dietary restriction can alter normal age-related patterns of cell loss in the striatum.

Our finding that there was significant elevation of TH activity in adrenal gland of DR mice is consistent with the concept that caloric restriction by intermittent feeding stimulates the secretion of adrenal epinephrine. Previous studies have shown that lipolytic and glycongenolytic actions of epinephrine result in the mobilization of fuels to counteract the onset of hypoglycemia during fasting (Tepperman and Tepperman 1987) and that adrenal TH activity is increased in response to systemic insulin injections (Ulus and Wurtman 1979; Fluharty *et al.* 1983). Our data are also consistent with the recent study by Moore *et al.* (1988) who reported an increase in TH activity as well as TH messenger RNA in adrenals from rats maintained on a calorically restricted diet. These data suggest that the effects of caloric restriction by either intermittent feeding or by restriction of total calories produces similar effects on the upregulation of catecholamine synthesis in the adrenal gland. In addition, the study of Moore *et al.* (1988) supports the notion that the increase in TH activity in DR rodents results from the induction of new enzyme protein rather than an increased activation of the existing enzyme pool.

Our finding of a positive correlation between the adrenal TH activity and plasma insulin levels is most interesting and worthy of further investigation. However, it is uncertain whether there is a causal relationship between these findings. Previous studies have shown that insulin can increase adrenal TH activity (Ulus and Wurtman 1979; Fluharty *et al.* 1983) in response to hypoglycemia and that gene probes derived from recombinant clones containing either human TH or insulin cross-hybridized and are physically linked on chromosome 11 (O'Malley and Rotwein 1988). However, the significance of such a linkage is presently unclear since the distribution gene expression for TH and INS are mutually exclusive in the endocrine and nervous systems.

Previous studies have shown that while insulin expression is high in the beta cells of the endocrine pancreas, gene expression for insulin has been reported to be absent in the brain (Baskin *et al.* 1988). Similarly, while message for TH is expressed within many nuclei of the brain, the adrenal medulla, and sympathetic ganglia, it is absent from peripheral endocrine tissues.

SUMMARY

Our data suggest that the beneficial effects of caloric restriction on slowing age-related changes in motor function are not mediated through morphological alterations of MSI neurons of the striatum. This finding is somewhat surprising since MSI neurons are the principal postsynaptic cell population for afferent dopaminergic fibers and a major component of the basal ganglia motor circuit. In contrast, our data suggest that the effects of caloric restriction may be mediated through alterations in other dopamine-receptive cell types in the striatum such as large aspiny cholinergic neurons. Previous studies have reported that afferent dopaminergic fibers synapse on cholinergic interneurons of the striatum and that the age-related loss of cholinergic markers in the striatum may be slowed by dietary restriction. Furthermore, our data provide support for the notion that the beneficial effects of caloric restriction may in some way be induced through alterations in the basic pattern of secretion of selective metabolic hormones which promote both the production and utilization of glucose. Our data suggest that both the amount and pattern of caloric intake are important contributors to extending life span and that caloric restriction, whether by decreasing total calories or by intermittent feeding promotes a similar alteration in the normal age-related pattern of glycogen and fat metabolism found in mice fed an *ad libitum* diet.

Although the mechanisms which underlie the modulation of aging by caloric restriction remain unknown, we hypothesize that part of these effects may be mediated through the neuromodulatory action of peripheral hormones or growth factors on selected neurotransmitter-containing regions of the brain, in particular, the striatum, hippocampus and hypothalamus. Previous studies have shown that peripheral hormones such as insulin may enter the brain at circumventricular organs such as the median eminence of the hypothalamus (Van Houten *et al.* 1983; Goodner and Berrie 1977), as well as through the blood CSF barrier in the choroid plexsus (Pardridge 1986; Duffy and Pardridge 1987). In addition, recent studies have shown that the brain has the highest concentration of insulin-like growth factor 2 (IGF-II) messenger RNA of all major organs (Murphy *et al.* 1987) and suggest that IGF-II is synthesized in the CNS. A recent study has also found that insulin receptors are selectively localized within specific regions of the brain including the hippocampus, as well as on selective neurotransmitter-containing neurons such as somatostatin neurons of the hypothalamus and cholinergic neurons of the striatum and nucleus basalis (Unger *et al.* 1989). Although the exact role for insulin and insulin-like growth factors in the modulation of aging by caloric restriction are unclear, it may be suggested that the presence of these molecules in the CNS provides a means for the brain to assess alterations in peripheral metabolic status through the selective interaction of these molecules with their receptors on specific populations in neurotransmitter neurons in the CNS.

ACKNOWLEDGMENTS

Supported by UPS Grants AG05445, AG07194, and NS22103. Dr. McNeill is a recipient of a Research Career Development Award from the National Institute on Aging (AG00300).

The authors wish to thank Sally Brown, Jeff Davis, Steven Hawes, Barbara Schroeder and Ed Spangler for their expert technical assistance and Lisa Gilbert for typing this manuscript.

REFERENCES

BARROWS, JR., C. H. and KOKKONEN, G. C. 1984. Nutrition and aging: Human and animal laboratory studies. *In* Nutrition in Gerontology, J. M. Ordy, D. Harman and R. Alfin-Slater (eds.). Raven Press, New York.

BASKIN, D. G., WILCOX, B. J., FIGLEWICZ, D. P. and DORSA, D. M. 1988. Insulin and insulin-like growth factors in the CNS. Trends Neurosci. *11*, 107–111.

BERTRAND, H. A., ANDERSON, W. R., MASORO, E. J. and YU, B. P. 1987. Action of food restriction on age-related changes in adipocyte lipolysis. J. Gerontol. *42*, 666–673.

BLACK, I. B. 1975. Increased tyrosine hydroxylase activity in frontal cortex and cerebellum after reserpine. Br. Res. *95*, 170–176.

BUELL, S. J. and COLEMAN, P. D. 1981. Quantitative evidence for selective dendritic growth in normal human aging but not in senile dementia. Br. Res. *214*, 23–41.

CHAKRÅBARTY, K. and LEVEILLE, G. A. 1969. Influence of periodicity of eating on the activity of various enzymes in adipose tissue, liver and muscle of the rat. J. Nut. *96*, 76–82.

COLEMAN, P. D. *et al.* 1986. Stability of dendrites in cortical barrels of C57BL/6N mice between 4 and 45 months. Neurobiol. Aging *7*, 101–105.

COLEMAN, P. D. and FLOOD, D. G. 1986. Dendritic proliferation in the aging brain as a compensatory repair mechanism. Prog. Br. Res. *70*, 227–237.

COLEMAN, P. D. and FLOOD, D. G. 1987. Neurons numbers and dendritic extent in normal aging and Alzheimer's disease. Neurobiol. Aging *8*, 521–545.

COLEMAN, P. D. and RIESEN, A. E. 1978. Environmental effects on coritical dendritic fields. I. Rearing in the dark. J. Anat. *102*, 363.

CONNOR, JR., J. R., DIAMOND, M. C. and JOHNSON, R. E. 1980. Occipital cortical morphology of the rat: Alterations with age and environment. Exp. Neurol. *68*, 158–170.

COOPER, J. R., BLOOM. F. E. and ROTH, R. H. 1986. The biochemical basis of neuropharmacology, 5th Ed. Oxford University Press, New York.

COSPITO, J. and KULTAS-ILINSKY, K. 1981. Synaptic organization of motor corticostriatal projections in the rat. Exp. Neurol. *72*, 257–266.

CUTLER, R. G. 1981. Lifespan extension. *In* Aging: Biology and Behavior, J. L. McGaugh, and S. B. Kiesler (eds.). Academic Press, New York.

DAVIS, B. J. *et al.* 1990. Neuroendocrine effects of lifelong dietary restriction by intermittent feeding in mice. Biochem. Adv. Aging (In press.)

DELONG, M. and ALEXANDER, G. 1986. Organization of the basal ganglia. *In* Diseases of the Nervous System, A. K. Asbury, G. M. McKhann and W. I. McDonald (eds.). William Heinemann Medical Books, London.

DIFIGLIA, M., PASIK, P. and PASIK, T. 1976. A Golgi study of neuronal types in the neostriatum of monkeys. Br. Res. *114*, 245–256.

DUFFY, K. and PARDRIDGE, W. 1987. Blood-brain barrier transcytosis of insulin developing rabbits. Br. Res. *420*, 32–38.

FALLON, J. H. and MOORE, R. Y. 1978. Catecholamine innervation of the basal forebrain. IV. Topography of the dopamine projection to the basal forebrain and neostriatum. J. Comp. Neurol. *180*, 545–580.

FALLON, J. H., RILEY, J. N. and MOORE, R. Y. 1978. Substantia nigra dopamine neurons: separate populations project to neostriatum and allocortex. Neurosci. Lett. *7*, 157–162.

FLOOD, D. G. *et al.* 1985. Age-related dendritic growth in the "oldest old." Br. Res. *345*, 366–368.

FLUHARTY, S. J., SNYDER, G. L., STRICKER, E. M. and ZIGMOND, M. J. 1983. Short-and-long-term changes in adrenal tyrosine hydroxylase activity during insulin-induced hypoglycemia and cold stress. Br. Res. *267*, 384–387.

FREUND, T. F., POWELL, J. F. and SMITH, A. D. 1984. Tyrosine hydroxylase-immunoreactive boutons in synaptic contact with identified striatonigral neurons, with particular reference to dendritic spines. Neurosci. *13*, 1189–1215.

GERFEN, C. R. 1984. The neostriatal mosaic: compartmentalization of corticostriatal input and striatonigral output systems. Nature *311*, 461–464.

GERFEN, C. R. 1985. The neostriatal mosaic. I. Compartmental organization of projections from the striatum to the substantia nigra in the rat. J. Comp. Neurol. *236*, 454–476.

GOODNER, C. and BERRIE, M. 1977. The failure of rat hypothalamic tissues to take up labeled insulin in vitro or to respond to insulin in vitro. Endocrinol. *101*, 605–612.

GOODRICK, C. L. 1984. Effects of lifelong restricted feeding on complex maze performance in rats. Age *7*, 1–2.

GRAYBIEL, A. M. 1983. Compartmental organization of the mammalian striatum. *In* Molecular and Cellular Interactions Underlying Higher Brain Function, J. P. Changeux, J. Glowinski, M. Imbert and F. E. Bloom (eds.). Prog. Br. Res. 586, 247–256, Elsevier, New York.

GRAYBIEL, A. M. and RAGSDALE, C. W. 1983. Biochemical anatomy of the striatum. *In* Chemical Neuroanatomy, P. C. Emson (ed.). Raven Press, New York.

HAZZARD, W. R. *et al.* 1968. A double antibody immunoassay for glucagon. Diabetes *17*, 179–186.

HINDS, J. W. and MCNELLY, N. A. 1977. Aging of the rat olfactory bulb: Growth and atrophy of constituent layers and changes in size and number of mitral cells. J. Comp. Neurol. *171*, 345–368.

INGRAM, D. K. 1991. Effects of caloric restriction on brain and behavioral function in aging rodents. *In* The Potential for Nutritional Modulation of Aging Processes, D. K. Ingram, N. W. Shock and G. T. Baker (eds.). Food and Nutrition Press, Trumbull, CT.

INGRAM, D. K. *et al.* 1987. Dietary restriction benefits learning and motor performance of aged mice. J. Gerontol. *42*, 78–81.

IP, M., IP, C., TEPPERMAN, H. M. and TEPPERMAN, J. 1977. Effect of adaptation to meal feeding on insulin, glucagon and the cyclic nucleotide-protein kinase system in rats. J. Nutr. *107*, 746–757.

JONES, W. J. and THOMAS, D. B. 1962. Changes in the dendritic organization of neurons in the cerebral cortex following deafferentation. J. Anat. Lond. *96*, 375.

JOSEPH, J. A., WHITAKER, J., ROTH, G. S. and INGRAM, D. K. 1983. Lifelong dietary restriction affects striatally mediated behavioral responses in aged rats. Neurobiol. Aging *4*, 191–196.

KEMP, J. M. and POWELL, T. P. S. 1970. The cortico-striate projection in the monkey. Brain *93*, 525.

KEMP, J. M. and POWELL, T. P. S. 1971. The termination of fibers from the cerebral cortex and thalamus upon dendritic spines in the caudate nucleus: A study with the Golgi method. Philos. Trans. R. Soc. London, Ser. B. *262*, 429.

LEHMAN, J. and LANGER, S. Z. 1983. The striatal cholinergic interneuron: Synaptic target of dopaminergic terminalis? Neuroscience *10*, 1105.

LEVIN, P. *et al.* 1982. Dietary restriction retards the age-associated loss of rat striatal dopaminergic receptors. Science *21*, 561–562.

LONDON, E. D., WALLER, S. B., ELLIS, A. T. and INGRAM, D. K. 1985. Effects of intermittent feeding on neurochemical markers in aging rat brain. Neurobiol. Aging *4*, 191–196.

MASORO, E. J. 1984a. Food restriction and the aging process. J. Am. Geriatrics Soc. *32*, 296–300.

MASORO, E. J. 1984b. Nutrition as a modulator of the aging process. The Physiologist *27*, 98–101.

McNEILL, T. H. and KOEK, L. 1990. Differential effect of advancing aging on neurotransmitter cell loss in the substantia nigra and striatum of the C57 BL/6N mouse. Brain Res. *521*, 107–118.

McNEILL, T. H., KOEK, L. L., BROWN, S. A. and RAFOLS, J. A. 1988b. Age-related changes in the nigrostriatal system. Ann. N. Y. Acad. Sci. *515*, 239–248.

McNEILL, T. H., KOEK, L. L., BROWN, S. A. and RAFOLS, J. A. 1990. Quantitative analysis of age-related dendritic in medium spiny I (MSI) striatal neurons C57BL/6N mice. Neurobiol. Aging (In press.)

MELVIN, J. and HAMILL, R. W. 1986. Gonadal hormonal regulation of neurotransmitter synthesizing enzymes in developing hypogastric ganglia. Br. Res. *383*, 38–46.

MORGAN, C. R. and LAZAROW, A. 1963. Immunoassay of insulin two antibody system. Plasma levels of normal, subdiabetic and diabetic rats. Diabetes *12*, 115–126.

MOORE, M. A. *et al.* 1988. Age-related changes in adrenal tyrosine hydroxylase expression and catecholamine content: Effects of dietary restriction. Soc. Neurosci. *14*, 403.

MOYER, A., MOYER, U. and COLEMAN, P. D. 1985. An inexpensive PC based system for quantification of neuronal processes. Soc. Neurosci. *11*, 261.

MURPHY, L., BELL, G. and FRIESEN, H. 1987. Blood-brain barrier transcytosis of insulin in developing rabbits. Endocrine *120*, 1279–1282.

NADAKAVUKAREN, M. J., FITCH, K. L. and RICHARDSON, A. 1987. Dietary restriction retards age-related decrease in cell population of rat corneal endothelium. Proc. Soc. Exp. Biol. Med. *184*, 98–101.

O'MALLEY, K. L. and ROTWEIN, P. 1988. Human tyrosine hydroxylase and insulin genes are contiguous on chromosome 11. Nucleic Acid Res. *16*, 4437–4446.

OSTERBURG, H. H., DONAHUE, H. G., SEVERSON, J. A. and FINCH, C. E. 1981. Catecholamine levels and turnover during aging in brain regions of male C57BL/6J mice. Br. Res. *161*, 303–310.

PARDRIDGE, W. M. 1986. Receptor-mediated peptide transport through the blood-brain barrier. Endocrine Rev. *7*, 314–330.

RAGSDALE, JR., C. W. and GRAYBIEL, A. M. 1981. The fronto-striatal projection in the cat and monkey and its relationship to inhomogeneities established by acetylcholinesterase histochemistry. Br. Res. *208*, 259–266.

RANDALL, P. K., SEVERSON, J. A. and FINCH, C. E. 1981. Aging and the regulation of striatal dopaminergic mechanisms in mice. J. Pharmacol. Exp. Ther. *219*, 690–700.

ROGERS, J., ZORNETZER, S. F., BLOOM, F. E. and MERVIS, R. E. 1984. Senescent microstructural changes in rat cerebellum. Br. Res. *292*, 23.

ROTH, G. S., INGRAM, D. K. and JOSEPH, J. A. 1984. Delayed loss of striatal dopamine receptors during aging of dietarily restricted rats. Br. Res. *300*, 27–32.

SEVERSON, J. A. and FINCH, C. E. 1980. Reduced dopaminergic binding during aging in the rodent striatum. Br. Res. *192*, 147–162.

STRONG, R. *et al.* 1980. Age-related alterations in the rodent brain cholinergic system and behavior. Neurobiol. Aging *1*, 59–63.

STRONG, R., SAMORAGJSKI, T. and GOTTESFELD, Z. 1982. Regional mapping of neostriatal neurotransmitter systems as a function of aging. J. Neurochem. *39*, 831–836.

TEPPERMAN, J. and TEPPERMAN, H. M. 1987. Metabolic and Endocrine Physiology, 5th Ed. Yearbook Medical Publishers, Chicago.

ULUS, I. H. and WURTMAN, R. J. 1979. Selective response of rat sympathetic nervous system to various stimuli. J. Physiol. *293*, 513–523.

UNGER, J. *et al.* 1989. Distribution of insulin receptor-like immunoreactivity in the rat forebrain. Neuroscience *31*, 143–157.

VAN DER LOOS, H. 1956. Une conbinaison de deux vieilles methodes histologiques pour le systeme nerveux central. Mschr. Psychiat. Neurol. *132*, 330–334.30.50.

VAN HOUTEN, M., NANCE, D., GAUTHIER, S. and POSNER, B. 1983. Origin of insulin-receptive nerve terminals in rat median eminence. Endocrinology *113*, 1393–1399.

WALFORD, R. L. *et al.* 1974. Long term dietary restriction and immune function in mice: response to sheep red blood cells and to mitogenic agents. Mech. Ageing Dev. *2*, 447–454.

WEINDRUCH, R. 1984. Dietary restriction and the aging process. *In* Free Radicals in Molecular Biology, Aging, and Disease, D. Armstrong, R. S. Sohal, R. G. Cutler and T. F. Slater (eds.). Raven Press, New York.

WEINDRUCH, R. and WALFORD, R. L. 1982. Life span and spontaneous cancer incidence in mice dietarily restricted beginning at one year of age. Science *215*, 1415–1418.

WILSON, C. J. and GROVES, P. M. 1980. Fine structure and synaptic connections of the common spiny neuron of the rat neostriatum: A study employing intracellular injection of horseradish perioxidase. J. Comp. Neurol. *194*, 599.

YU, B. P. *et al.* 1984. Age changes in hepatic metabolic characteristics and their modulation by dietary manipulation. Mech. Aging Dev. *24*, 67–81.

CHAPTER 20

EFFECTS OF LONG-TERM ALTERATIONS OF DIETARY CALCIUM AND MAGNESIUM ON INDICES OF RAT BRAIN AGING AND BONE STRUCTURE

P. LANDFIELD, L. CADWALLADER, S. VINSANT, D. FLEENOR, S. KERR and L. CAMPBELL
Bowman Grey School of Medicine
Winston-Salem, North Carolina
and
P. ETIENNE, M.D.
CIBA-GEIGY US
Summit, New Jersey

INTRODUCTION

There is increasing evidence that alterations in calcium homeostasis may play an important role in the mammalian brain aging process (cf. reviews in Khachaturian 1984; Gibson and Peterson 1987; Landfield 1988a; Roth 1988).However, the specific aspect of altered calcium homeostasis that is most critical in aging phenomena has not been defined. A number of studies suggest that aging in nonneural (Roth 1988) or neural (Gibson and Peterson 1987) systems is associated with decreased calcium (Ca) availability, whereas other studies indicate that Ca availability or influx in brain neurons may be increased with aging (cf. reviews in Khachaturian 1984; Landfield 1988a). Since there is considerable evidence that elevated levels of intracellular Ca are toxic to excitable cells (cf. Schlaepfer and Hasler 1979; Siesjo 1981; Nayler *et al.* 1979), the findings of increased Ca availability or influx through voltage-sensitive Ca channels may have implications for mechanisms of age-related neuronal loss.

Moreover, there is increasing evidence that the excitotoxic effects of some amino acids may be mediated by receptor-operated ion channels (e.g., N-methyl-D-aspartate channels) that admit Ca ions but are blocked by magnesium (Mg) ions. The neurotoxic effects of ischemia, for example, may be mediated by these channels (cf. reviews in Fagg *et al.* 1986; Meldrum 1987; Schwarcz *et al.* 1984).

These considerations suggested that long-term alteration in Ca or Mg dietary intake, if they were able to influence brain levels of Mg and Ca, might provide an intervention method for testing the Ca-alteration hypothesis of brain aging. This chapter outlines in greater detail the underlying rationale and describes the methods and results of a long-term experiment to test the effects of chronically altering dietary Mg and Ca.

Age-related Changes in Brain Calcium Homeostasis

Hippocampal synaptic physiology is characterized by both a highly robust form of frequency potentiation (FP) (growth of postsynaptic responses during repetitive presynaptic stimulation) (Andersen and Lomo 1967; MacVicar and Dudek 1979; Schwartzkroin 1975; Pitler and Landfield 1987), and an extremely long-lasting form of postactivation potentiation, termed long-term potentiation (LTP) (Bliss and Lomo 1973; cf. reviews in Landfield and Deadwyler 1988). We have consistently observed a deficit in FP in the hippocampus of aged rats (Landfield *et al.* 1978a, 1986; Landfield 1980), which is correlated with impairment of some aspects of behavioral plasticity in aging animals (Landfield 1980; Landfield and Morgan 1984). Consequently, frequency potentiation could well be a mechanism through which biologically meaningful information is amplified and through which LTP or other long-lasting changes underlying memory are induced.

Studies using Mg, a well-established competitive inhibitor of Ca actions on neurons, have indicated that elevation of the extracellular Mg/Ca ratio in the bathing medium improves frequency potentiation in hippocampal slices, but particularly in slices from aged animals (Landfield 1981; Landfield *et al.* 1986). Conversely, a high Ca bathing medium impairs FP in young rat hippocampal slices. In addition, a high Mg diet (2.0%) for 4 days was found to strengthen maze reversal learning and FP in intact rats. Again, the effect was greater for aged animals (Landfield and Morgan 1984).

The studies with high Mg/Ca ratios suggested that the impairment of hippocampal FP in aged rats might be due to increased Ca influx through voltage-sensitive Ca channels, leading to impaired function by a number of possible mechanisms (e.g., transmitter depletion, Ca current inactivation, afterhyperpolarizations, etc.) (Landfield *et al.* 1986). However, the effect could also be accounted for by a number of other processes, including changes in non-Ca-dependent processes or in the amount of Ca buffering or extrusion (cf. Michaelis *et al.* 1984; Smith 1988). Therefore, we tested the Ca influx hypothesis more directly, by measuring Ca dependent afterhyperpolarization, and Ca spikes in hippocampal neurons. Each of these processes were found to be prolonged in hippocampal neurons in aged rats, following a controlled depolarization (Landfield and Pitler 1984; Pitler and Landfield 1987). Based on these observations, we have proposed that an increase in membrane Ca conductance is one of the initiating factors in the development of age-related changes in neuronal Ca homeostasis and, consequently, in neuronal function and structure (Landfield 1988a).

Current Views about the Physiology and Role of NMDA Receptors in Aging

The NMDA (N-methyl-D-aspartate) receptor, one of the classes of glutamate receptor-mediating excitatory synaptic transmission, is being found to play a critical role in many complex neurophysiological and "plastic" events which underlie central neural development and function in vertebrates. In the present context, it appears of considerable interest because it is associated with an ion channel that is highly permeable to Ca ions, as well as Na ions (the NMDA receptor complex).

The NMDA receptor is comprised of distinct domains whose interactions form the basis of the initiation and regulation of receptor activity. That is, the NMDA receptor complex is not simply a ligand-gated ion channel (as are many fast-acting transmitter receptors), but is subject to additional regulation by the amino acid glycine and, uniquely, by voltage-dependent binding of magnesium ions inside the channel. Another binding site for psychoactive drugs such as phenylcyclidine (PCP) and MK-801 is also located within the channel. The NMDA receptor complex has evolved a unique form of receptor- and voltage-dependent gating, involving binding of Mg inside the channel. Hence switching on NMDA receptor mechanisms requires at the minimum: (1) binding of transmitter to its recognition site and (2) relief of the channel blockade (for example, by local depolarization of the postsynaptic membrane by other excitatory inputs). In addition, receptor function may be subject to rapid up- or down-regulation by changes in the levels of glycine and/or Mg in the local extracellular environment. (See Fagg 1986 for review.)

The NMDA receptor complex is involved in long-term potentiation and some forms of learning in mature animals (cf. reviews in Landfield and Deadwyler 1988), burst firing and the generation of patterned activity in neuronal networks, use-dependent stabilization of synaptic connectivity in young animals and pathologies such as epilepsy, spasticity, ischemic neuronal death and neurodegeneration. (See Meldrum 1987 for review.) Ca entry is essential in the multiple roles of the NMDA receptor complex. The role of the NMDA receptor complex in ischemic neuronal death is now well established, but its role in neurodegeneration is still controversial.

The endogenous neurotoxin quinolinic acid acts as an agonist to excitatory amino acid receptors, and its level is increased in senescent rats. It has been speculated that it may play a role in the genesis of the neuronal destruction seen in degenerative diseases such as Huntington's Disease (Shoulson 1983) and Alzheimer's Disease (Schwarcz *et al.* 1984). Some of the inherited ataxias are related to glutamate dehydrogenase deficiency (Plaitakis *et al.* 1980) perhaps leading to a relative overactivity of excitatory amino acid functions (due to enhanced levels of glutamate) in certain parts of the brain. Lynch *et al.* (1986) have suggested that Ca-activated proteases (calpains) may play a role in brain cell death during aging, and Etienne and Baudry (1987) have postulated that excitatory amino acid transmission is an important trigger for the Ca entry and activation of the calpains. Proteases are thought to play a role in the irreversible neuronal cytoskeleton changes which underlie some forms of neuronal pathology (e.g., Lynch *et al.* 1986; Schlaepfer and Hasler 1979).

Thus, there are two lines of evidence that raise the possibility that increased Ca influx through, on one hand, voltage-sensitive Ca channels and, on the other, receptor-operated (NMDA) Ca channels may play a role in aging-related loss of neurons or in lasting electrophysiological impairments. Magnesium appears capable of reducing Ca influx through both types of channels and, as noted, elevated dietary Mg can affect brain neurophysiology in intact animals (Landfield and Morgan 1984). Brain Mg can be raised through dietary means, even though Mg concentration in the brain's extracellular space is tightly regulated by barrier and transport mechanisms (Katzman 1975; Mordes and Wacker 1978); i.e., while brain Mg does not rise appreciably during acute plasma elevations of Mg, the Mg concentration in brain or cerebrospinal fluid can be changed by chronically altering plasma Mg over several hours or days (Pritchard 1955; Buck *et al.* 1979; Chutkow 1974). Equilibrium of brain and plasma Mg or Ca appears to develop after 24 h (Katzman 1975).

In the present studies, therefore, we tested the hypothesis that the rate of brain aging can be modulated by long-term manipulation of dietary Mg and Ca intake. However, because of side effects (e.g., gastrointestinal disturbances, hair balls, etc.) the amount of Mg in the diet could not be as high as the 2.0% used in the relatively short (4 day) feeding periods in the prior study (e.g., Landfield and Morgan 1984).

To assess brain aging at the end of the 9 month intervention experiment, a series of brain morphometric and electrophysiological correlates of aging in the hippocampus of rats were used. These have been shown previously to separate young from aged rats very consistently and to, therefore, provide suitable biomarkers of brain aging (cf. Landfield 1982, 1988b). They include pyramidal cell density in field CA1 (Landfield *et al.* 1981), frequency potentiation, field EPSP amplitude and population spike threshold (Landfield *et al.* 1978, 1986; McNaughton *et al.* 1981). In addition, measures of bone density, adrenal gland weight (e.g., Landfield *et al.* 1987b) and overall incidence of pathology were obtained.

METHODS

General Design

Six different dietary regimens were compared, which were enriched or restricted in Mg and/or Ca. Groups of aging male Fischer 344 rats (n = 13 each) received different experimental diets in which Ca and Mg were varied in the drinking water and food, between the ages of 16–25 months. (The rats were obtained from the germfree colony of the National Institute on Aging at age 15 months, and the experiment was begun approximately one month later after they had been acclimated to their new housing conditions). A control group of 5 month rats (n = 12) received the control diet (Normal Mg, Normal Ca). No animals with overt pathology present at the start were included in the study. All animals were housed behind a laminar flow air-barrier unit in an isolated room throughout the study and were approached only by investigators in clean lab coats and gloves. No instances of respiratory infection were found during the experiment. The six aged groups with their corresponding daily Ca and Mg intake (range of mean values in mg/rat/day), the number of animals who survived to the end in each group and the number of animals found free of serious pathology at sacrifice are presented in Table 20.1. The concentrations of Ca and Mg in the drinking water that would represent high, low or normal values of intake were obtained from studies in the literature (cf. Mordes and Walker 1978) and from normal contents of standard rat lab chow. All animals were fed a diet largely free of Ca and Mg (Teklad), and Ca and Mg were replaced or elevated by addition to the drinking water. Water intake was measured routinely to determine levels of intake. However, the Very High Mg group could not be given all of its Mg in the drinking water (due to depression of water intake); therefore, its diet was supplemented with food containing sufficient Mg to provide approximately half of that group's Mg intake. The effects of the Mg-enriched diets had been tested in a pilot experiment. The high Mg diet was nearly as high as could be sustained without diarrhea or other apparent detrimental effects. Throughout the study, animals were monitored for food and water consumption and weight levels. Ten days before the end of the study, all animals were placed back on the control diet. After these 10 days, electrophysiological measurements were carried out (lasting about 3

TABLE 20.1
MG/CA DIETARY INTAKE AND SURVIVING ANIMALS IN AGED GROUPS

Mg	Ca	Mg Intake[1] (Range)	Ca Intake[1] (Range)	Survivors to Sacrifice	Healthy at Sacrifice
Normal	normal	5.5–9.0	3.7–6.6	12/13	9/13
Very high	normal	50.9–87.5	3.8–7.3	6/13	6/13
High	normal	16.9–33.3	3.9–6.5	10/13	9/13
Low	normal	0.7–1.0	5.3–6.7	10/13	9/13
Low	low	0.7–1.0	0.9–2.0	11/13	10/13
Normal	high	3.9–6.5	23.4–49.5	12/13	9/13

[1]Values are group means in mg/animal/day.

h/animal). At the end of the electrophysiologial studies, the animals were perfused with mixed aldehyde fixative for neuroanatomical studies. Because only a few animals could be studied electrophysiologically each day, the termination of the diet was staggered over a period of about one month, and animals from the different groups were studied alternately.

Electrophysiological Measurements

The stereotaxic and physiological methods for placing stimulating and recording electrodes in hippocampus to elicit the typical monosynaptic Schaffer collateral-commissural response (recorded in field CA1) were described previously (Landfield *et al.* 1978a; Landfield and Morgan 1984). The properties of this response have also been described earlier by others in some detail. The present studies focused on measures of the population spike and population (or field) EPSP, which are extracellular summations of synchronous action potentials, and individual dendritic EPSPs, respectively (Andersen and Lomo 1967). In urethane-anesthetized rats, a bipolar stimulation electrode was lowered into the Schaffer collateral fibers in the CA3 region, while recordings were obtained from the CA1 region of the hippocampus, using an extracellular microelectrode. Stimulation intensity was set at a level needed to produce a control population spike of one half the maximum spike. The ratio of the second to the first population spike in a paired-pulse paradigm was then measured in the pyramidal cell somal layer after a 100 msec and a 200 msec interpulse interval. The recording electrode was then lowered to the dendritic field in which the Schaffer collaterals terminate (Swanson *et al.* 1978) and the field EPSP was measured after single, paired and repetitive pulses. For repetitive stimulation, a train of 7 Hz was applied to the Schaffer-commissural fibers and the field EPSP amplitude in CA1 was measured (percent of control) after 5, 15, and 30 s stimulation. Data were excluded from any animal exhibiting seizure activity during stimulation.

Fixation, Tissue Preparation and Sampling

Under deep urethane anesthesia, the abdomen was opened and the descending abdominal aorta clamped with a hemostat, to direct fixative solution toward the upper body. The rib cage and diaphragm were then cut, and the right auricle was cut to allow drainage of the fixative solution, while the left ventricle was catheterized and perfused at a rate of 50–60 mL/minute. A 2% glutaraldehyde and 2% paraformaldehyde fixative solution in 0.15-M sodium cacodylate buffer containing 1.0 mM Ca was used as the fixative solution. Perfusion of the fixative solution was maintained for 10–15 minutes, after which the brain was removed and stored in fixative overnight. Standard criteria for acceptable fixation quality were followed.

The brain was blocked, glued to a chuck, and cut in 250-μm-thick coronal sections on a Pelco vibratome. Sections were taken beginning at the frontal tip of the hippocampus and throughout the part of the brain containing hippocampus. These sections were compared under a dissecting microscope, and the slice that was either 2000 μm or 2250 μm from the front of the hippocampus was selected for analysis (depending upon which of the 2 conformed more closely to a particular configuration of cell layer patterns). The hippocampal slice was then dehydrated, embedded in Araldite 502 and stained according to standard EM procedures. The embedded tissue was subsequently trimmed such that semithin sections (1 μm thick) were cut perpendicular to the medial-lateral axis of the section, and parallel to the CA1 apical dendrites. The block face was trimmed on a line through CA1 and the dentate gyrus, at a consistent point based on the shapes of the ventral and dorsal leaves of the granule cell layer of the dentate gyrus.

Quantitative Neuroanatomy

For each animal, the nucleoli of pyramidal cells were counted blind (from coded slides) on 5 randomly selected, semithin sections (1 μm-thick) of the stratum pyramidale. The width of this cell layer (stratum pyramidale) on each section (approximately 250 μm) was also measured with a calibrated eyepiece. Total nucleoli were then divided by total cell layer width, and data were expressed as neurons/100 μm stratum pyramidale width. Only neurons that were clearly within the pyramidal somal layer were counted. Nucleolar diameters also were measured in all cells on one or two sections for each animal, in order to ensure that nucleolar diameter was not changed by a treatment (since large diameter particles are more likely to be counted.).

The depth of stratum radiatum (e.g., length of apical dendrites) was also measured in all animals, in order to determine whether overall structural growth, which can reduce cell density, had occurred. (These data were not significant and are not reported here).

Adrenal Weight Measurements

Adrenal weights for the pair of adrenals from each animal were obtained following trimming of all fat and connective tissue. They were measured both wet and dry (after 2 days in a low-heat oven).

Bone Measurements

Femurs were boiled for several hours and most of the soft tissues were removed after this first step. Remaining soft tissues were removed after immersion in a mild acid bath followed by drying. Volume was measured by water displacement.

Pathology

A complete pathological examination was performed by a veterinary pathologist in all animals that died or showed unusual forms of major pathology during the study. The probable cause of death or pathology is presented in Table 20.2 by group, with the number of animals for each diagnosis indicated in parentheses.

TABLE 20.2
CAUSES OF DEATH AND INCIDENCE OF PATHOLOGY AT SACRIFICE IN AGED GROUPS

(1) Normal Mg, Normal Ca	
Deaths:	wasting (1)[1]
Pathology:	gastric aneurism (1); abdominal or neck tumor (2)
(2) High Mg, Normal Ca (Very High and High Combined)	
Deaths:	wasting (4); abscess on ear (*Staphylococcus aureus*); (2) internal hemorrhage (1); trichobezoar (hair balls) (2); abdominal abscess (1)
Pathology:	pituitary tumor (1)
(3) Low Mg, Normal Ca	
Deaths:	wasting (2); brain tumor (1)
Pathology:	pituitary tumor (1)
(4) Low Mg, Low Ca	
Deaths:	wasting (1); pericardial tumor (1)
Pathology:	pituitary tumor (1)
(5) Normal Mg, High Ca	
Deaths:	wasting(1);
Pathology:	brain tumor (1); adrenal tumor (2)

[1]Wasting is a common precursor of death in aging Fischer rats, and appears to result from leukemia and/or renal failure.

Statistical Methods

Analyses of variance followed by post hoc tests (Bonferroni method) were used to examine differences between the experimental groups. Because of loss of animals and generally similar patterns, the High and Very High Mg groups were combined into one High Mg group for most analyses. A probability level of $P < 0.05$ was used for determining statistical significance.

RESULTS

Mortality and Weight Patterns

Comparatively more animals die in the Very High Mg, Normal Ca group, which did not exhibit normal weight gain after the first 2–3 months, than in any of the other age groups (no animals died in the young group). Figure 20.1 shows the mean weight of all surviving animals in each group at approximately biweekly intervals during the study. The mean weight accordingly is affected by the contribution of animals who died later in the course of the study. Only the Very High Mg group differed statistically from the others on mean weight values.

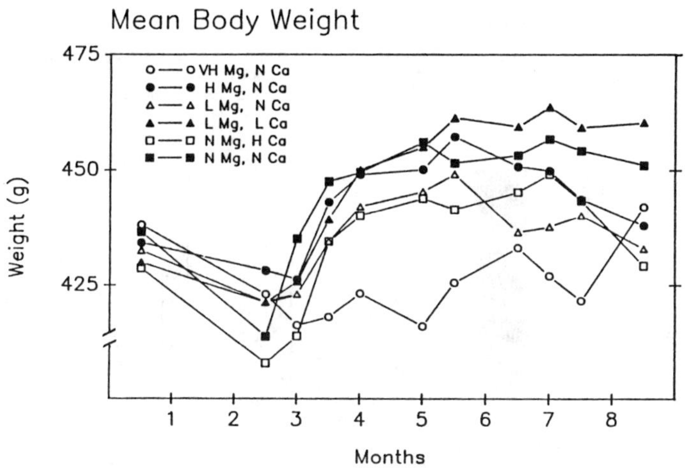

FIG. 20.1. MEAN WEIGHT OF ALL SURVIVING ANIMALS IN THE AGED GROUPS AT APPROXIMATELY BIWEEKLY INTERVALS DURING THE STUDY
N Mg, N Ca = Normal Mg, Normal Ca (control); VH Mg, N Ca = Very High Mg, Normal Ca; H Mg, N Ca = High Mg, Normal Ca; L Mg, N Ca = Low Mg, Normal Ca; L Mg, L Ca = Low Mg, Low Ca; N Mg, H Ca = Normal Mg, High Ca.

Electrophysiological Measurements

As anticipated from the literature, several electrophysiological measures showed significant age differences, including frequency potentiation. However, there were no significant differences between any aged dietary groups on any of these variables. Figure 20.2 shows the results for FP at 30 s of 7 Hz stimulation, which illustrate the lack of significant differences between aged dietary groups. The other electrophysiological variables exhibited similar patterns and are not illustrated here.

Neuronanatomical Measurements

CA1 pyramidal cell density showed the significant differences between young and aged animals that have been reported previously (Landfield *et al.* 1981). Again, however, there were no significant differences between aged dietary groups (Fig. 20.3). There was a trend for the Low Mg, Normal Ca group to show higher pyramidal cell counts than the other aged groups, but this effect was not statistically significant.

Adrenal Gland Weight

As reported previously (cf. Landfield *et al.* 1978b), aged animals exhibited substantially larger adrenal glands than young controls (about 75% increase in weight).

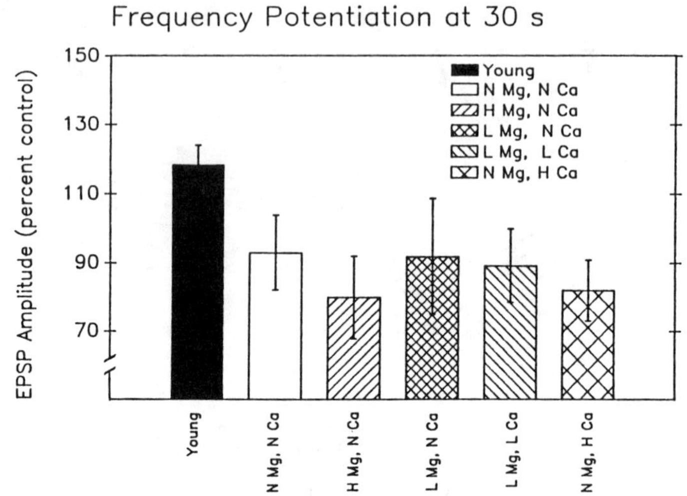

FIG. 20.2. GROUP MEANS ± S.E. OF CA1 POPULATION EPSP AMPLITUDE (PERCENT OF CONTROL) AT 30 S DURING A TRAIN OF 7 HZ STIMULATION OF THE SCHAFFER-COMMISSURAL FIBERS (VERY HIGH MG AND HIGH MG GROUPS COMBINED)

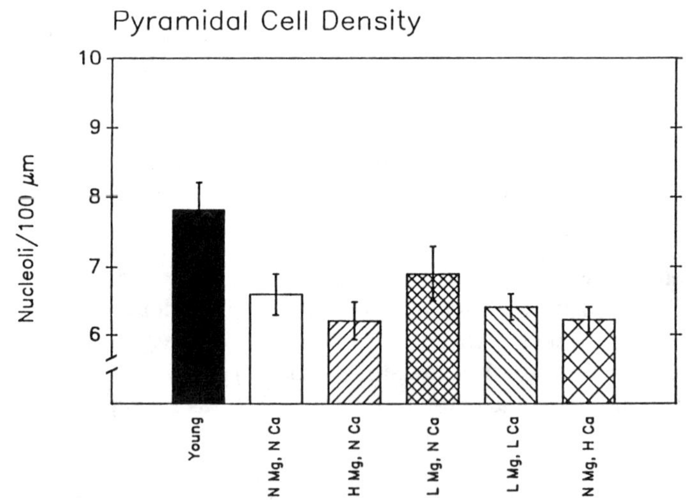

FIG. 20.3. GROUP MEANS ± S.E. OF CA1 PYRAMIDAL NEURON DENSITY (NUCLEOLI/100 μm OF STRATUM PYRAMIDALE WIDTH) IN THE EXPERIMENTAL AND CONTROL DIETARY GROUPS

Again, however, there were no significant differences among the aged dietary groups (Fig. 20.4). The Low Mg, Low Ca group tended nonsignificantly to exhibit lower adrenal gland weight than the other aged groups.

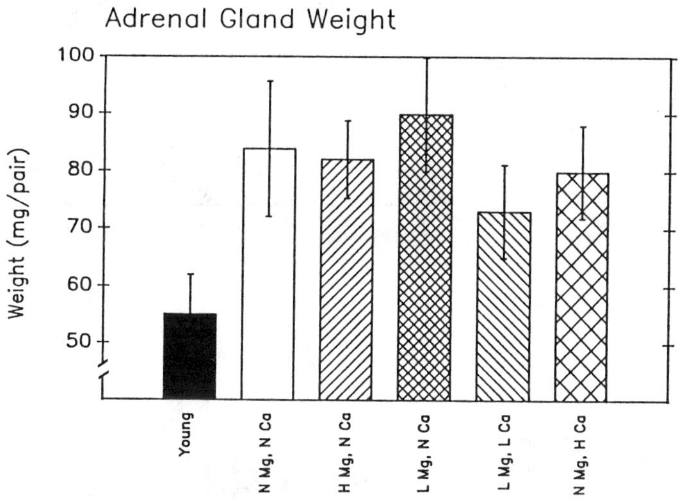

FIG. 20.4. GROUP MEANS ± S.E. OF ADRENAL GLAND WET WEIGHT (MG/PAIR), IN THE EXPERIMENTAL AND CONTROL DIETARY GROUPS

Bone Measurements

Bone measures could not be obtained for the Low Mg, Normal Ca group due to inadvertent loss of some tissues. Nevertheless, bone measurements for the other groups showed significant effects of diet: Both the Low Mg, Low Ca and High Mg, Normal Ca groups exhibited significant lower bone mass and density then did aged controls (Normal Mg, Normal Ca). The High Ca group also tended to exhibit lower bone density, but this effect was not significant (Fig. 20.5C).

Pathology

Two forms of pathology that are relatively unusual for aged Fischer rats were found with some frequency in the High Mg groups. These were trichobezoar (hair balls) with resulting impaction of the gastrointestinal tract, and abscesses in the vicinity of the ear canal. We have also observed hair balls in previous experiments with rats on a high Mg diet. The reason why rats lick or eat their fur while on a high Mg diet is unclear but it is possible that, by so doing, they attempt to compensate for a perceived deficit in a food ingredient (e.g., Ca). With regard to the abscesses in the region of the ear (which contained *Staphylococcus aureus*), it was difficult to

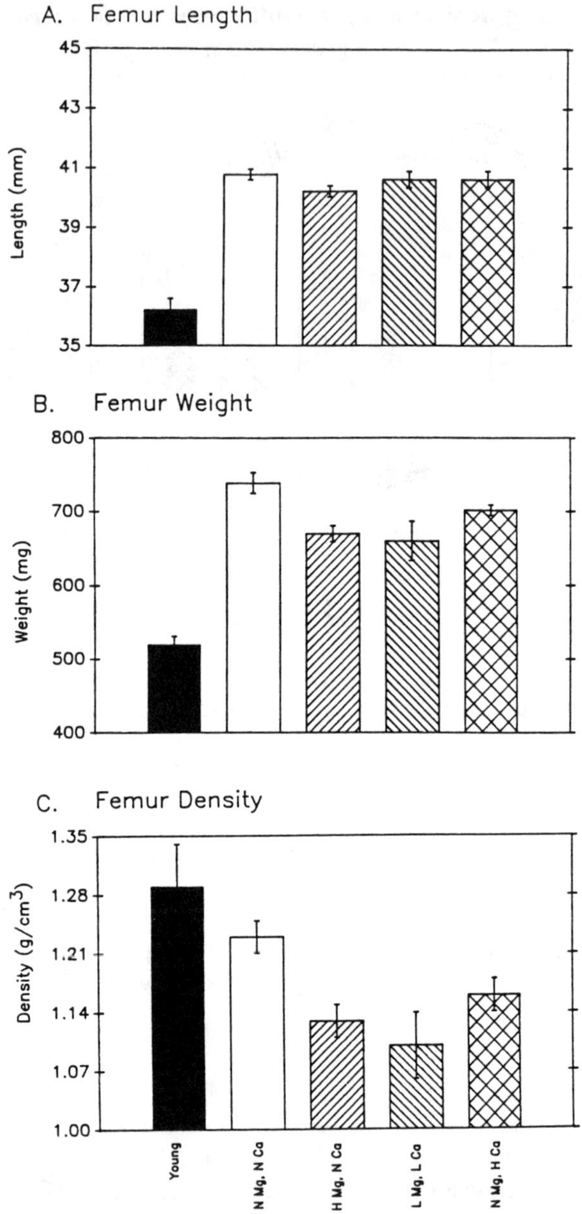

FIG. 20.5. A: GROUP MEANS ± S.E. OF BONE (FEMUR) LENGTH (MM), IN THE EXPERIMENTAL AND CONTROL DIETARY GROUPS; B: GROUP MEANS ± S.E. OF BONE (SINGLE FEMUR) MASS (MG); C: GROUP MEANS ± S.E. OF BONE (FEMUR) DENSITY (MG/CC)

determine whether cancer in the ear canal region preceded the infection, or whether the infection caused inflammatory, anaplastic changes that appeared positive for cancer of the ear canal.

Apart from these aspects of pathology in the High Mg animals, there appeared to be no major differences in the overall rate of pathology. The Low Mg, Low Ca group contained the highest number of animals with no obvious pathology at the termination of the experiment, but apart from the High Mg group, the differences in pathology incidence in these groups were slight and not significant.

DISCUSSION

The results of this study did not support the hypothesis that altered availability of brain Mg or Ca can influence brain aging. However, as is often the case for negative results, the data do not rule out the original hypothesis, because it is not clear that the interventions altered brain Ca homeostasis effectively, or that they did not affect some other processes which counteracted the effects of dietary interventions on aging changes. One clearly possible explanation is that animals on the Mg-enriched diet, and particularly those on the very high Mg diet, were affected by some deleterious actions of the dietary manipulation that were independent of potential actions of the diet on brain Ca availability. That the animals on the high Mg diet were not healthy in general is suggested by the weight data (Fig. 20.1) and by the high incidence of deaths in the Very High Mg group. In addition, the high number of ear abscesses in the high Mg groups and the high incidence of hair balls suggests that some unusual forms of pathology were present in these animals. Conceivably, the high Mg diet used (0.3–0.5%), which was close to the highest feasible without inducing substantial diarrhea, was high enough to disrupt peripheral functions but was not high enough to influence Ca/Mg balance in the brain.

Thus, is seems clear that further tests of the altered Ca homeostasis hypothesis of brain aging will be necessary, although such tests will apparently require a greater effect on brain Ca availability relative to effects on peripheral Ca and Mg metabolism.

Although not significant statistically, there was a consistent trend for animals in one of the other of the two groups with lower than normal totals of Mg + Ca intake (i.e., the Low Mg, Normal Ca and the Low Mg, Low Ca groups) to exhibit somewhat lower values for age-related changes across several variables. One possible direction for future investigation may be to examine the possibility that lowering the overall intake of these divalent cations may in some way reduce the development of brain or nonneural aging changes; i.e., even levels that we term "normal" may be relatively high for this rat strain, and high levels of one or the other or both of these cations may somehow stress neural or nonneural systems essential to the maintenance of function during aging. It should be emphasized, however, that alterations in dietary Ca and Mg of the degree used here were able to affect measures of bone density in aging rats (Fig. 20.5). Thus, it seems clear that until the implications of various levels of dietary Ca/Mg for osteoporosis and other bone disorders are better understood, caution should be used in the recommended levels of Ca or Mg intake for aging humans. Even the High Ca group exhibited a trend to reduced bone mass, suggesting that the *balance* of Mg and Ca may be as important as absolute values in this context. Although the relevance of these studies in rats to humans is, of course, not yet clear, the data suggest the need for more extensive studies on the relations of Ca and Mg intake to bone density and to other aspects of health and function in aging humans.

ACKNOWLEDGMENTS

These studies were supported in part by grants from CIBA-GEIGY and from the National Institute on Aging. We appreciated the excellent and skilled assistance of members of the Department of Comparative Medicine in assessing animal health, and we thank the Document Preparation Center for their valuable assistance in preparing the manuscript.

REFERENCES

ANDERSEN, P. and LOMO, T. 1967. Control of hippocampal output by afferent volley frequency. Progr. Brain Res. *27*, 400–412.

BLISS, T. V. P. and LOMO, T. 1973. Long-lasting potentiation of synaptic transmission in the dentate area of the anesthetized rabbit following stimulation of the perforant path. J. Physiol. (Lond.) *232*, 331–356.

BUCK, D. R., MAHONEY, A. W. and HENDRICKS, D. F. 1979. Effects of cerebral intraventricular magnesium injections and a low magnesium diet on nonspecific excitability level, audiogenic seizure susceptibility and serotonin. Pharmacol. Biochem. Behav. *10*, 487–491.

CHUTKOW, J. G. 1974. Metabolism of magnesium in central nervous system. Neurology *24*, 780–787.

ETIENNE, P. and BAUDRY, M. 1987. Calcium-dependent aspects of synaptic plasticity, excitatory amino acid neurotransmission, brain aging and schizophrenia: a unifying hypothesis. Neurobiol. Aging *8*, 362–366.

FAGG, G. E. 1985. L-glutamate, excitatory amino acid receptors and brain function. TINS, May, 207–210.

FAGG, G. E., FOSTER, A. C. and GANON, A. H. 1986. Excitatory amino acid synaptic mechanisms and neurological function. TINS, Sept., 357–363.

GIBSON, G. E. and PETERSON, C. 1987. Calcium and the aging nervous system. Neurobiol. Aging *8*, 329–344.

KATZMAN, R. 1975. Cerebrospinal fluid physiology: Role of secretory and medicated transport systems. *In* The Nervous System, Vol. 1: The Basic Neurosciences, D. B. Tower (ed.). Raven Press, New York.

KHACHATURIAN, Z. S. 1984. Towards theories of brain aging. *In* Handbook of Studies on Psychiatry and Old Age, D. Kay and G. D. Burrows (eds.). Elsevier, Amsterdam.

LANDFIELD, P. W. 1980. Correlative studies of brain neurophysiology and behavior during aging. *In* The Psychobiology of Aging, D. G. Stein (ed.). Elsevier, Amsterdam.

LANDFIELD, P. W. 1981. Age-related impairment of hippocampal frequency potentiation: Evidence of an underlying deficit in transmitter release from studies of Mg^{2+}-bathed hippocampal slices. Soc. Neurosci. Abstr. *7*, 371.

LANDFIELD, P. W. 1982. Measurement of brain aging: conceptual issues and neurobiological indices. *In* Endocrine and Neuroendocrine Mechanisms of Aging, R. Adelman and G. Roth (eds.). CRC Press, Boca Raton.

LANDFIELD, P. W. 1988a. Increased calcium currents in rat hippocampal neurons during aging. *In* The Calcium Channel: Structure, Function and Implications, Bayer AG Centenary Symposium, M. Morad, W. Nayler, S. Kazda and M. Schramm (eds.). Springer-Verlag, Berlin.

LANDFIELD, P. W. 1988b. Commentary on biomarkers of aging in the nervous system. Exp. Gerontol. *23*, 413–416.

LANDFIELD, P. W., BASKIN, R. K. and PITLER, T. A. 1981. Brain aging correlates: Retardation by hormonal-pharmacological treatments. Science *214*, 581–584.

LANDFIELD, P. W. and DEADWYLER, S. A. 1988. Long-Term Potentiation: From Biophysics to Behavior. Alan R. Liss, New York.

LANDFIELD, P. W., McGAUGH, J. L. and LYNCH, G. 1978a. Impaired synaptic potentiation in the hippocampus of aged, memory-deficient rats. Brain Res. *150*, 85–101.

LANDFIELD, P. W. and MORGAN, G. 1984. Chronically elevating plasma Mg^{2+} improves hippocampal frequency potentiation and reversal learning in aged and young rats. Brain Res. *322*, 167–171.

LANDFIELD, P. W. and PITLER, T. A. 1984. Prolonged Ca^{2+}-dependent afterhyperpolarizations in hippocampal neurons of aged rats. Science *226*, 1089–1092.

LANDFIELD, P. W., PITLER, T. A. and APPLEGATE, M. D. 1986. The effects of high Mg^{2+}-to-Ca^{2+} ratios on frequency potentiation in hippocampal slices of young and aged rats, J. Neurophysiol. *56*, 797–811.

LANDFIELD, P. W. and PITLER, T. A. 1987. Calcium spike duration: prolongation in hippocampal neurons of aged rats. Soc. Neurosci. Abstr. *13*, 718.

LANDFIELD, P. W., WAYMIRE, J. L. and LYNCH, G. S. 1978b. Hippocampal aging and adrenocorticoids: Quantitative correlations. Science *202*, 1098–1102.

LYNCH, G., LARSON, J. and BAUDRY, M. 1986. Proteases, neuronal stability, and brain aging: An hypothesis. *In* Treatment Development Strategies for Alzheimer's Disease, T. Crook, R. Bartus, S. Ferris and S. Gershon (eds.). Mark Powley Assoc., Madison, CT.

McNAUGHTON, B. L., BARNES, C. A. and ANDERSEN, P. 1981. Synaptic efficacy and EPSP summation in granule cells of rat fascia dentata studied in vitro. J. Neurophysiol. *46*(5), 952–966.

MacVICAR, B. A. and DUDEK, F. E. 1979. Intracellular recordings for hippocampal CA3 pyramidal cells during repetitive activation of mossy fibers *in vitro*. Brain Res. *168*, 377–381.

MELDRUM, B. 1987. Excitatory amino acid antagonists as potential therapeutic agents. *In* Neurotoxins and their Pharmacological Implications, P. Jenner (ed.). Raven Press, New York.

MICHAELIS, M. L., JOHE, K. and KITOS, T. E. 1984. Age-dependent alterations in synaptic membrane systems for Ca^{2+} regulation. Mech. Ageing Dev. *25*, 215–225.

MORDES, J. P. and WACKER, W. E. C. 1978. Excess magnesium. Pharmacol. Rev. *29*, 273–299.

NAYLER, W. G., POOLE-WILSON, P. A. and WILLIAMS, A. 1979. Hypoxia and calcium. J. Molec. Cell Cardiol. *11*, 683–706.

PITLER, T. A. and LANDFIELD, P. W. 1987. Postsynaptic membrane shifts during frequency potentiation of the hippocampal EPSP. J. Neurophysiol. *58*, 866–882.

PLAITAKIS, A., NICKLAS, W. J. and DESNICK, R. J. 1980. Glutamate dehydrogenase deficiency in three patients with spinocerebellar syndrome. Ann. Neurol. *7*, 297–303.

PRITCHARD, J. A. 1955. The use of the magnesium ion in the management of eclamptogenic toxemias. Surg. Gynecol. Obstet. *100*, 131–140.

ROTH, G. S. 1988. Mechanisms of altered hormone and neurotransmitter action during aging: the role of impaired calcium mobilization. Ann. N.Y. Acad. Sci. *521*, 170–176.

SCHLAEPFER, W. W. and HASLER, M. B. 1979. Characterization of the calcium-induced disruption of neurofilaments in rat peripheral nerve. Brain Res. *168*, 299–309.

SCHWARCZ, R. *et al.* 1984. Excitotoxic models for neurodegenerative disorders. Life Sci. *35*, 19–32.

SCHWARTZKROIN, P. A. 1975. Characteristics of CA1 neurons recorded intracellularly in the hippocampal *in vitro* slice preparation. Brain Res. *85*, 423–436.

SHOULSON, I. 1983. Huntington's disease: anti-neurotoxic therapeutic strategies. *In* Excitotoxins, K. Fuxe, P. Roberts and R. Schwarcz (eds.). Plenum Press, New York.

SIESJO, B. K. 1981. Cell damage in the brain: a speculative synthesis. J. Cereb. Blood Flow Metab. *1*, 155–185.

SMITH, D. O. 1988. Muscle-specific decrease in presynaptic calcium dependence and clearance during neuromuscular transmission in aged rats. J. Neurophysiol. *59*, 1069–1082.

SWANSON, L. W., WYSS, J. M. and COWAN, W. M. 1978. An autoradiographic study of the organization of intrahippocampal association pathways in the rat. J. Comp. Neurol. *181*. 681–716.

CHAPTER 21

THE INVOLVEMENT OF GLUCOSE AND GLUCOSE REGULATION IN MEMORY IN RODENTS AND HUMANS

PAUL E. GOLD, Ph.D
Department of Psychology and Neuroscience Program
University of Virginia
Charlottesville, Virginia

A growing body of evidence suggests that carbohydrate consumption possibly influences a broad range of behaviors, such as mood, activity and aggression (cf. Spring *et al.* 1987). In addition, there is clear evidence that performance on neuropsychological tests, particularly in diabetics, is influenced by blood glucose levels (Holmes *et al.* 1986; Holmes 1986). Ideas about the underlying bases for these relationships include possible influences of circulating glucose on brain energy metabolism (Siebert *et al.* 1986), as well as the possibility that high carbohydrate meals increase tryptophan availability to augment serotonin synthesis (e.g., Fernstrom and Wurtman 1971).

With specific relevance to aging research, there is evidence suggesting that decreases in brain glucose metabolism may occur during Alzheimer's disease (cf. Hoyer 1986; Hoyer *et al.* 1988), and that cerebral glucose metabolism is correlated with memory performance in individual elderly subjects (Riege *et al.* 1985). In addition, circulating glucose may be involved in acetylcholine synthesis, particularly during age-related decreases in brain oxidative metabolism (Gibson and Peterson 1980, 1981). The possible relationship between blood glucose levels and cholinergic function is particularly interesting in light of the evidence that cholinergic dysfunctions, as well as many other brain changes which are likely to contribute also to declines in memory during senescence (cf. Zornetzer 1984), are evident in individuals with age-related cognitive impairments (e.g., Davies and Maloney 1977; Perry 1980;

Coyle *et al.* 1983). Also, pharmacological manipulations of cholinergic functions in young subjects indicate that cholinergic antagonists generally interfere with memory processes while agonists enhance such performance (e.g., Baratti *et al.* 1979; Flood and Cherkin 1986; Flood *et al.* 1981; Drachman 1981; Fuld 1984).

This chapter will review recent evidence in animals and humans that glucose administration enhances memory processing and, in particular, attenuates memory impairments which appear during normal aging. Interestingly, this research did not evolve from studies of nutritional influences on memory and aging but, rather, was derived from the extensive information that neuroendocrine status at the time of an experience regulates memory storage for that experience. The next section of this chapter will discuss this background information and will describe recent findings which suggest that some of the neuroendocrine influences on memory appear to act through a mechanism which includes an important contribution of increases in circulating glucose levels. The subsequent section will discuss glucose enhancement of memory in relation to aging.

HORMONAL REGULATION OF MEMORY STORAGE PROCESSES

Many treatments impair memory when administered soon after an experience. In animals, for example, an early study by Duncan (1949) demonstrated that electroconvulsive shock impaired later memory when administered soon after training. Importantly, the extent of impairment decreased as the time between training and treatment increased—i.e., electroconvulsive shock produced retrograde amnesia. During the 25 years which followed this demonstration, comparable results were obtained in many species, tasks and with many additional treatments (cf. McGaugh and Herz 1972).

In addition to further demonstrations of retrograde amnesia, there was a parallel and remarkable series of studies which indicated that some treatments, mostly pharmacological stimulants, would enhance later memory if administered soon, but not at long delays, after training (McGaugh 1983). Thus, the general findings of this research indicated that memory storage processes were susceptible to modification, both impairment and enhancement, for some time after the to-be-remembered experience was over.

These findings presented the possibility that there were endogenous physiological responses to an experience which might themselves enhance or impair memory, in a sense selecting on the basis of posttraining responses those events which are significant and therefore worth committing to storage (Gold and McGaugh 1975). This view leads to the following neurobiological scenario. If an animal is trained with footshock as the motivational stimulus, the strength of memory assessed later will vary with the intensity of the footshock. In addition, the hormonal consequences (e.g., epinephrine release from the adrenal medulla) will also vary with the footshock intensity. The question is whether such differences in neuroendocrine responses regulate memory storage and, thereby, affect later performance of learned responses.

To determine whether the hormonal responses to training contribute to later memory performance, we trained animals with a mild footshock and administered epinephrine shortly after training. When tested for memory on the next day, the rats which received epinephrine performed better than did control animals (Gold and van Buskirk 1975). Memory enhancement with epinephrine follows an inverted-U dose-response curve and the optimal epinephrine dose for memory enhancement is a dose which results in circulating epinephrine levels quite close to those seen in rats which had received a more intense footshock during training (McCarty and Gold 1981).

It is now quite clear that epinephrine enhances memory in a wide range of conditions (McGaugh and Gold 1989). Furthermore, the effects of epinephrine are blocked in the presence of peripherally administered adrenergic receptor antagonists (e.g., Gold and van Buskirk 1978; Sternberg *et al.* 1986). Similarly, the effects of many other treatments which enhance or impair memory are also blocked by these treatments (Gold and Sternberg 1978), suggesting that epinephrine effects on memory may explain many of the actions of other treatments as well. Thus, epinephrine enhances memory in a manner which suggests strongly that the hormone acts normally to regulate the brain mechanisms which underlie memory storage processes. Additional findings suggest that other hormones, including ACTH, and several neurotransmitter systems also contribute to regulation of memory storage processing (cf. Gold and Zornetzer 1983; McGaugh and Gold 1988).

Evidence such as that described above suggests that epinephrine regulates the brain processes responsible for memory storage. However, in determining the neurobiological mechanisms which might underlie memory regulation, it is important to note that epinephrine does not appear to enter the central nervous system from the circulation (Axelrod *et al.* 1959). Therefore, it seems likely that epinephrine effects on memory are indirect and may be mediated by peripheral actions of the hormone. One of the major physiological consequences of epinephrine release into blood is an increase in circulating glucose levels in response to an interaction of epinephrine effects on glucagon, insulin and on hepatic glucose stores (Ellis *et al.* 1967; Chideckel *et al.* 1977).

Recent findings indicate that glucose injections mirror many of the effects of epinephrine on memory, providing initial evidence that circulating glucose levels may modify memory storage processes and may mediate epinephrine effects on memory (cf. Gold 1988; Gold and Stone 1988). Like epinephrine, glucose injections administered immediately after training enhance memory in an inverted-U dose-response manner (Fig. 21.1) (Messier and White 1987; Gold 1986; Gold *et al.* 1986). Injections delayed after training by an hour or more do not affect later memory retention. Moreover, the blood glucose levels produced by epinephrine injections and by glucose injections at doses which enhance memory are comparable, and match well the glucose levels seen after training with a stronger footshock intensity (Fig. 21.2) (Hall and Gold 1986).

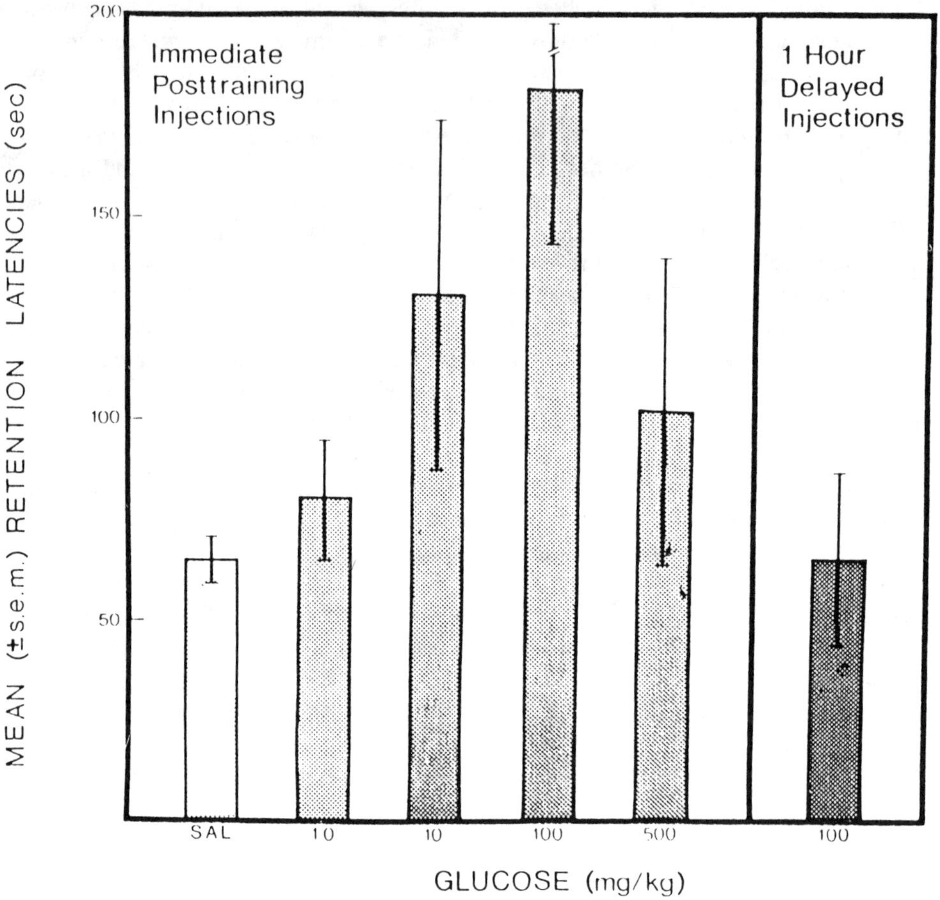

From Gold 1986

FIG. 21.1. EFFECTS OF POSTTRAINING GLUCOSE ON MEMORY TESTED 24 H LATER

Note that glucose-enhanced memory in an inverted-U dose-response manner. Also, glucose injections delayed by 1 h after training did not significantly alter later performance.

There is one major difference in the results obtained with glucose and epinephrine. Epinephrine effects on memory are not evident in animals treated with adrenergic receptor antagonists, such as propranolol or phenoxybenzamine, prior to training. However, glucose effects on memory remain intact in animals pretreated in this manner (Gold *et al.* 1986). These results are therefore consistent with the view that glucose effects on memory reflect a step subsequent to epinephrine activation of peripheral adrenergic receptors. The possibility that circulating glucose acts directly on CNS functions is suggested by findings that posttraining intracerebroventricular injections of glucose also enhance memory (Lee *et al.* 1988).

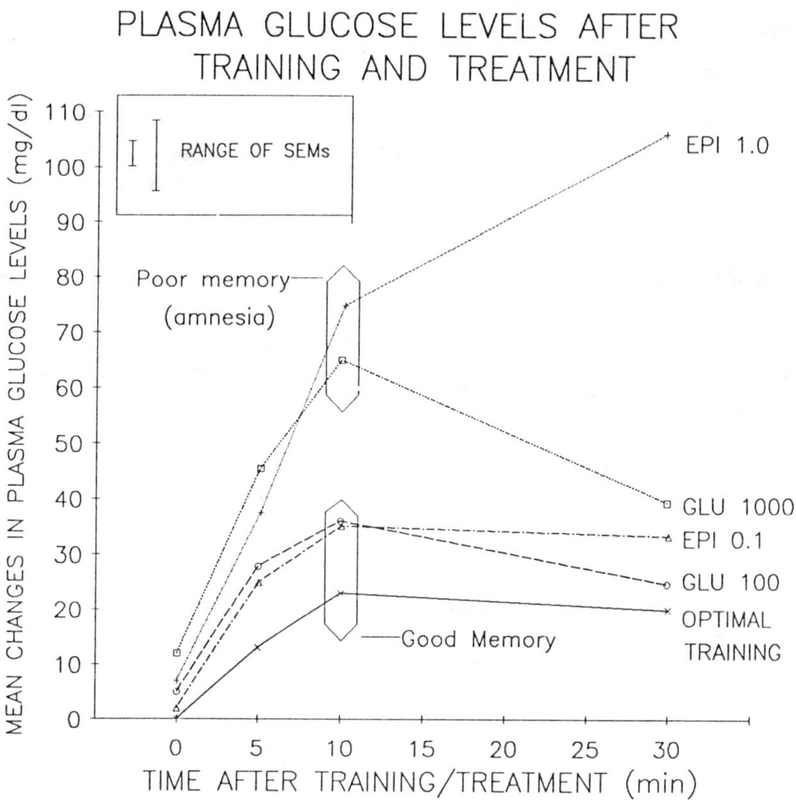

From Hall and Gold 1986

FIG. 21.2. PLASMA GLUCOSE LEVELS MEASURED AT SEVERAL TIMES BEFORE AND AFTER AVOIDANCE TRAINING AND EPINEPHRINE OR GLUCOSE INJECTIONS

Note that the training condition and epinephrine and glucose doses which enhance memory all result in roughly comparable posttraining increases in circulating glucose. Amnestic treatments (high doses of epinephrine or glucose) resulted in blood glucose increases well beyond that typically seen after footshock.

MECHANISM OF GLUCOSE EFFECTS ON MEMORY

We have recently begun to examine some of the pharmacological mechanisms through which glucose acts. In addition, the findings of these experiments have identified additional glucose actions on brain functions.

Glucose Interactions With Cholinergic Functions

There is considerable evidence that memory storage is impaired by treatments which interfere with central cholinergic systems and enhanced by treatments which augment these systems. For example, scopolamine, a muscarinic antagonist, impairs memory in both animals and humans (e.g., Flood and Cherkin 1986; Piercy *et al.* 1987; Rush 1986; Introini-Collison and McGaugh 1988; Drachman 1981; Fuld 1984). In mice, we found that scopolamine-induced amnesia is attenuated in animals that receive posttraining injections of epinephrine or glucose. In one experiment (Stone *et al.* 1990c) mice received scopolamine, or scopolamine plus epinephrine or glucose, prior to testing in a spontaneous alternation task. As shown in Fig. 21.3, scopolamine treatment resulted in significantly impaired performance on this task. Epinephrine and glucose reversed this behavioral deficit. Similar results were seen in mice trained in an inhibitory avoidance task as described above (Stone *et al.* 1988b).

On the basis of these findings, we examined other possible interactions of glucose with cholinergic functions. In each case, the findings indicate that glucose attenuates the effects of cholinergic antagonists and augments the effects of cholinergic agonists. Scopolamine-treated mice exhibit marked hyperactivity (Bushnell 1987), and additional treatment with glucose blocks this effect (Fig. 21.4.)(Stone *et al.* 1987, 1988a).

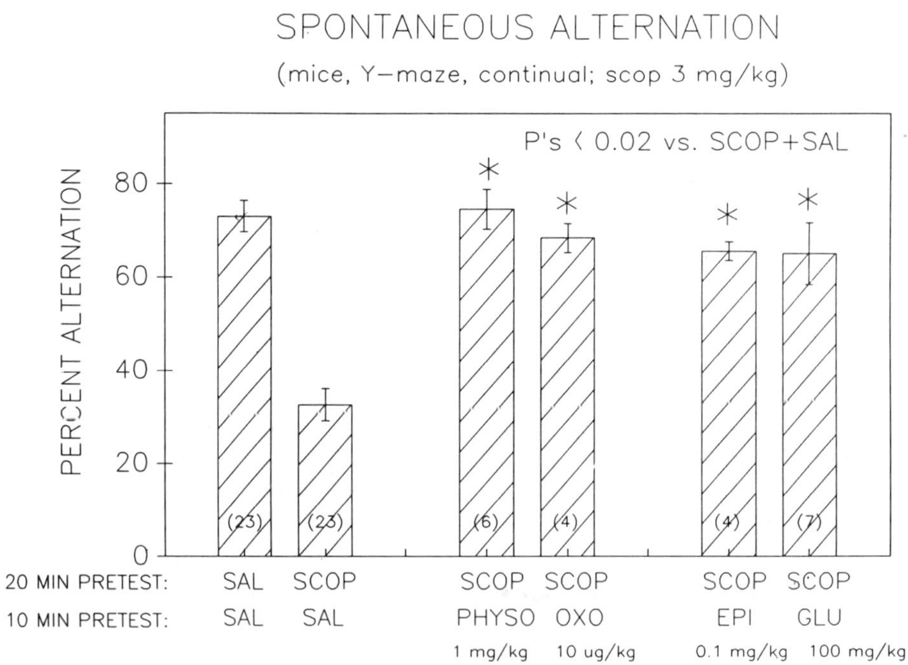

From Stone et al. 1990c

FIG. 21.3. SCOPOLAMINE IMPAIRMENT OF SPONTANEOUS ALTERNATION BEHAVIOR IN MICE

Note that scopolamine-treated mice exhibited a significant deficit in this task. The deficit was blocked by cholinergic agonists (physostigmine or oxotremorine) as well as by epinephrine or glucose.

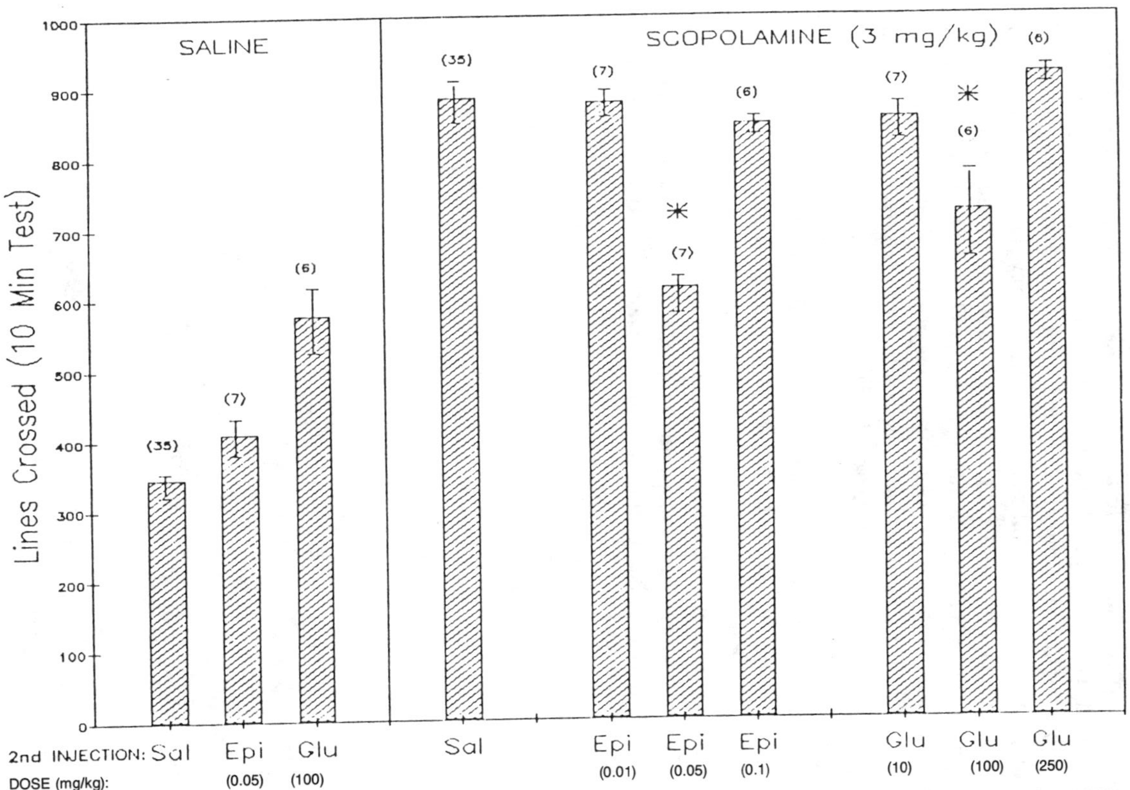

From Stone et al. 1988b

FIG. 21.4. EPINEPHRINE AND GLUCOSE ATTENUATION OF SCOPOLAMINE-INDUCED HYPERACTIVITY IN MICE

Note that the increased activity levels observed in scopolamine-treated mice were attenuated, in an inverted-U dose-response manner, by epinephrine and glucose.

Note that the reversal of the hyperactivity by glucose follows an inverted-U dose-response relationship, as seen also in studies of memory enhancement. Similarly, the cholinergic antagonist, atropine, impairs spontaneous alternation performance, and this effect too is reversed by glucose treatment. Atropine treatment also impairs electrographic sleep, particularly interfering with paradoxical sleep measures. Glucose reverses this deficit as well (Fig. 21.5)(Stone *et al.* 1990a).

In addition to having memory impairments and other behavioral changes, animals treated with scopolamine also exhibit reduced brain 2-deoxyglucose uptake (Piercy *et al.* 1987). As in behavioral studies, glucose injections attenuate the decrease in brain 2-DG uptake seen after scopolamine (Stone and Gold 1990a). Mice received scopolamine or scopolamine plus glucose 10 minutes prior to injection of ^{3}H-2-/DG (10 μCi/mouse, s.c.). Forty minutes later, the brains were removed, dissected into eight brain regions solubilized and assessed for radioactive content. The results indicate that scopolamine produced a significant decrease in 2-DG uptake in most brain regions. This significant decrease was not observed in the animals which received additional treatment with glucose. Total brain results are shown in Fig. 21.6. Thus, in addition to reversing behavioral effects of scopolamine, the present findings indicate that glucose also reverses a neurobiological consequence of scopolamine administration. These findings are consistent with others which demonstrate that cholinergic systems may regulate brain metabolism (Dam and London 1983; London *et al.* 1985; London *et al.* 1988).

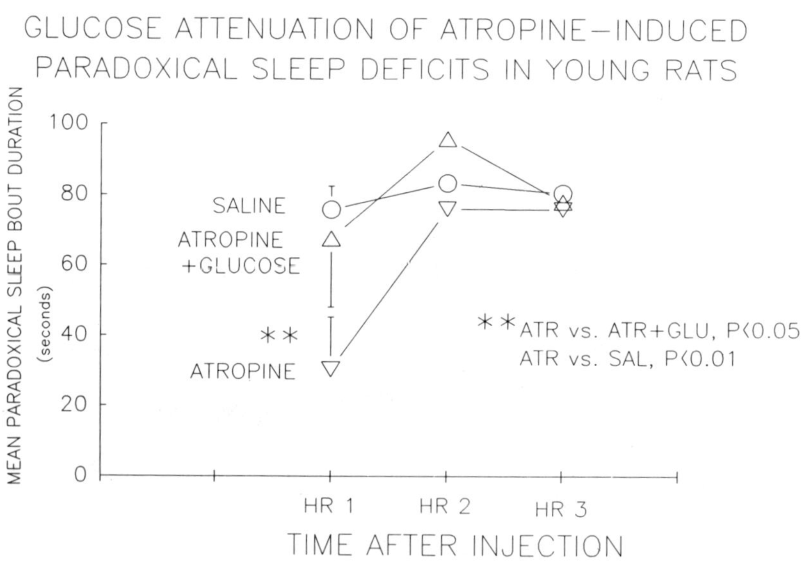

From Stone et al. 1990a

FIG. 21.5. ATROPINE EFFECTS ON PARADOXICAL SLEEP BOUT DURATION
Note that atropine reduced the duration of paradoxical sleep bouts during the first hour after injection. This impairment was blocked by additional treatment with glucose.

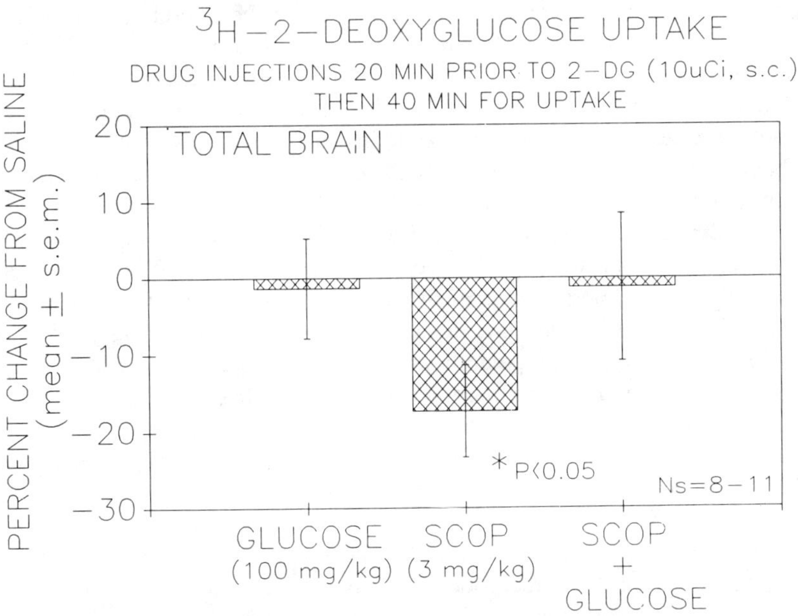

From Stone and Gold 1990a

FIG. 21.6. SCOPOLAMINE EFFECTS ON BRAIN ^{3}H-2-DEOXYGLUCOSE UPTAKE (2-DG)

At a dose which impairs memory, scopolamine produces a marked decrease in brain 2-DG uptake. Additional treatment with glucose (IP), at a dose which reverses memory impairment after scopolamine, also blocks the decrease in 2-DG uptake.

Glucose Interactions With Opioid Functions

In addition to interactions of glucose with cholinergic drugs, recent evidence also suggests that glucose interacts with opioid functions. In many situations, opioid agonists produce behavioral effects (e.g., memory impairment, hyperactivity) similar to those seen with cholinergic antagonists. Conversely, opioid antagonists have some behavioral effects similar to those of cholinergic agonists. These reciprocal actions support the view that opioid systems, e.g., in the medial septum (Moroni *et al.* 1977; Krnjevic and Ropert 1981), inhibit cholinergic neurons. Consistent with this view, several findings provide evidence for important interactions between opioids and cholinergic systems in modulating memory. In most experiments, memory is enhanced by opioid antagonists and impaired by agonists (cf. Martinez *et al.* 1981; Martinez *et al.* 1988). Scopolamine-induced amnesia is attenuated by additional treatment with the opioid antagonist, naloxone (Rush 1986). Conversely, enhancement of memory with naloxone, an opioid antagonist, is blocked by additional treatment with the cholinergic antagonist, atropine (Barrati *et al.* 1984). In addition, memory impairment produced by β-endorphin is blocked by the cholinergic agonists oxotremorine and physostigmine (Introini and Barrati 1984).

If glucose augments cholinergic function, glucose should attenuate the actions of opioid agonists. We recently found that morphine impairs memory in the spontaneous alternation task described above and that additional treatment with glucose restores this behavior to values comparable to those of control mice (Stone *et al.* 1990c). Similarly, glucose attenuates hyperactivity elicited by morphine (Stone *et al.* 1990b) as well as morphine-induced analgesia (Raz *et al.* 1988; Brase and Dewey 1988).

Thus, early indications are that glucose may influence the functions of opioid systems as well as cholinergic systems. It may be relevant here to mention that many other treatments, including cholinergic agonists as well as "noncholinergic" drugs, also attenuate the effects of scopolamine on memory (Flood and Cherkin 1986; Itoh *et al.* 1988). One such treatment is cholecystokinin octapeptide (CCK-8)(Itoh *et al.* 1988). In addition to blocking scopolamine effects on memory, this hormone itself enhances memory (in an inverted-U dose-response manner), an effect which is abolished by subdiaphragmatic vagotomy (Itoh and Katsuura 1986; Flood *et al.* 1987). In the periphery, CCK-8 releases acetylcholine from the ileum (Vizi 1973). In addition, peripheral CCK-8 injections stimulate acetylcholine release from neocortex (Magnani *et al.* 1984); this effect follows an inverted-U dose-response curve which is modified in the presence of opioid antagonist, naloxone.

Figure 21.7 summarizes a current working hypothesis which integrates our current information regarding glucose actions on the central nervous system. Although the model shows glucose and opioids acting in parallel (with opposing effects) on cholinergic function, we are unable at this time to determine whether the glucose actions are at or before the level of the opioid neurons or at the later cholinergic step. Nonetheless, the pharmacological findings are consistent throughout with the view that injections of glucose, at doses which result in relatively small increases in blood glucose levels, attenuate opioid and augment cholinergic actions.

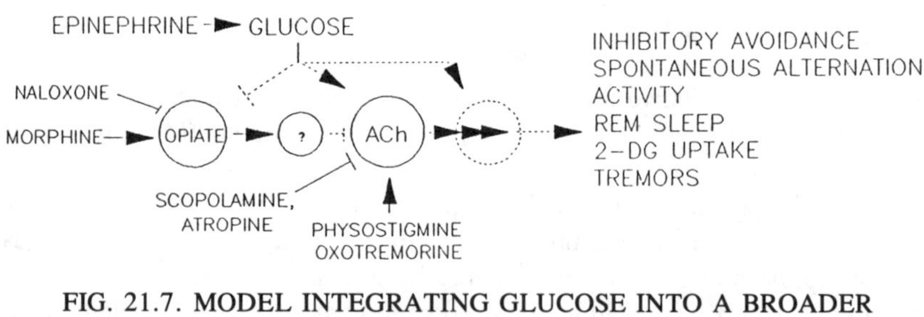

FIG. 21.7. MODEL INTEGRATING GLUCOSE INTO A BROADER PHARMACOLOGICAL SCHEME

This pattern of interaction between peripheral and central systems is quite consistent across a wide range of behaviors, including memory, activity, tremors, and sleep.

AGING AND MEMORY

In a wide range of species, including man, aging is accompanied by diminished capacity to store new memories (cf. Kubanis and Zornetzer 1981). There are two major categories of neurobiological explanations for age-related memory deficits. One is that the neural substrates—perhaps anatomical (Greenough and Bailey 1988) or biochemical (Abrams and Kandel 1988; Gustafsson and Wigstrom 1988) changes in response to experience—are no longer effective memory storage processes. For example, there is evidence of decreased cell numbers in several specific populations of neurons (cf. Coleman and Flood 1987) and loss of neurotransmitter functional integrity (i.e., decreases in transmitter levels or in activity of key enzymes in acetylcholine, biogenic amine systems)(cf. Zornetzer 1984; Severson 1987). Thus, it is possible that the memory dysfunctions seen in aged animals reflect the loss of neural systems which function to store new information.

A second possibility, based on the results of studies of memory modulation, is that the neural substrates are relatively intact but the modulatory events which regulate these substrates (turn them on or off) are not present in aged animals. Perhaps the aging brain has difficulty in storing new information, not only because of absent or diminished memory substrate mechanisms but because of loss of the regulatory processes which enable storage mechanisms to work optimally. This latter possibility has some support from studies which demonstrate that plasma epinephrine responses to relatively minor stressors (e.g., footshock such as might be used in avoidance training) are decreased in aged compared to young animals (McCarty 1981). It is with this in mind that we examined the effects of epinephrine and glucose on memory in elderly rodents and humans.

Animals

Rodents, like other animals, exhibit a marked deficit in memory storage (cf. Kubanis and Zornetzer 1981; Gold and Stone 1988). For example, if 2-year-old rats are trained and tested in a one-trial inhibitory avoidance task, the animals exhibit forgetting as early as several hours after training (Gold *et al.* 1981). This contrasts sharply with the performance of young (2–3-month-old) rats which retain good performance as long as 3 weeks after training. One-year-old rats show intermediate rates of forgetting. These findings are quite similar to those obtained in mice (Zornetzer *et al.* 1982) and do not differ in major respects from those obtained in several other species.

If decreased neuroendocrine activation by experience accompanies old age, it is possible that appropriate treatments at the time of training would attenuate age-related memory impairments. In rats and mice, epinephrine injections administered immediately after training results in performance in old animals comparable to that seen in untreated young animals. Figure 21.8 shows the results of one such study

(Sternberg *et al.* 1985). Rats were trained in a one-trial inhibitory avoidance task and were tested one week later, i.e., at a time when there is clear evidence of age-related memory deficits. The results indicate that those 1- or 2-year-old animals which received epinephrine injections immediately after training had retention performance a week later similar to that of young untreated animals. Similarly, glucose reversed the age-related impairment seen in mice tested for spontaneous alternation performance (Fig.21.9)(Stone and Gold 1988c). These findings therefore suggest that injections of epinephrine or glucose ameliorate age-related memory impairments in rodents.

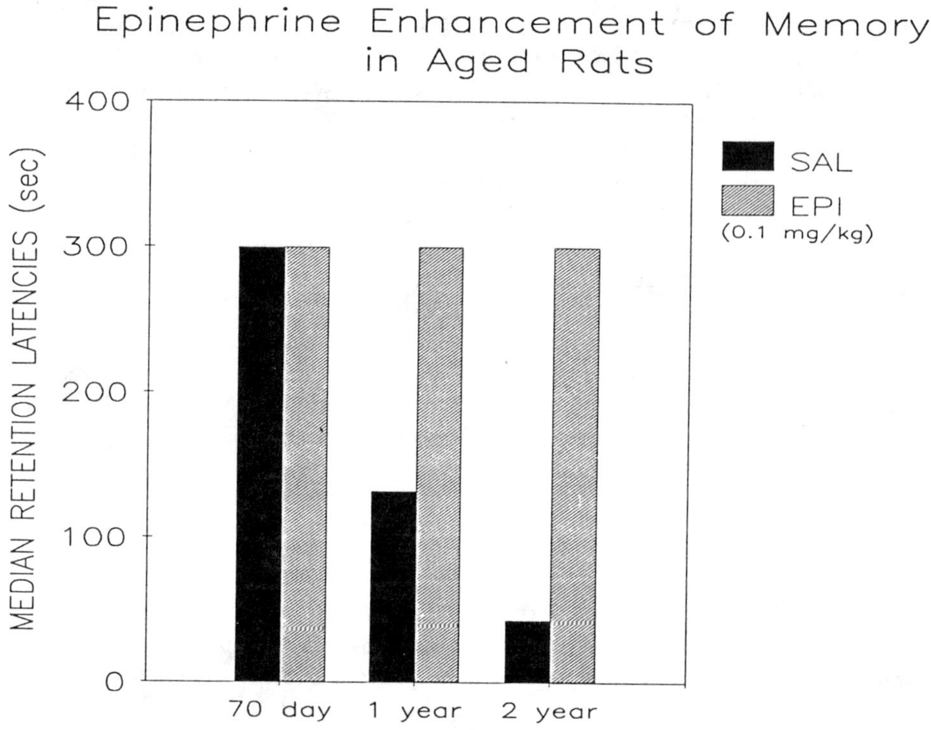

From Sternberg et al. 1985

FIG. 21.8. EPINEPHRINE EFFECTS ON MEMORY IN OLD RATS

Rats were trained in a one-trial inhibitory avoidance task and tested for memory one week later. Note first that the saline groups exhibit clear age-related differences at this training-testing interval. One- and two-year-old rats which received an immediate posttraining injection of epinephrine showed enhanced retention on the one week tests.

An additional age-related change in brain function is evident in disruption of electrographic sleep patterns (Prinz 1977; Prinz *et al.* 1982a, 1982b; Stone and Gold 1988b), which may be related to impaired cholinergic functions (cf. Sitaram and Gillin 1979). Stone *et al.* (1989) found that 2-year-old rats exhibit a change in sleep

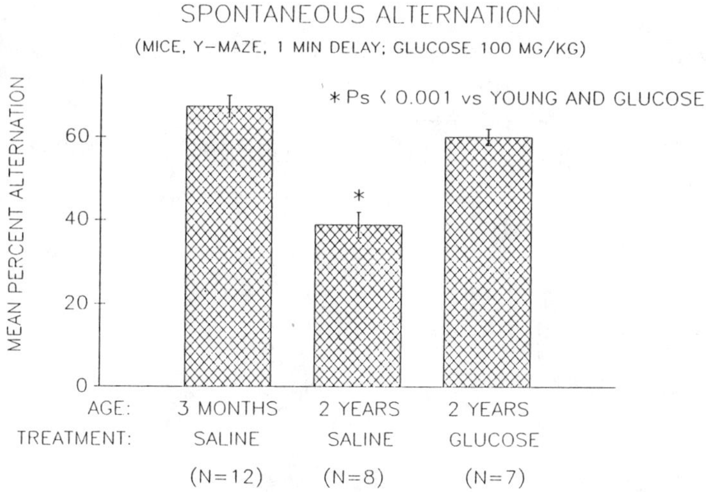

Stone and Gold 1990b

FIG. 21.9. SPONTANEOUS ALTERNATION BEHAVIOR IN YOUNG AND OLD MICE
Note that 2-year-old mice exhibit a significant deficit in spontaneous alternation behavior. This deficit is attenuated in mice pretreated with glucose.

patterns which particularly involves decreases in the amount of time spent in paradoxical sleep. Of particular interest here, the findings indicate that the extent of deficit in paradoxical sleep is tightly correlated with individual animals' memory performance in several tasks (Stone *et al.* 1989; Markowska *et al.* 1989). Recent findings indicate that glucose, at doses which enhance memory, also enhances sleep in aged animals, restoring paradoxical sleep to values near those of young animals (Fig. 21.10)(Stone *et al.* 1990e). It may be important also to note that glucose was most effective in reversing the age-related sleep deficits in those animals in which hippocampal choline acetyltransferase activity was highest, i.e., in the individual animals in which this marker of forebrain cholinergic function was near that of young animals. This correlation is consistent with the evidence presented above suggesting that glucose acts, at least in part, by augmenting CNS cholinergic functions.

Humans

Because of the relative safety of the treatment, Hall *et al.* (1988) began examinations of glucose effects on memory in elderly humans. The subjects in these experiments were healthy volunteers, aged 60–75 years. In the first experiment, each subject arrived in the laboratory on three consecutive mornings with instructions to abstain from all food and beverages except water after midnight preceding the testing procedures. Upon arrival, each subject completed a questionnaire requesting information about health, and completed a simple test of mental competency. Of

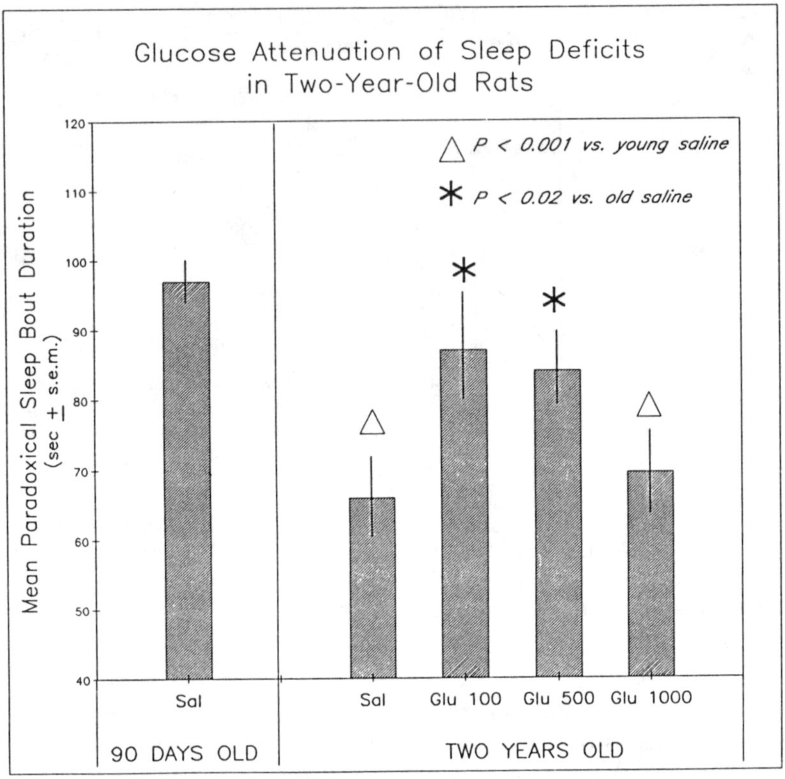

From Stone et al. 1990e

FIG. 21.10. PARADOXICAL SLEEP BOUT DURATION IN YOUNG AND OLD RATS
Note that 2-year-old rats have a substantial decrease in this measure of paradoxical sleep. Glucose injections reverse this sleep deficit in an inverted-U dose-response manner consistent with that observed in memory and activity studies.

the subjects tested, four were excluded from analyses on the basis of this information. An initial blood glucose level was determined for each person, and the subjects then received one of two beverages (powdered lemonade prepared with glucose [50 g] or saccharin [23.5 mg]). The glucose or saccharin condition was counterbalanced across Days 1 and 2. Blood glucose assessments were made at several points through the 2-h testing procedure.

The subjects then received a battery of tests taken from the Wechsler (1945) series. These included digit span (forward and backward), logical memory (narrative passage), and paired-associate word lists. Two standardized versions of each test were used; these were counterbalanced by day and treatment. Performance was assessed for most tests on the same day, and for the paired-associate test 24 h later (prior to the Day 2 treatment and without additional tests on Day 3). The counterbalanced design enabled use of each subject as his or her own control, thus reducing variability across subjects. The results indicated that glucose significantly enhanced performance on the logical memory test, but not on other tests.

These encouraging results provided the basis for a subsequent experiment (Manning *et al.* 1990) which included digit span and logical memory and, in addition, examined performance on a verbal selective reminding test (Buschke and Fuld 1974) and tests of attention (letter cancellation), overall cognitive function (Ammons and Ammons 1962), and motor performance (finger tapping). The results of this second experiment (Fig. 21.11) again clearly demonstrated that glucose treatment enhanced performance on the logical memory test but not the digit span test as before. In addition, glucose significantly enhanced performance on the selective reminding test. No glucose effects were observed on the other tests.

These findings are remarkably consistent with predictions made on the basis of the animal studies. Furthermore, it appears that the glucose enhances performance on tests of long-term memory (logical memory and selective reminding tests) but not short-term memory (digit span). Thus, glucose appears to have its largest ef-

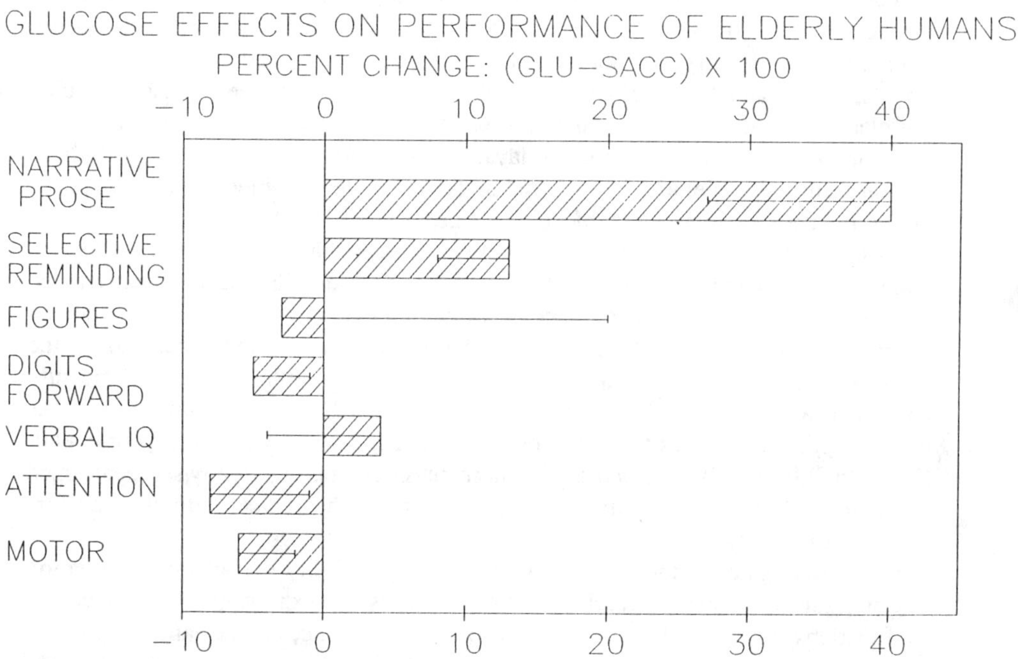

From Manning et al. 1990

FIG. 21.11. GLUCOSE EFFECTS ON MEMORY AND OTHER TESTS IN ELDERLY HUMANS

The results are shown here as percent change to accommodate all test results in a single figure. Note that glucose ingestion significantly enhanced performance on logical (narrative) memory and on a verbal selective reminding test. The enhancement was not evident in tests of overall cognitive function (quick IQ), attention, or motor performance.

fects on those memory tests on which elderly subjects have the greatest deficit, although this generalization requires additional testing before being confirmed.

GLUCOSE REGULATION AND MEMORY

In the experiments on human memory, blood glucose levels were assessed during testing to determine whether glucose ingestion in this manner led to increases in blood glucose levels. Subjects exhibited a significant increase in blood glucose levels after ingesting glucose but not saccharin. However, evaluation of the individual increases in blood glucose levels in relation to performance on the memory tests revealed an unexpected, and potentially important, finding. Those elderly subjects who had relatively poor glucose regulation (i.e., relatively high peak increases in blood glucose levels during the 2 h after ingestion) had poor memory when compared to the elderly subjects who had good glucose regulation (i.e., relatively low peak increases in blood glucose levels). Remarkably, the correlation between glucose regulation and memory in individual subjects was evident not only on the glucose treatment day but also on the saccharin control day; a similar relationship between glucose regulation and memory was not evident in individual young (20-year-old) subjects. The results obtained with elderly subjects are illustrated in Fig. 21.12, in which it is clear that blood glucose regulation predicts memory performance in elderly subjects on control as well as treatment days. These findings are consistent with those demonstrating that memory is impaired in diabetic elderly subjects when compared to age-matched nondiabetic subjects (Perlmuter *et al.* 1984).

On the basis of these results, we tested the relationship between glucose regulation and memory in aged rats as well (Stone *et al.* 1990d). The rats had been trained and tested in an inhibitory avoidance task one month earlier. The animals received an injection of glucose (500 mg/kg) and blood glucose was measured during the next hour. As observed previously in humans, glucose regulation was significantly correlated with 2-year-old rats' memory performance assessed 30 days earlier. As in humans, no evidence of a comparable relationship was observed in young adult (2-month-old) rats. Thus, glucose toleration measurements apparently segregate aged populations, both rats and humans, in a manner which predicts individual performance on memory tests.

These findings open the potentially important possibility that glucose regulation in young subjects may predict which of those subjects will exhibit age-related memory dysfunctions. In our studies, there were no large differences in the range of glucose tolerance scores in young and old subjects; yet, the correlations between glucose tolerance and memory were observed only in elderly subjects. It is likely that the individual differences in glucose tolerance are maintained from young adulthood into old age. If so, glucose tolerance may provide a premorbid marker of the subpopulation of individuals likely to demonstrate age-related memory impairments. Such findings would provide an opportunity to target chronic manipulations intended to retard age-related cognitive deficits to those individuals which would otherwise have the problems.

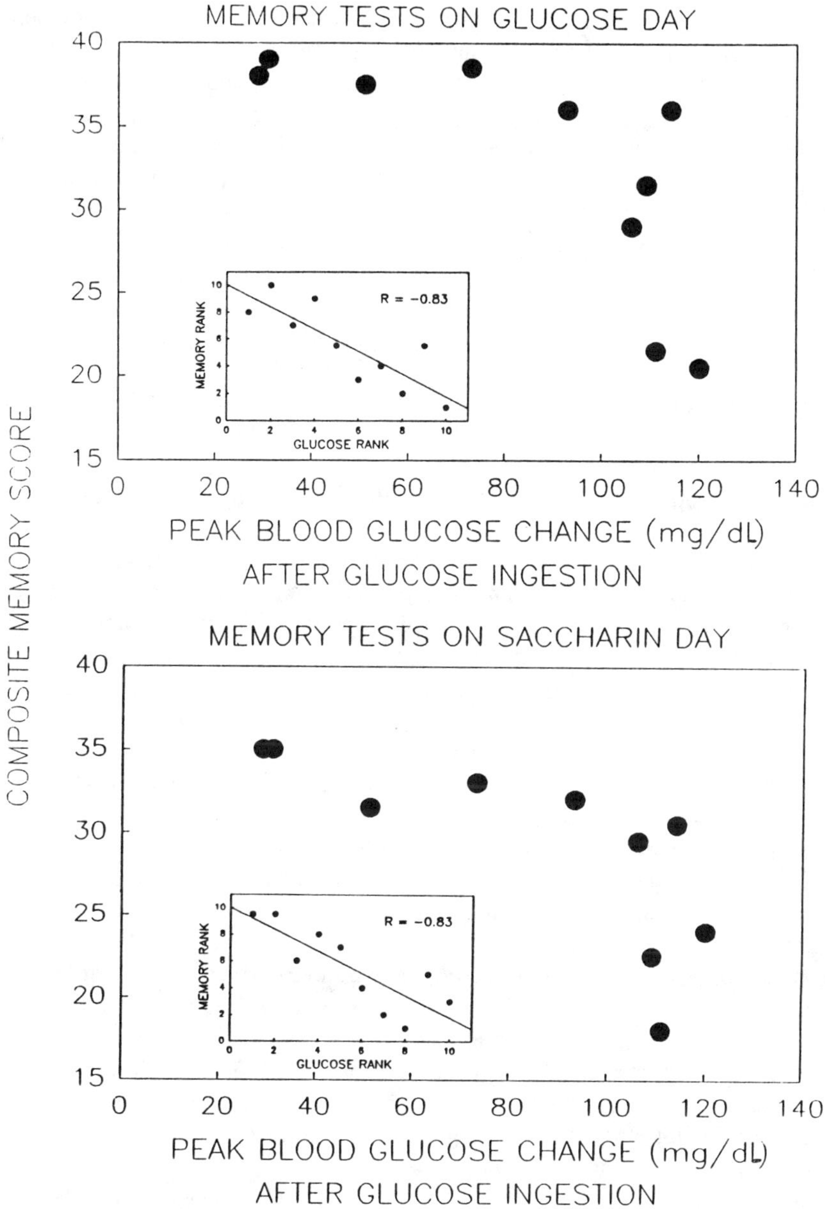

Hall et al. 1989

FIG. 21.12. RELATIONSHIP BETWEEN PEAK GLUCOSE INCREASES, WITHIN 2 H OF GLUCOSE (50 MG) INGESTION, AND INDIVIDUAL PERFORMANCE ON THE LOGICAL MEMORY TEST

Note that the glucose responses were obtained on the glucose test day (upper graph), but a significant relationship between poor glucose regulation and poor memory was observed on both glucose and saccharin (control) days (upper and lower graphs).

Moreover, it is possible that dietary and pharmacological control may be useful manipulations with which to delay the onset of memory dysfunctions. To the extent that such treatments can improve glucose regulation in young subjects, it is possible, though entirely untested, that such chronic manipulations could reduce the memory problems which accompany aging. An unresolved paradox then arises: Acute glucose treatment enhances memory in both young and old animals, but reduced chronic glucose consumption during young adulthood might improve memory during aging.

CONCLUSIONS

The findings presented here indicate that acute glucose treatment enhances memory in humans and in animals, perhaps acting as a step in biological regulation of memory subsequent to epinephrine release. More to the point of this meeting, glucose treatment enhances memory in elderly subjects. Evidence obtained in animal studies suggests that glucose also ameliorates sleep deficits in aged rats, a physiological measure which is highly correlated with individual memory performance in these animals. Furthermore, glucose also influences several additional behaviors, in a manner suggesting that glucose augments cholinergic function and inhibits opioid functions.

The findings also demonstrate that memory and brain 2-deoxyglucose uptake are both impaired by scopolamine treatment; both are also reversed by additional treatment with glucose. These findings are generally consistent with reports by Riege *et al.* (1985), who found that brain glucose metabolism and memory decrease together in individual subjects, and reports by Gibson and Peterson (1980, 1981), who noted that circulating glucose and brain oxidative metabolism may contribute to age-related changes in cholinergic function.

An additional finding is that memory performance is particularly deficient in those individual aged, but not young, subjects with relatively poor blood glucose regulation. These findings are similar to those observed in comparisons of elderly diabetics and nondiabetics. Chronic hyperglycemia can modify the dynamics of blood-brain glucose transfer processes, resulting in diminished brain glucose uptake (Gjedde and Crone 1981). Aging has also been associated with alterations in blood-brain transport leading to decreased glucose influx (cf. Mooradian 1988). Whether poor glucose regulation can be used as a premorbid marker of later age-related memory dysfunction, and whether early control of glucose tolerance can ameliorate later deficits during aging, remain to be studied.

ACKNOWLEDGMENTS

This work was supported by research grants from ONR (N0001489-J-1216), NIA (AG07648) and NIH (NSS-2-S07-RR07094).

REFERENCES

ABRAMS, T. W. and KANDEL, E. R. 1988. Is contiguity detection in classical conditioning a system or cellular property? Learning in *Aplysia* suggests a possible molecular site. Trends Neurosci. *11*, 128–135.

AMMONS, R. B. and AMMONS, C. H. 1962. The Quick Test (QT): Provisional Manual. Psychol. Rep. *11*, 434–449.

AXELROD, J., WEIL-MALHERBE, H. and TOMCHICK, R. 1959. The physiological disposition of ^{3}H-epinephrine and its metabolite metanephrine. J. Pharmacol. Exp. Ther. *127*, 251–256.

BARATTI, C. M. *et al.* 1979. Memory facilitation with post-trial injection of oxotremorine and physostigmine in mice. Psychopharmacology *64*, 85–88.

BARATTI, C. M., INTROINI, I. B. and HUYGENS, P. 1984. Possible interaction between central cholinergic muscarinic and opioid peptidergic systems during memory consolidation in mice. Behav. Neural Biol. *40*, 155–169.

BRASE, D. A. and DEWEY, W. L. 1988. Glucose and morphine-induced analgesia. *In* Nutritional Modulation of Neural Function, J. E. Morley, M. B. Sterman and J. H. Walsh (eds.). Academic Press, New York.

BUSCHKE, H. and FULD, P. A. 1974. Evaluating storage, retention, and retrieval in disordered memory and learning. Neurology *24*, 1019–1025.

BUSHNELL, P. H. 1987. Effects of scopolamine on locomotor activity and metabolic rate in mice. Pharmacol. Biochem. Behav. *26*, 195–198.

CHIDECKEL, E. W. *et al.* 1977. Role of glucagon in mediating metabolic effects of epinephrine. Am. J. Physiol. *232*, E464–E470.

COLEMAN, P. D. and FLOOD, D. G. 1987. Neuron numbers and dendritic extent in normal aging and Alzheimer's disease. Neurobiol. Aging *8*, 521–545.

COYLE, J. T., PRICE, D. L. and DELONG, M. R. 1983. Alzheimer's disease: a disorder of cortical cholinergic innervation. Science *219*, 1184–1190.

DAM, M. and LONDON, E. D. 1983. Effects of cholinomimetics on glucose utilization in rat brain optic systems. Eur. J. Pharmacol. *87*, 137–140.

DAVIES, P. and MALONEY, A. J. F. 1976. Selective loss of central cholinergic neurons in Alzheimer's Disease. Lancet *2*, 1043.

DRACHMAN, D. A. 1981. The cholinergic system, memory, and aging. *In* Aging, Vol. 17: Brain Neurotransmitters and Receptors in Aging and Age-Related Disorders, S. J. Enna, T. Samarajski and B. Beer (eds.). Raven Press, New York.

DUNCAN, C. P. 1949. The retroactive effect of electroshock on learning. J. Comp. Physiol. Psychol. *42*, 32–44.

ELLIS, S., KENNEDY, B. L., EUSEBI, A. J. and VINCENT, N. H. 1967. Autonomic control of metabolism. Ann. N.Y. Acad. Sci. *139*, 826–832.

FERNSTROM, J. D. and WURTMAN, R. J. 1971. Brain serotonin content: Increase following ingestion of carbohydrate diet. Science *174*, 1023–1025.

FLOOD, J. F. and CHERKIN, A. 1986. Scopolamine effects on memory retention in mice: A model of dementia? Behav. Neural Biol. *45*, 169–184.

FLOOD, J. F., LANDRY, D. W. and JARVIK, M. E. 1981. Cholinergic interactions and their effects on long-term memory processing. Brain Res. *215*, 177–185.

FLOOD, J. F., SMITH, G. E. and MORLEY, J. E. 1987. Modulation of memory processing by cholecystokinin: Dependence on the vagus nerve. Science *236*, 745–747.

FULD, P. A. 1984. Test profile of cholinergic dysfunction and of Alzheimer-type dementia. J. Clin. Neuropsychol. *6*, 380–392.

GIBSON, G. E. and PETERSON, C. 1980. Acetylcholine metabolism in senescent mice. Age *3*, 116.

GIBSON, G. E. and PETERSON, C. 1981. Aging decreases oxidative metabolism and the release and synthesis of acetylcholine. J. Neurochem. *37*, 978–984.

GJEDDE, A. and CRONE, C. 1981. Blood-brain glucose transfer: Repression in chronic hyperglycemia. Science *214*, 456–457.

GOLD, P. E. 1986. Glucose modulation of memory storage processing. Behav. Neural Biol. *45*, 342–349.

GOLD, P. E. 1988. Plasma glucose modulation of memory storage processes. *In* Cellular Mechanisms of Conditioning and Behavioral Plasticity, C. D. Woody (ed.). Plenum Press, New York.

GOLD, P. E. and McGAUGH, J. L. 1975. A single-trace, two process view of memory storage processes. *In* Short-term Memory, D. Deutsch and J. A. Deutsch (eds.). Academic Press, New York.

GOLD, P. E. *et al.* 1981. Age-dependent changes in retention in rats. Exp. Aging Res. *8*, 53–58.

GOLD, P. E. and STERNBERG, D. B. 1978. Retrograde amnesia produced by several treatments. Evidence for a common neurobiological mechanism. Science *201*, 367–369.

GOLD, P. E. and STONE, W. S. 1988. Neuroendocrine factors in age-related memory dysfunctions: Studies in animals and humans. Neurobiol Aging *9*, 709–717.

GOLD, P. E. and VAN BUSKIRK, R. B. 1975. Facilitation of time-dependent memory processes with posttrial epinephrine injections. Behav. Biol. *13*, 145–153.

GOLD, P. E. and VAN BUSKIRK, R. B. 1978. Effects of alpha- and beta-adrenergic receptor antagonists on posttrial epinephrine modulation of memory: Relationship to posttraining brain norepinephrine concentrations. Behav. Biol. *24*, 1168–1184.

GOLD, P. E., VOGT, J. and HALL, J. L. 1986. Posttraining glucose effects on memory: Behavioral and pharmacological characteristics. Behav. Neural Biol. *46*, 145–155.

GOLD, P. E. and ZORNETZER, S. F. 1983. The mnemon and its juices: Neuromodulation of memory processes. Behav. Neural Biol. *38*, 151–189.

GREENOUGH, W. T. and BAILEY, C. H. 1988. The anatomy of a memory: Convergence of results across a diversity of tests. Trends Neurosci. *11*, 142–146.

GUSTAFSSON, B. and WIGSTROM, H. 1988. Physiological mechanisms underlying long-term potentiation. Trends Neurosci. *11*, 156–162.

HALL, J. L. and GOLD, P. E. 1986. The effects of training, epinephrine, and glucose injections on plasma glucose levels in rats. Behav. Neural Biol. *45*, 156–176.

HALL, J. L. *et al.* 1989. Glucose enhancement of memory in young and aged humans. Neuropsychologia *27*, 1129–1138.

HOLMES, C. S. 1986. Neuropsychological profiles in men with insulin dependent diabetes. J. Consult. Clin. Psychol. *54*, 386–389.

HOLMES, C. S., KOEPKE, K. M. and THOMPSON, R. G. 1986. Simple versus complex performance impairments at three blood glucose levels. Psychoneuroendocrinology *11*, 353–357.

HOYER, S. 1986. Senile dementia and Alzheimer's diseases. Brain blood flow and metabolism. Prog. Neuropsychopharmacol. Biol. Psychiatry *10*, 447–478.

HOYER, S., OESTERREICH, K. and WAGNER, O. 1988. Glucose metabolism as the site of the primary abnormality in early-onset dementia of Alzheimer type? J. Neurol. *235*, 143–148.

INTROINI, I. and BARATTI, C. M. 1984. The impairment of retention induced by B-endorphin in mice may be mediated by reduction of central cholinergic activity. Behav. Neural Biol. *41*, 152–163.

INTROINI-COLLISON, I. and McGAUGH, J. L. 1988. Modulation of memory by post-training epinephrine: Involvement of cholinergic mechanisms. Psychopharmacology *94*, 379–385.

ITOH, S. and KATSUURA, G. 1986. Behavioral effect of cholecystokinin octapeptide in vagotomized rats. Can. J. Physiol. Pharmacol. *64*, 745–747.

ITOH, S., TAKASHIMA, A. and KATSUURA, G. 1988. Preventive effect of cholecystokinin octapeptide on scopolamine-induced memory impairment in the rat. Drug Dev. Res. *12*, 63–70.

KRNJEVIC, K. and ROPERT, N. 1981. Septohippocampal pathway modulates hippocampal activity by a cholinergic mechanism. Can. J. Physiol. Pharmacol. *59*, 911–914.

KUBANIS, P. and ZORNETZER, S. F. 1981. Age-related behavioral and neurobiological changes: A review with emphasis on memory. Behav. Neural Biol. *31*, 115–172.

LEE, M. K., GRAHAM, S. and GOLD, P. E. 1988. Memory enhancement with posttraining intraventricular glucose injection in rats. Behav. Neurosci. *102*, 591–595.

LONDON, E. D., CONNOLLY, R. J., SZIKSZAY, M. and WAMSLEY, J. K. 1985. Distribution of cerebral metabolic effects of nicotine in the rat. Eur. J. Pharmacol. *110*, 391–392.

LONDON, E. D., DAM, M. and FANELLI, R. J. 1988. Nicotine enhances cerebral glucose utilization in central components of the rat visual system. Brain Res. Bull. *20*, 381–385.

MAGNANI, M., MANTOVANI, P. and PEPEU, G. 1984. Effect of cholecystokinin octapeptide and ceruletide on release of acetylcholine from cerebral cortex of the rat *in vivo*. Neuropharmacology *23*, 1305–1309.

MANNING, C., HALL, J. L., and GOLD, P. E. 1990. Glucose and memory in elderly humans: Effects on verbal memory. Psychol. Sci. (In press).

MARKOWSKA, A. L. *et al.* 1989. Individual differences in aging: Behavioral and neurobiological correlates. Neurobiol. Aging *10*, 31–44.

MARTINEZ, J. L. *et al.* 1981. Endogenous Peptides and Learning and Memory Processes. Academic Press, New York.

MARTINEZ, J. L., WEINBERGER, S. B. and SCHULTEIS, G. 1988. Enkephalins and learning and memory: A review of evidence for a site of action outside the blood-brain barrier. Behav. Neural Biol. *49*, 192–221.

McCARTY, R. 1981. Aged rats: Diminished sympathetic-adrenal medullary response to acute stress. Behav. Neural Biol. *33*, 204–212.

McCARTY, R. and GOLD, P. E. 1981. Plasma catecholamines: Effects of footshock level and hormonal modulators of memory storage. Horm. Behav. *15*, 168–182.

McGAUGH, J. L. 1983. Hormonal influences on memory. Annu. Rev. Psychol. *34*, 297–323.

McGAUGH, J. L. and GOLD, P. E. 1989. Hormonal modulation of memory. *In* Psychoendocrinology, R. Brush and S. Levine (eds.). Academic Press, New York.

McGAUGH, J. L. and HERZ, M. J. 1972. Memory Consolidation. Albion, San Francisco.

MESSIER, C. and WHITE, N. M. 1987. Memory improvement by glucose, fructose and two glucose analogs: A possible effect on peripheral glucose transport. Behav. Neural Biol. *48*, 104–127.

MOORADIAN, A. D. 1988. Effect of aging on the blood-brain barrier. Neurobiol. Aging *9*, 31–39.

MORONI, F., CHENEY, D. L. and COSTA, E. 1977. Inhibition of acetylcholine turnover in rat hippocampus by intraseptal injections of β-endorphin and morphine. Naunyn-Schmiedeberg's Arch. Pharmacol. *299*, 149–153.

PERLMUTER *et al.* 1984. Decreased cognitive function in aging non-insulin-dependent diabetic patients. Am. J. Med. *77*, 1043–1048.

PERRY, E. K. 1980. The cholinergic system in old age and Alzheimer's disease. Age Aging *9*, 1–8.

PIERCY, M. F., VOGELSANG, G. D., FRANKLIN, S. R. and TANG, A. H. 1987. Reversal of scopolamine-induced amnesia and alterations in energy metabolism by the nootropic piracetam: Implications regarding identification of brain structures involved in consolidation of memory traces. Brain Res. *424*, 1–9.

PRINZ, P. N. 1977. Sleep patterns in the healthy aged, interrelationships with intellectual function. J. Gerontol. *32*, 179–186.

PRINZ, P. N. *et al.* 1982a. Sleep, EEG and mental function changes in dementia. Neurobiol. Aging *3*, 361–370.

PRINZ, P. N. *et al.* 1982b. Changes in the sleep and waking EEG in non-demented and demented elderly. J. Am. Geriatr. Soc. *30*, 86–93.

RAZ, I., HASDAI, D., SELTZER, Z. and MELMED, R. N. 1988. Effect of hyperglycemia on pain perception and on efficacy of morphine analgesia in rats. Diabetes *37*, 1253–1259.

RIEGE, W. H., METTER, E. J., KUHL, D. E. and PHELPS, M. E. 1985. Brain glucose metabolism and memory functions: Age decrease in factor scores. J. Gerontol. *40*, 459–467.

RUSH, D. K. 1986. Reversal of scopolamine-induced amnesia of passive avoidance by pre- and post-training naloxone. Psychopharmacology *89*, 296–300.

SEVERSON, J. A. 1987. Synaptic regulation of neurotransmitter function in aging. Rev. Biol. Res. Aging *3*, 191–206.

SIEBERT, G., GESSNER, B. and KLASSER, M. 1986. Energy supply of the central nervous system. Bibl. Nutr. Dieta *38*, 1–26.

SITARAM, N. and GILLIN, J. C. 1979. Acetylcholine: Possible involvement in sleep and analgesia. *In* Brain Acetylcholine and Neuropsychiatric Diseases, K. L. Davis and P. A. Berger (eds.). Plenum Press, New York.

SPRING, B., CHIODO, J. and BOWEN, D. J. 1987. Carbohydrates, tryptophan, and behavior: A methodological review. Psychol. Bull. *102*, 234–256.

STERNBERG, D. B., KOROL, D., NOVACK. G. D. and McGAUGH, J. L. 1986. Epinephrine-induced memory facilitation: Attenuation by adrenergic receptor antagonists. Eur. J. Pharmacol. *129*, 189–203.

STERNBERG, D. B., MARTINEZ, J., McGAUGH, J. L., and GOLD, P. E. 1985. Age-related memory deficits in aged mice and rats: Enhancement with peripheral epinephrine. Behav. Neural Biol. *44*, 213–220.

STONE, W. S., COTTRILL, K. L. and GOLD, P. E. 1987. Glucose and epinephrine attenuation of scopolamine-induced increases in locomotor activity in mice. Neurosci. Res. Commun. *1*, 105–111.

STONE, W. S., COTTRILL, K. L., WALKER, D. and GOLD, P. E. 1988a. Blood glucose and brain function: Interactions with CNS cholinergic systems. Behav. Neural Biol. *50*, 325–343.

STONE, W. S., CROUL, C. and GOLD, P. E. 1988b. Attenuation of scopolamine-induced amnesia in mice. Psychopharmacology *96*, 417–420.

STONE, W. S. *et al.* 1989. Association of sleep parameters and memory in intact old and nucleus basalis-lesioned young rats. Behav. Neurosci. *103*, 755–764.

STONE, W. S. and GOLD, P. E. 1988. Sleep and memory relationships in intact old and amnestic young rats. Neurobiol. Aging *9*, 719–727.

STONE, W. S. and GOLD, P. E. 1990a. Glucose attenuation of scopolamine-induced deficits in spontaneous alternation behavior and in regional brain [^{3}H]2-deoxyglucose uptake. (Submitted).

STONE, W. S. and GOLD, P. E. 1990b. Glucose enhances both memory and 2-deoxyglucose uptake in 2-year-old mice. (Submitted).

STONE, W. S., RUDD, R. R. and GOLD. P. E. 1990a. Glucose injections attenuate atropine-induced sleep and memory deficits: Possible effects of atropine on peripheral glucose regulation. (In preparation).

STONE, W. S., RUDD, R. R. and GOLD, P. E. 1990b. Glucose and physostigmine effects on morphine- and amphetamine-induced increases in locomotor activity in mice. Behav. Neural Biol. *54*, 146–155.

STONE, W. S., WALSER, B., GOLD, S. D. and GOLD, P. E. 1990c. Scopolamine- and morphine-induced impairments of spontaneous alternation performance in mice: Reversal with glucose and with cholinergic and adrenergic agonists. (Submitted).

STONE, W. S., WENK, G. L., OLTON, D. S. and GOLD, P. E. 1990d. Poor glucose regulation predicts sleep and memory deficits in normal aged rats. J. Gerontol. *45*, B169–B173.

STONE, W. S., WENK, G. L., STONE, S. M. and GOLD, P. E. 1990e. Glucose attenuation of sleep deficits in old rats and possible relationships between circulating glucose and neurochemical functions. (Submitted).

VIZI, E. S. 1973. Acetylcholine release from guinea pig ileum by parasympathetic ganglion stimulation and gastrin-like polypeptide. Br. J. Pharmacol. *47*, 765–777.

WECHSLER, D. A. 1945. A standardized memory scale for clinical use. J. Psychol. *19*, 87–95.

ZORNETZER, S. F. 1984. Brain substrates of senescent memory decline. *In* The Neuropsychology of Memory, L. Squire and N. Butters (eds.). Guilford Press, New York.

ZORNETZER, S. F., THOMPSON, R. and ROGERS, J. 1982. Rapid forgetting in aged rats. Behav. Neural Biol. *36*, 49–60.

CHAPTER 22

DIETARY MANIPULATIONS OF BRAIN AGING

K. NANDY, M.D., Ph.D.
Department of Anatomy
Boston University School of Medicine
Boston, Massachusetts
and
S. NANDY, L. BLATT, Ph.D., and L. NANDY
Department of Psychology
Boston University School of Medicine
Boston, Massachusetts

INTRODUCTION

Dietary manipulation is probably the most reliable method used so far to alter the mammalian aging process (McCay *et al.* 1939; also, McCay and Crowell 1934). The studies of McCay and Crowell (1934) demonstrated that increases in both mean and maximum life span of rodents could be achieved by extending the animal's growth period by dietary restriction. Different dietary regimens have been used by different investigators to extend life span in mammals (Fernandes *et al.* 1976; Goodrick 1978; Gerbase-DeLima *et al.* 1975; Barrows and Kokkonen 1978), and these include either feeding 60% rats at *ad libitum* intake levels (Bertrand *et al.* 1980) or allowing rats free access to laboratory chow diet every other day (Goodrick *et al.* 1982). Ross (1961) and Ross and Brass (1973) observed that dietary restriction before maturity was most effective in extending life span of the animal, as compared to animals of the same age and sex fed on *ad libitum* diet, and that these animals showed a lower incidence of lung disease and spontaneous tumors (Jose and Good 1971). Age changes in the immune system were also retarded, and the animals showed lower spleen weight, reduced thymus growth, and higher proliferative responses of T-lymphocytes to mitogens and allogen as stimulation (Gerbase-DeLima *et al.* 1975). Undernourished mice exhibited reduced levels of brain-reactive antibody formation associated with aging (Nandy and Nandy 1986; Nandy 1985).

Based on data in two papers published by Ross (1959, 1961), Sacher (1977) analyzed relations between longevity and metabolism to observe a near constancy of kcal/g lifetime in both dietary and control groups. He concluded that the undernutrition appeared to work by reducing the metabolic rate per gram of rat. This view was contradicted by Masoro *et al.* (1980), who found an increase in kcal/g lifetime in the restricted animals. The latter authors concluded that the diet did not slow the rate of aging by slowing the metabolic rate.

Other studies reported that dietary restriction reduced *in vitro* peroxidation (malondialdehyde formation) in liver homogenates, lipofuscin accumulation in heart and brain, and free lysosomal activity in liver and brain homogenates (Chipalkatti *et al.* 1983; Nandy *et al.* 1987). It was suggested that the diet is likely to work by reducing the free-radical mediated damage.

It has been observed that vitamin E deficiency may produce a number of pathological conditions, identified in both animals and man, and can cause the deposition of darkish pigment in sex glands and uterine muscles in rats (Majaj *et al.* 1963; Oski and Barness 1967; Martin and Moore 1936, 1939; Einarsen and Ringsted 1938). The metabolic role of vitamin E is primarily as an antioxidant which scavenges and destroys the free radicals formed by the interaction of polyunsaturated fatty acids with molecular oxygen. These free radicals generate a chain of reactions, leading to the production of lipid peroxides, and finally to the formation of the lipofuscin pigment (Tappel 1965, 1970, 1972). Several other investigators also examined tissues, including adipose tissue, cardiac and uterine muscles in rats following diets supplemented with or deficient in vitamin E (Filer *et al.* 1946; Dam and Granados 1945; Mason and Emmel 1945). These authors found increased pigmentation in rats deficient in vitamin E and less so in animals fed on supplemental vitamin E. Sulkin and Srivanij (1960) found more lipofuscin in the nerve tissue of vitamin E deficient rats than controls, using histochemical methods. Using fluorescence microscopy, Wegliecki *et al.* (1968) found increased lipofuscin in different layers of the adrenal glands in the deficient animals. Katz *et al.* (1978) studied the fluorescent pigment in the eye and other tissues of rats fed on normal chow diet, and diets deficient in or rich in vitamin E. These authors also observed less pigment in animals fed on chow diet and supplemented diet than those on deficient diet in retinal pigmented epithelium, testes, kidney, intestine and heart muscle.

LIPOFUSCIN AND ITS PROPERTIES

One of the most consistent cytological changes associated with mammalian aging is the deposition of the lipofuscin age pigment in the neurons of the CNS (Brody 1960; Gatenby 1953; Lillie *et al.* 1941). The pigment has been described in the literature with different names by different investigators; these include: ceriod, wear and tear pigment, and chromolipid (Pearse 1964; Samorajski *et al.* 1964; Sulkin and Sulkin 1967; Siakotos *et al.* 1977). Lipofuscin is identified commonly by its autofluorescence, histochemical, and ultrastructural characteristics. The pigment has been studied most extensively in the neurons of rodents. It begins to develop around 2–3 months of age in C57BL/6 mice, and thereafter increases progressively as a function of age. The pigment formation appears to occur in two stages, and these show different fluorescence, staining, and chemical properties (see Table 22.1) (Nandy 1971).

TABLE 22.1
TWO STAGES OF NEURONAL LIPOFUSCIN AGE PIGMENT FORMATION

Properties	Early Stage	Late Stage
Distribution	Scattered granules	Perinuclear or polar clumps (unipolar or bipolar)
Staining properties	Easily stained by PAS and Sudan Black B	Easily stained by Nile blue, ferricferricyanide methods
Autofluorescence	Greenish-yellow with emission spectrum of 4000–4600A° and peak at 4400A°	Orange-yellow with emission spectrum of 4200–5000A° and a peak at 4800A°
Extraction by lipid solvents	Partial	Less so
Digestion by lipase and trypsin	Partial	Less so
Ultra-structure	Fine granules associated with lysomes and vacuoles	Large masses of the materials surrounded by lysosomal membranes containing vacuoles of varying sizes

Two different methods have been used for quantitation of lipofuscin in normal aging, as well as following manipulations by drugs and diet. The biochemical method includes spectrofluorometric assay of the pigment spectra of a chloroform-methanol extraction of the tissue (Fletcher *et al.* 1973). This method is lacking in several respects: it does not measure any nonextracted pigment, and cannot determine any relation of the pigment with different cell types. The other method, known as the morphometric method, is based on the counts of the intersections overlying pigment particles of an external grid placed in the ocular of a microscope. Although the method is laborious, and somewhat subjective to a less experienced examiner, the method correlates well with the pigment in different cell types, and can detect any qualitative change in the pigment as well (Nandy 1971; Mann and Yates 1974; Riga and Riga 1974; Reichel *et al.* 1968).

The mode of formation of lipofuscin is not clearly understood, and it has been suggested by a number of investigators that free radicals might play a major role by causing lipid peroxidation in the cells (Tekeuchi *et al.* 1976; Tappel 1965, 1968; Harman 1956). The possible correlations between lipid peroxidation product, lipofuscin, and the thiobarbituric acid reactant (malondialdehyde) have been studied in different laboratories. In our laboratory, lipofuscin pigment and malondialdehyde content were measured in retinal pigmented epithelium and frontal cortex in mice of different ages (3,12 and 24 months). The study exhibited a positive correlation between the two substances in both tissues, and a significant age-related difference in the values of lipofuscin and malondialdehyde was noted ($P < 0.05$) (Nandy 1984) (Table 21.2.).

EFFECTS OF DIETARY MANIPULATIONS

Vitamin E Deficient Diet

A number of studies were conducted to assess the effects of vitamin E deficient diets in different tissues, including the brain (Wegliecki 1968; Dam and Granados 1945; Martin and Moore 1936, 1939; Mason and Emmel 1945; Sulkin and Sulkin 1967). Lal *et al.* (1973) studied the effects of vitamin E deficient diets in rats for 14 months, starting at the age of 45 days. Vitamin E deficient diets increased body weight and reduced brain weight. Tests for short term and long term memory showed both learning and memory deficits. There were impairments of retention of one-trial learning, acquisition and retention of conditional avoidance response, and performance of delayed-alternation response. The experimental animals also showed a significantly increased accumulation of lipofuscin in the neurons of the frontal cortex.

TABLE 22.2
COMPARISON OF LIPOFUSCIN PIGMENT (LP) AND MALONDIALDEHYDE (MDA)[1] IN THE RETINAL PIGMENT EPITHELIUM (RPE) AND FRONTAL CORTEX (FC) IN MICE OF DIFFERENT AGES

	RPE		FC	
Age (Months)	LP	MDA	LP	MDA
3	37.25 ± 25.9	2.3 ± 0.2	66.29 ± 41.22	3.4 ± 0.4
12	223.31 ± 32.4	4.7 ± 0.6	375.77 ± 73.31	5.1 ± 0.9
24	602.37 ± 63.7	9.6 ± 0.8	835.17 ± 90.32	9.8 ± 1.2

[1]MDA is expressed as μg/mg of tissue using thiobarbituric acid assay. The values of LP represent the number of intersections in the ocular grid overlying the pigment particles in RPE and the neurons in the frontal cortex. The differences between age groups (3–12, 12–24 months) are statistically significant ($P < 0.05$).

The effects of vitamin E deficient diet on the pigment in the neurons of the hippocampus, frontal cortex, and Purkinje cells of the cerebellum in C57BL/6 mice have been recently studied in our laboratory. Three-month-old female mice were fed on vitamin E deficient diet (Nutritional Biochemical) for a period of 3–24 months, and the pigment was quantified by the morphometric method in frozen sections of the brain. Lipofuscin was significantly increased in the neurons as early as three months in mice on the diet, compared to the control animals of the same age and sex. It was noted that pigment increased progressively with age in both dietary and control mice, but there was significantly more pigment in the dietary group than the control group (Table 22.3) (Nandy 1984; Nandy *et al.* 1987).

TABLE 22.3
EFFECTS OF VITAMIN E DEFICIENT DIET ON LIPOFUSCIN PIGMENT IN THE NEURONS OF HIPPOCAMPUS AND FRONTAL CORTEX IN MICE (C67BL/6)

Dietary Period and (Age in Months)[1]	Control		Vitamin E Deficient	
	HC	FC	HC	FC
3(6)	7.2 ±3.1	8.3 ±3.0	12.7 ±3.2	13.1 ±4.2
6(9)	20.6 ±6.0	16.3 ±4.2	36.5 ±8.2	30.1 ±7.3
12(15)	28.6 ±6.2	30.7 ±7.2	52.6 ±9.4	56.3 ±7.7
24(27)	47.4 ±9.8	45.9 ±9.2	74.0 ±10.8	76.9 ±9.3

[1]Three-month-old mice were fed on vitamin E deficient diet and Purina mouse chow (control) for 3, 6, 12 and 24 months. The figures represent the numbers of intersections overlying pigment granules using an ocular grid in a fluorescence microscope.
HC = Hippocampal neurons.
FC = Frontal cortical neurons.

Vitamin E Excess Diet

Although studies on the effects of Vitamin E deficient diet are numerous, the effects of vitamin E excess diet on brain aging are not well documented. Recently, a study has been completed in our laboratory on the effects of vitamin E excess diet on the CNS. Three-month-old female mice were fed on a diet supplemented with vitamin E (0.2 g/100 g Purina Mouse Chow). Animals were fed on the diet for 3–24 months, and control animals were given Purina Mouse Chow without supplement. It was observed that lipofuscin was significantly reduced in the neurons of the frontal cortex and hippocampus, compared to the controls after 6 months on the diet. The results were even more pronounced after 12 and 24 months on the diet (Table 22.4) (Nandy 1985).

TABLE 22.4
EFFECTS OF SUPPLEMENTAL VITAMIN E ON LIPOFUSCIN PIGMENT IN THE NERVE CELLS OF HIPPOCAMPUS AND FRONTAL CORTEX OF C57BL/6 MICE

Dietary Period and (Age in Months)[1]	Control		Vitamin E Supplement	
	HC	FC	HC	FC
3(6)	8.2 ±3.1	6.2 ±3.0	6.3 ±4.1	6.6 ±3.2
6(9)	20.6 ±6.0	16.3 ±4.2	14.6 ±5.7	12.1 ±3.9
12(15)	38.6 ±6.2	40.7 ±7.2	24.3 ±10.1	25.2 ±9.7
24(27)	57.4 ±10.4	55.9 ±9.6	39.2 ±12.7	36.9 ±9.1

[1]Three-month-old female mice were fed on vitamin E excess diet (0.2 g/100 g of chow) for 3, 6, 12 and 24 months. The figures represent the numbers of intersections overlying pigment granules using an ocular grid in a fluorescence microscope.

HC = Hippocampal neurons.
FC = Frontal cortical neurons.

Dietary Restriction

Although there are numerous studies in the literature on the effects of dietary restriction on the mammalian aging process, its effects on the aging of the brain have not been investigated thoroughly. The effects of undernutrition on the lipofuscin pigment of CNS neurons have recently been investigated in our laboratory. Both young (3 months) and old (24 months) female mice were used in this study. Young mice were fed on a diet of 2–3 g of chow per day with supplemental vitamins. Animals were weighed weekly, and their body weights were maintained at 16–18 g. Controls consisted of mice of the same age and sex, fed *ad libitum* on Purina mouse chow, with consumption averaging about 4–6 g/day. The body weights of the control animals were 22–26 g. Animals were sacrificed after 3, 6, 12, and 24 months, and the frozen sections of the brain were examined morphometrically to quantify the lipofuscin pigment in a fluorescent microscope. Compared to the controls, there was a significant reduction of the pigment in neurons of the hippocampus, frontal cortex and Purkinje cells of the cerebellum of the dietary animals. The reduction of the pigment was significant after 6 months on the diet, and this difference was even greater after 12 and 24 months. On the other hand, the old mice did not show any significant change in the pigment after 6 months on the diet. Therefore, it appears that the dietary restriction is equally effective in retarding both general aging and brain aging (Table 22.5).

TABLE 22.5
EFFECTS OF DIETARY RESTRICTION ON LIPOFUSCIN PIGMENT IN THE NEURONS OF HIPPOCAMPUS (HC) AND THE FRONTAL CORTEX (FC) OF AGING MICE[1]

Dietary Period and (Age in Months)	Control Group		Dietary Group	
	HC	FC	HC	FC
Onset	5.2	4.6		
(3)	±3.2	±3.5		
6	15.1	14.2	10.6	10.2
(9)	±3.1	±3.0	±3.6	±3.8
12	32.2	30.4	22.4	24.3
(15)	±6.6	±7.1	±7.2	±7.9
24	52.5	46.7	36.3	29.1
(27)	±13.2	±10.1	±12.1	±10.2
Onset at 24 Months of Age				
3	52.5	46.7	50.6	50.0
(27)	±13.2	±10.1	±16.1	±13.3
6	62.7	56.7	61.9	59.3
(30)	±15.7	±14.7	±16.9	±17.3

[1]The numbers represent those of the intersections overlying pigment granules in the neurons using an ocular grid in a fluorescence microscope.

When young mice (3 months) on the diet for 12 months and the controls were trained in a radial maze learning paradigm, diet-restricted mice exhibited faster learning and higher asymptotic performance relative to the control mice fed *ad libitum*. This was correlated with lower lipofuscin content in neurons of the hippocampus and frontal cortex in the the experimental group.

SIGNIFICANCE OF DIETARY MANIPULATIONS

Gerontologists have described the aging changes in mammals as being intrinsic, progressive, universal and deleterious. Among the aging changes observed in the mammalian nervous system, lipofuscin deposition in the cytoplasm of the neuron is the most conspicuous. It is also progressive and shows a consistent pattern, and presents the potential for deleterious effects. Therefore, it appears that lipofuscin formation correlates well with both brain aging and the general aging process.

The relation between lipofuscin and learning has been studied by several investigators. Following certain experimental manipulations such as nutritional changes and drugs, the learning ability was enhanced, and this was correlated with reduced lipofuscin deposition in the neurons. The converse was also demonstrated: reduced learning performance correlates with increased pigmentation. Dietary restriction has been shown to reduce lipofuscin accumulation (Nandy *et al.* 1987; Enesco and Kruk 1981). Recently, restricted diet has been associated with enhanced radial maze performance, as well as reduced pigment accumulation in the neurons of mice (Idrabo *et al.* 1987). Prolonged caloric restriction has been shown to affect motor performance (Joseph *et al.* 1983; Ingram *et al.* 1987), as well as complex maze performance (Ingram *et al.* 1987; Goodrick 1984). However, lipofuscin accumulation was not examined in these studies.

Enhanced pigment formation following vitamin E deficient diet has also been associated with an impaired ability to learn a conditioned stimulus and a delayed-alternation response (Lal *et al.* 1973; Nandy and Lal 1978). Although animals fed a vitamin E deficient diet performed significantly worse than the controls, their nonassociative behaviors, such as exploratory and spontaneous locomotor activity were not affected.

Previous studies have also demonstrated a significant improvement in learning in mice following treatment with centrophenoxine, and this was also associated with reduced lipofuscin in the neurons of hippocampus and frontal cortex (Nandy 1978; Nandy and Lal 1978). Although a definite pathophysiological correlation of lipofuscin with nervous system functioning has not been clearly established, its excess or depletion appears to be correlated with certain functions associated with neuronal senescence. The morphological data tend to suggest strongly that lipofuscin pigment may be considered as a marker of neuronal aging. It may only be suggested here that dietary manipulations may exert their effect on neuronal aging, either directly due to alteration of the pigment formation or by causing changes in the process underlying pigmentogenesis.

Several theories have been proposed to explain the aging process in mammals. Of all the theories, one most applicable to our findings is the free-radical theory of aging, originally proposed by Harman (1956). Free radicals may initiate lipid peroxidation reactions, producing malondialdehyde, which, in turn, reacts with amines to form fluorescent conjugated Schiff bases with spectral properties similar to those found with lipofuscin pigment. Vitamin E acts as an antioxidant by scavenging free radicals formed in the tissues. Several parameters appear to correlate with each other in both *in vitro* and *in vivo* systems: polyunsaturated fatty acid levels, oxygen uptake, malondialdehyde production, lipofuscin formation, and vitamin E levels (Dillard and Tappel 1971). Despite the correlation between the levels of polyunsaturated lipids and vitamin E in tissues *in vitro*, animal studies have not been conclusive to date. It appears that free radicals play an important role in the biological aging process, including lipofuscin formation in the neurons. It is also quite likely that the dietary manipulations which alter biological aging processes, including brain aging, act by influencing the free radical formation in tissues during aging.

SUMMARY

The most successful method applied so far in altering life span in mammals is dietary manipulation started early in life. One of the consistent cytological changes associated with mammalian aging is the deposition of lipofuscin age pigment in the cytoplasm of neurons. The pigment is commonly demonstrated by its characteristic autofluorescence, histochemical and ultrastructural properties. Lipofuscin may be quantified morphometrically by using an ocular grid in a fluorescence microscope. The pigment formation in the neurons may be altered by various dietary manipulations and these are associated with changes in learning and memory as well. The effects of antioxidants on lipofuscin formation in neurons have been studied in different laboratories including ours. It has been observed that a vitamin E deficient diet may enhance pigment formation as well as lipid peroxidation in neurons. On the other hand, diet containing excess vitamin E was accompanied by reduced lipid peroxidation and lipofuscin formation in the neurons. Furthermore, animals subjected to dietary (caloric) restriction exhibited both improved learning and memory, and reduced lipofuscin in the neurons of hippocampus and frontal cortex. It has been suggested that the dietary manipulations affect aging processes by influencing the free radical formation in the tissues during aging, and the accumulation of lipofuscin may be a valuable index of these effects.

REFERENCES

BARROWS, C. H. and KOKKONEN, G. C. 1978. Diet and life extension in animal model systems. AGE *1*, 131–148.

BERTRAND, H. A., LYND, F. T., MASORO, E. J. and YU, B. P. 1980. Changes in adipose mass and cellularity through the adult life of rats fed *ad libitum* or life-prolonging diet. J. Gerontol. *35*, 827–835.

BIERI, J. G. and ANDERSON, A. A. 1960. Peroxidation of lipids in tissue homogenates as related to vitamin E. Arch. Biochem. *90*, 105–110.

BRODY, H. 1960. The deposition of aging pigment in human cerebral cortex. J. Gerontol. *15*, 258–281.

CHIPALKATTI, S., DE, A. K., and AIYAR, A. S. 1983. Effects of diet restriction on some biochemical parameters related to aging in mice. J. Nutr. *113*, 944–950.

DAM, M. and GRANADOS, H. 1945. Peroxidation of body fat in vitamin E deficiency. Acta Physiol. Scand. *10*, 162–171.

DILLARD, C. J. and TAPPEL, A. L. 1971. Fluorescent products of lipid peroxidation of mitochondria and microsomes. Lipids *6*, 715–721.

DYLEWSKI, D. P., NANDY, S., NANDY, K. 1983. Effects of centrophenoxine on the retinal pigment epithelium of old mice. Neurobiol. Aging *4*, 89–95.

EINARSON, L. and RINGSTED, A. 1938. Effects of Chronic Vitamin E Deficiency on the Nervous System and Skeletal Musculature in Adult Rats. Levin and Munksgaard, Copenhagen.

ENESCO, H. E. and KRUK, P. 1981. Dietary restriction reduces fluorescent accumulation in aging mice. Exp. Gerontol. *16*, 357–361.

FERNANDES, G., YUNIS, E. J. and GOOD, R. A. 1976. Influence of diet on the survival of mice. Proc. Natl. Acad. Sci. USA *73*, 1279–1283.

FILER, L. G., RUMERY, R. E. and MASON, K. E. 1946. Specific unsaturated fatty acids in the production of acid fast pigment in the vitamin E deficient rat and the specific action of tocopherols. *In* Transactions of the First Conference on Biological Antioxidants.

FLETCHER, B. L., DILLARD, C. J. and TAPPEL, A. L. 1973. Measurement of fluorescent lipid peroxidation products in biological systems and tissues. Analyt. Biochem. *52*, 1–9.

GATENBY, J. B. 1953. The Golgi apparatus in the living sympathetic ganglion cells of the mouse. J. Roy. Microsc. Soc. *73*, 61–81.

GERBASE-DELIMA, M. *et al.* 1975. Immune function and survival in a long-lived mouse strain subjected to undernutrition. J. Gerontol. *21* 154–202.

GOODRICK, C. L. 1978. Body weight increment and length of life: the effect of genetic constitution and dietary protein. J. Gerontol. *23*, 184–190.

GOODRICK, C. L. 1984. Effect of lifelong restricted feeding on complex maze performance in rats. AGE *7*, 1–2.

GOODRICK, C. L. *et al.* 1982. Effects of intermittent feeding upon growth and life span in rats. Gerontol. *28*, 233–241.

GRINNA, L. S. 1976. Effects of dietary tocopherol on liver microsomes and mitochondria of aging rats. J. Nutr. *106*, 918–929.

HARMAN, D. 1956. Aging: A theory based on free radical and radiation chemistry. J. Gerontol. *11*, 298–300.

HARMAN, D. 1987. Free radical theory of aging: Current status. *In* Lipofuscin-1987: State of the Art, I. Zs.-Nagy (ed.). Excerpta Medica, New York.

IDRABO, F. *et al.* 1987. Dietary restriction: Effects on radial maze learning and lipofuscin pigment deposition in the hippocampus and frontal cortex. Arch. Gerontol. Geriatr. *6*, 355–362.

INGRAM, D. K. *et al.* 1987. Dietary restriction benefits learning and motor performance of aged mice. J. Gerontol. *42*, 72–81.

JOSE, D. G. and GOOD, R. A. 1971. Absence of enhancing antibody in cell mediated immunity to tumor heterografts in protein deficient rats. Nature *231*, 323–325.

JOSEPH, J., WHITTAKER, J., ROSS, G. S. and INGRAM, D. K. 1983. Lifelong dietary restriction affects striatially mediated behavioral responses in aged rats. Neurobiol. Aging *4*, 191–196.

KATZ, M. L., STONE, W. L. and DRATZ, E. A. 1978. Fluorescent pigment accumulation in retinal pigmented epithelium of antioxidant deficient rats. Invest. Opthalmol. Vision Sci. *17*, 1049–1058.

LAL, H., POGAKAR, S., DALY, P. and PURI, S. 1983. Behavioral and neuropathalogical manifestions of nutritionally induced central nervous system aging in the rat. *In* Progress in Brain Research, D. Ford (ed.). Elsevier, New York.

LILLIE, R., DRAFT, F. S. and SEBREL, W. H. 1941. Cirrhosis of the liver in the rat on deficient diet and effects of alcohol. Publ. Health Rept. (Wash.) *56*, 1255–1256.

MAJAJ, A. S., DINNING, J. S., AZZAM, S. and DARBY, W. J. 1963. Vitamin E responsive megaloblastic anemia in infants with protein-caloric malnutrition. Am. J. Clin. Nutr. *12*, 374–379.

MANN, D. N. A. and YATES, P. O. 1974. Lipoprotein pigments—Their relationship to aging in the human nervous system. I. Lipofuscin content of nerve cells. Brain *97*, 481–488.

MARTIN, A. G. P. and MOORE, T. 1936. Changes in the uterus and kidneys in rats kept on vitamin E free diet. Chem. Ind. *55*, 236–238.

MARTIN, A. G. P. and MOORE, T. 1939. Some effects of prolonged vitamin E deficiency in the rat. J. Hyg. (London) *39*, 643–650.

MASORO, E. J., YU, B. P., BERTRAND, H. A. and LYND, F. T. 1980. Nutritional probe of the aging process. Fed. Proc. *39*, 3178–3182.

MASON, K. E. and EMMEL, A. F. 1945. Vitamin E and muscle pigment in the rat. J. Anat. Res. *92*, 33–59.

McCAY, C. M. and CROWELL, M. F. 1934. Prolonging the life span. Sci. Mon. *39*, 405–414.

McCAY, C. M., MAYNARD, L. A., SPERLING, G. and BARNES, L. L. 1939. Retarded growth, life span, ultimate body size, and age changes in the albino rat after feeding diets restricted in calories. J. Nutr. *18*, 1–13.

NANDY, K. 1971. Properties of lipofuscin age pigment in neurons. Acta Neuropathol. *19*, 25–32.

NANDY, K. 1978. Centrophenoxine: Effects on aging brain. J. Am. Geriatr. Soc. *26*, 74–81.

NANDY, K. 1984. Effects of antioxidants on neuronal lipofuscin pigment. *In* Free Radicals in Molecular Biology, Aging, and Diseases, D. Armstrong, R. S. Sohal, R. G. Cutler and T. F. Slater (eds.). Raven Press, New York.

NANDY, K. 1985. Immunopathology of aging and dementia. *In* Senile Dementia of the Alzheimer's Type. J. T. Hutton and J. E. Kenney (eds.). Allen R. Liss, New York.

NANDY, K. and BOURNE, G. H. 1966. Effects of centrophenoxine on neuronal lipofuscin pigment. Nature (London) *210*, 313–314.

NANDY, K. and BOURNE, G. H. 1968. Further studies on the effects of centrophenoxine on lipofuscin pigment in the neurons of senile guinea pigs. J. Gerontol. *23*, 82–92.

NANDY, K. *et al.* 1987. Experimental manipulations of lipofuscin formation in aging mammals. *In* Lipofuscin—1987: State of the Art, I. Zs.-Nagy (ed.). Excerpta Medica, New York.

NANDY, K. and LAL, H. 1978. Neuronal lipofuscin and learning deficits in aging mammals. *In* Neuropsychopharmacologicum, P. Denniker (ed.). Pergamon Press, New York.

NANDY, K. and NANDY, L. 1986. Immunological and autoimmune phenomena in senile brain disease. *In* Biological Substrates of Alzheimer's Disease, A. Sheibel and A. F. Wechsler (eds.). Academic Press, New York.

NANDY, K. and SCHNEIDER, F. H. 1976. Lipofuscin pigment formation in neruoblastoma cells in culture. *In* Neurobiology of Aging, R. D. Terry and S. Gershon (eds.). Raven Press, New York.

OSKI, F. A. and BARNESS, L. A. 1967. Vitamin E deficiency: A previously unrecognized cause of hemolytic anemia in the premature infant. J. Pediatr. *70*, 210–220.

PEARSE, A. G. E. 1964. Histochemistry, Theoretical and Applied. Little, Brown, and Co., Boston.

REICHEL, W., HOLLANDER, J., CLARK. J. H. and STREHLER, B. L. 1968. Lipofuscin pigment accumulation as a function of age and distribution in rodent brain. J. Gerontol. *23*, 71–78.

RIGA, S. and RIGA, D. 1974. Effects of centrophenoxine on the lipofuscin pigment in the nervous system of old rats. Brain Res. *72*, 265–275.

ROSS, M. H. 1959. Protein, calories and life expectancy. Fed. Proc. *18*, 1190–1207.

ROSS, M. H. 1961. Length of life and nutrition in the rat. J. Nutr. *75*, 197–210.

ROSS, M. H. and BRASS, G. 1973. Influence of protein under- and over-nutrition on spontaneous tumor prevalence in the rat. J. Nutr. *103*, 944–963.

ROYCHAUDHURI, C. and DESAI, I. D. 1971. Ceroid pigment formation and irreversible sterility in vitamin E deficiency. Science *173*, 1028–1029.

RUDRA, D. N., DICKERSON, J. W. T. and WALKER, R. 1975. The effects of some antioxidants on lipofuscin accumulation in rat brain. Proc. Nutr. Soc. *34*, 122.

SACHER, G. A. 1977. Life table modification and life prolongation. *In* The Biology of Aging, C. A. Finch and L. Hayflick (eds.). Van Nostrand Reinhold, New York.

SAMORAJSKI, T., KEEFE, J. R. and ORDY, J. M. 1964. Intracellular localization of lipofuscin age pigment in the nervous system. J. Gerontol. *19*, 262–276.

SIAKOTOS, A. N., ARMSTRONG, D., KOPPANG, N. and MILLER, J. 1977. Biochemical significance of age pigment in neurons. *In* The Aging Brain and Senile Dementia, K. Nandy and I. Sherwin (eds.). Plenum Press, New York.

SULKIN, N. M. and SRIVANIJ, P. 1960. The experimental production of senile pigments in the nerve cells of young rats. J. Gerontol. *15*, 2–9.

SULKIN, D. and SULKIN, N. M. 1967. An electron microscopic study of the autonomic ganglion cells in guinea pigs during ascorbic acid deficiency. Lab. Invest. *16*, 142–152.

TAPPEL, A. L. 1965. The free radical lipid peroxidation damage and its inhibition by vitamin E and selenium. Fed. Proc. *24*, 73–78.

TAPPEL, A. L. 1968. Will antioxidant nutrient slow aging process? Geriatrics *23*, 97–105.

TAPPEL, A. L. 1970. Biological antioxidant protection against lipid peroxidation damage. Am. J. Clin. Nutr. *23*, 1137–1139.

TAPPEL, A. L. 1972. Vitamin E and free radical peroxidation of lipids. Ann. N. Y. Acad. Sci. *203*, 12–28.

TAPPEL, A. L., FLETCHER, B. and DEAMER, D. 1973. Effects of antioxidants and nutrients on lipid peroxidation fluorescent products and aging in the mouse. J. Gerontol. *28*, 415–424.

TOUBOLD, R. O., SIAKOTOS, A. N. and PERKINS, E. G. 1975. Studies on the chemical nature of lipofuscin age pigment isolated from normal human brain. Lipids *10*, 383–390.

TEKEUCHI, N. *et al.* 1976. Effects of alpha tocopherols on thiobarbituric acid reactive substances in serum and hepatic subcellular organelles and lipid metabolism. Exp. Gerontol. *11*, 179–185.

TINBURG, H. M. and BARBER, A. A. 1970. Studies on vitamin E action: Peroxidation inhibition in structural protein-lipid mycelle complexes derived from rat liver microsomes. J. Nutr. *100*, 413–418.

WEGLIECKI, W. B., REICHEL, W. and NAIR, P. P. 1968. Accumulation of lipofuscin-like pigment in the rat adrenal cortex as a function of vitamin E-deficiency. J. Gerontol. *21*, 469–475.

CHAPTER 23

DIETARY ANTIOXIDANTS AND BRAIN AGING: HOPES AND FACTS

IMRE ZS.-NAGY, M.D.
Verzár International Laboratory for Experimental Gerontology (VILEG)
Hungarian Section: University Medical School Debrecen, Hungary
and
Italian Section: Department of Gerontological Research, Italian National Institute of Geriatrics (INRCA) Ancona, Italy

INTRODUCTION

The membrane hypothesis of aging (MHA) attributes the age-dependent dehydration of the intracellular mass to a life-long, free radical induced cross-linking of the cell plasma membrane components, the consequence of which is a gradual decrease of the passive permeability of the membrane for potassium. This results in an increase of the intracellular potassium concentration, a condensation of the cell colloids and a loss of water content of the cells. The increasing intracellular density gradually inhibits all enzymic processes including the transcription, translation and decomposition of the damaged compounds and results in first a slowing down and then cessation of the growth in adulthood, and leads to aging later on. The MHA is consistent with numerous other aging concepts, such as the free radical and dysdifferentiation theories of aging. Testing of the MHA can be performed by pharmacological interventions. This possibility represents some hopes for a successful attempt of prolongation of life. The experimental evidence supporting the MHA is reviewed. It was found that the nootropic effects of centrophenoxine (CPH) and its derivative (BCE-001) can be interpreted on the basis of the $OH^{\cdot}$ radical scavenger properties of dimethylaminoethanol (DMAE) or 1,3-bis(dimethylamino)-2-propanol incorporated in the phospholipid pool of neuronal membranes of the brain. These drugs exert a protective role in the cell membrane against the $OH^{\cdot}$ radical attacks. These experiments support the view that properly designed dietary (or nondietary) antioxidant supplementations may be useful in retarding the aging process of the brain.

A Terminological Note

The term "dietary antioxidant" needs some clarification. Although it is used rather widely in the literature, it should be noted that it does not cover any well-defined concept. The term "antioxidant" in itself is confusing, since in a chemical sense, it should mean "reductant." As a matter of fact, some authors speak about the reducing power of antioxidants as a basis of their classification (Weber and Miquel 1986).

Historically, the term antioxidant was used for the designation of a series of compounds or enzymatic systems that are able to eliminate oxygen free radicals (= active oxygen species). For example, Weber and Miquel (1986) distinguished "exogenous antioxidants" (vitamin E and A, ascorbate, sulfur amino acids and selenium compounds) against the "endogenous antioxidants" and free radical scavenging systems (glutathione, superoxide dismutase = SOD, catalase = CA, glutathione peroxidase = GPO, and other peroxidases). The same authors use the term "dietary" antioxidants as a synonym of the exogenous ones. Nevertheless, it is clear now that these substances are not purely of an "antioxidant" (i.e., reductant) character in a chemical sense: e.g., (1) ascorbate is oxidized by two-electron acceptors via ascorbate free radical intermediates, and the latter can act as a one-electron reductant or also as a one-electron oxidant (Iyanagi *et al.* 1985); (2) superoxide anion radicals are basically of reductive nature against organic compounds (this reaction produces molecular oxygen and some reduced molecules); however, under certain circumstances, they can also behave as oxidants. Therefore, ascorbate itself or everything that is eliminating $O_2^{-\cdot}$ radicals may equally be termed as "antireductant" or "antioxidant." These examples are arbitrarily selected just to demonstrate that it is more appropriate to apply the term "radical scavenger" instead of the unclear "antioxidant." If one wishes to distinguish between the exogenous and endogenous scavengers by the term "dietary radical scavenger," it has to be considered that the exogenous scavengers are not only dietary, since a parenteral application of them is also possible. I accepted the use of the term "dietary antioxidants" in the title of my presentation as suggested by the organizers of these Proceedings; however, one should keep in mind these aforementioned considerations.

Historical Background

The question of whether dietary antioxidants may provide protective effects against aging is almost as old as the free radical theory of aging. As a matter of fact, one year after the implication of free radical reactions in biological processes such as aging was proposed (Harman 1956), rodent experiments were performed to test whether the empirically discovered radiation protection chemicals were able to prolong normal life span (Harman 1957), and numerous further attempts have been performed even thereafter (Harman 1960, 1961a, 1961b, 1980).

In a recent review, Weber and Miquel (1986) listed the available data on the effects of various compounds like butylated hydroxytoluene (BHT), 2-mercapto-ethylamine (2-MEA), cysteine, 2,2′-diaminodiethyldisulfide, santoquine, vitamin E, ascorbic acid, D,L-methionine, Na-selenite, quercetin, thiazolidine-4-carboxylic acid, tocopheryl-p-chlorophenoxyacetate, nordihydroguaiaretic acid (NDGA), folcysteine, propyl gallate, diludine, and α-tocopherolchinone. Their conclusions were as follows: (1) although some antioxidant supplementations are capable of extending the life span of experimental animals, the effects are not consistent when studying the same drug in various species: (2) some of the studies in the literature have not been designed carefully enough to exclude potential life-prolonging effects of reduced food intake during the antioxidant supplementations; (3) the hypothesis that antioxidants may prolong life by scavenging oxygen free radicals is still tenable, but the available data are insufficient for complete explanation.

The conclusions of Weber and Miquel (1986) are certainly acceptable. Regarding the inconsistency of known results, it is important to stress that all these data were obtained empirically, i.e., without having any clear idea about the molecular biology of the free radical induced events *in vivo*. One has to comment also on the fact that in spite of the relatively long history of the free radical theory of aging, no real breakthrough has been achieved so far in gerontology. The following issues may be of importance in this regard.

First, most biochemists have neglected the significance of free radicals in the biology, possibly because of their very low concentrations in living systems. This viewpoint has resulted in the fact that most of the biochemistry textbooks today do not have a chapter on free radicals. The real problem underlying this situation is the high reactivity of these radicals, explaining why one cannot expect any accumulation of them in the tissues. On the other hand, free radical studies in biological systems require specific, sophisticated techniques (e.g., electron spin resonance, ESR) which are not widely available yet. Therefore, even today a great part of the actual knowledge on the free radicals is based largely on circumstantial or indirect evidence. The free radical theory of aging has gained strong support with the discovery of superoxide dismutase (SOD) (McCord and Fridovich 1969a, 1969b); nevertheless, the general acceptance of this theory has not been achieved. What can safely be concluded at present is that oxygen free radicals do occur in biological systems and are involved in numerous biological phenomena such as cellular aging, mutagenesis, inflammation and other pathologies (Zs.-Nagy 1989a). Obviously, the uncertainties about the validity of the free radical theory of aging also exerted a negative feedback on the studies of the role of antioxidants in retarding aging.

Second, even the recognition of the biological role of oxygen free radicals cannot resolve all the existing contradictions. Living systems exhibit a paradoxical situation which needs explanation. Namely, young individuals consume considerably more oxygen per unit of mass and time (i.e., should produce more oxygen free radicals) as compared to older ones. Yet it is a fact that young cells and organisms are able to grow and differentiate, while older ones progressively deteriorate in their structure and functional performance. This apparent contradiction has also helped to discredit the free radical theory of aging and hindered the progress of antioxidant research as well. For this author it was always obvious that this apparent paradox must find its explanation in the biological structure itself. Theoretical evidence is available (Zs.-Nagy 1987) showing that this discrepancy can be explained with general validity based on the common properties of all living systems.

This chapter will attempt to summarize the most important theoretical points of the membrane hypothesis of aging (MHA) and some experimental data obtained on the basis of MHA. The MHA is a conceptual approach to cellular aging pursued in the author's laboratory over the last 12 years. The main conclusion is that a properly designed, efficient (probably multifactorial), nontoxic free radical defense system using dietary (or nondietary) oxy-radical scavengers added to the natural defense systems may represent a valid antiaging strategy.

SOME CHARACTERISTICS OF OXYGEN FREE RADICALS

Although many other sources of information are available regarding the physical and chemical characteristics of the oxygen free radicals, a brief survey of the most important points is necessary. There is no doubt that the monovalent reduction of molecular oxygen (performed by a number of various enzymes *in vivo*) leads to the formation of superoxide anion radicals ($O_2^{-\cdot}$). This radical is mostly a reductant agent. Superoxide radicals are dismutated very efficiently by the SOD (McCord and Fridovich 1969a, 1969b). The product of this reaction is hydrogen peroxide, which is a small, uncharged molecule expected to cross all cell membranes easily (Simon *et al.* 1981). It is much less harmful per se for the cells than the superoxide radicals. Nevertheless, two main systems have evolved to eliminate H_2O_2: (1) the catalases (wherever present) that are sensitive only for relatively high hydrogen peroxide concentrations, and also (2) glutathione peroxidase (GPO) (and some other peroxidases) reacting also with the low concentrations of H_2O_2. However, GPO requires glutathione for this reaction which may not always be available in the cells (Fridovich 1976). From these data, it can be assumed that some freely diffusing H_2O_2 is always present in living systems. As a matter of fact, Cutler (1985) has demonstrated that tissue homogenates do produce H_2O_2, and, moreover, the peroxide-producing potential of tissue homogenates is inversely correlated with the longevity of mammalian species.

One of the effects of the presence of H_2O_2 can be a direct lipid-peroxidation (Tappel 1975; Donato and Sohal 1981). However, probably more important is the Fenton-type reaction of H_2O_2 (Fenton 1894) with transition metals like iron (Zsupán *et al.* 1987), copper (Gutteridge 1988), cobalt or manganese (unpublished results). This type of reaction generates $OH^{\cdot}$ free radicals which are extremely reactive (Walling 1975; Czapski 1984; Dunford 1987), since they take an electron from any of the neighboring molecules within about two molecular collisions, i.e., they form intra- or intermolecular covalent cross-links. An important point to be emphasized is that due to the extremely high reactivity of the $OH^{\cdot}$ radicals, practically no enzymatic or any other protection is possible against them except that provided by the evolution of the life, i.e., the continuous replacement of the damaged components by resynthesis and concomitant degradation of the damaged molecules.

It has recently been emphasized that the deleterious effects of the $OH^{\cdot}$ radicals are enhanced if the the metal ion is bound to some organic molecule. In this case its carrier molecule becomes the "target" of the damage (Gutteridge and Xiao-Chang 1981; Czapski 1984; Samuni *et al.* 1983; Chiou *et al.* 1985; Goldstein and Czapski 1986; Stoewe and Prütz 1987).

The damaging effect of the $OH^{\cdot}$ radicals generated by the Fenton reaction has been demonstrated (1) *in vitro* by ESR spin trapping methods against all amino acids and some proteins (Floyd and Zs.-Nagy 1984; Zs.-Nagy and Floyd 1984a); (2)*in vivo* (Nagy *et al.* 1985; Zs.-Nagy 1988); and (3) in cultured cells (Scott *et al.* 1987; Larramendy *et al.* 1987; Zsupán *et al.* 1987). It has been shown that even *in vivo* a sufficient amount of Fe^{2+} is available (Floyd and Lewis 1983) for a Fenton reaction.

The short-living radical species, such as $OH^{\cdot}$ radicals, display an important characteristic usually neglected in biology. From polymer chemistry it is well known that the cross-linking efficiency of the $OH^{\cdot}$ radicals strongly depends on the physical density of the system in which the reaction is performed. If this system is of low density, such as the extremely diluted cytosol, intermolecular cross-linking cannot occur since the dissolved molecules are relatively far from each other, i.e., one radical will react with only one molecule. If the density of the system is larger such as in that of membranes, the probability of intermolecular cross-link formation will be considerably higher. In other words, the same rate of radical formation is much more efficient in damaging the molecular components in systems of higher density. Therefore, one can predict that a uniform $OH^{\cdot}$ radical attack will destroy the membrane components to a higher extent than the cytosolic ones. As a matter of fact, some membrane proteins of hepatocytes display tenfold shorter half-life than do the average proteins in the cytoplasm (Tauber and Reutter 1981). This situation forces very careful consideration of the physiological consequences of the cell membrane damage in all cellular systems.

How Free Radicals Can Damage Membranes

The most widely known mechanism of membrane damage induced by free radicals is lipid peroxidation. The age pigment (lipofuscin) accumulation has been explained by this reaction (Tappel 1975; Chio and Tappel 1969a, 1969b; Miquel *et al.* 1977; Donato and Sohal 1981). The main point of lipid peroxidation is that polyunsaturated fatty acids are decomposed by direct or indirect peroxidation processes resulting in malondialdehyde (MDA) as an end product. MDA is extremely reactive with primary amino groups of proteins and gives rise to the so-called Schiff-bases showing a characteristic fluorescence. It should be noted that several other chemical pathways of formation of the fluorescent compounds of lipofuscin have also been suggested recently (Eldred and Katz 1988; Kikugawa 1988).

It is well established that lipid peroxidation increases the rigidity of the lipid layer (Dobretsov *et al.* 1977; Shaw *et al.* 1980; Rice-Evans and Hochstein 1981; Yamaguchi *et al.* 1983). Data are available showing that lipid peroxidation decreases the activities of some membrane-bound enzymes (Pfeffer and Swislocki 1976, 1982), and the age-dependent decrease of the activities of numerous hormone-receptor complexes has also been ascribed to such phenomena (Adlin and Korenman 1980; Roth 1979a, 1979b). However, apart from these certainly important phenomena, it is impossible to disregard the capability of lipid peroxidation to alter the overall physicochemical properties of the cell membrane, primarily fluidity. Since the physicochemical state of the membrane lipids can directly determine basic functional parameters, such as permeability of the cell membrane for the monovalent ions and probably for water (Schroeder 1984; De Laat *et al.* 1984; Shinitzky 1984), a functional significance to the radical-induced physicochemical changes can be ascribed.

Apart from lipids the oxyradicals (mainly $OH^{\cdot}$) are capable of attacking membrane proteins (Zs.-Nagy 1979; Zs.-Nagy and Floyd 1984a) which results in their cross-linking (Nagy and Zs.-Nagy 1984; Davies 1987). It is reasonable to assume that this phenomenon is of greater importance than generally supposed. Given that the $OH^{\cdot}$ radicals are formed in the aqueous phase and have a very short lifetime, they will react with highest probability in the same phase. Thus, only a small portion of them will react with the deep, hydrophobic regions of the cell membrane.

The above data demonstrate that the life of the cells is accompanied by a continuous formation of lipid-lipid, lipid-protein or protein-protein cross-links. However, this type of damage occurs with considerably higher probability in the membranes than in the cytosol. In addition to the free radical induced damage, the cell plasma membrane is continuously exposed to an additional damaging factor. This is the residual heat created during each discharge of the resting transmembrane potential (Zs.-Nagy 1979). Membrane structure and function are continuously altered by these phenomena: obviously the asymmetric distribution of lipids across the cell membrane is also subject to changes in time (Schroeder 1984).

To maintain cellular homeostasis, damaged components must be replaced by newly synthesized ones and degraded by the lysosomal system. The degradation and replacement of the damaged components is in strict equilibrium at young and adult ages wherein no accumulation of the waste products (lipofuscin) occurs. Moreover, due to the higher metabolic rate in young tissues, an even higher amount of lipofuscin-like products are produced during the same time as compared to the old tissues. The rate of elimination of these products is highly efficient in that no accumulation can be observed in young cells (Zs.-Nagy 1987). This assumption has recently been verified. It was shown that young rat brain cells accumulate lipofuscin-like pigments if some of the lysosomal enzymes (e.g., thiol-proteases) were inhibited by leupeptin for a couple of days (Ivy *et al.* 1984; Ivy and Gurd 1988).

AN OUTLINE OF THE MEMBRANE HYPOTHESIS OF AGING

Theoretical Considerations

One of the most general characteristics of the cell membrane is its high passive permeability for potassium (P_K) and water (P_W). The ionic gradients between the intra- and extracellular spaces are maintained partly by these "passive" parameters of the membrane and by an active, energy-consuming pumping mechanism. Apart from the fact that the passive transport of ions across the cell membrane is not completely understood, it is safe to assume that the passive permeability should depend on the actual molecular structure of the cell membrane, including, among others, the liberty of motion of the components and the compactness. It is easy to show that a decrease in P_K involves an increased intracellular potassium concentration, if the resting potential of the cell remains invariate (Zs.-Nagy 1978). On the other hand, an increase of the intracellular ionic strength results in a considerable condensation (i.e., loss of water content) of the intracellular colloids. Considering the fact that the so-called maturation process of cells, tissues, organs and organisms represents a gradual increase of the intracellular dry mass content and this process is progressing even during aging, one cannot neglect the general significance of this phenomenon.

Taking into account the basic properties of the cell membrane, the MHA was outlined first as a working hypothesis (Zs.-Nagy 1978, 1979) and studied in detail thereafter (Zs.-Nagy 1986, 1987, 1988, 1989a). This concept proposes a cell physiological mechanism explaining the apparent paradox of the free radical theory of aging mentioned above. It is consistent with the dysdifferentiation hypothesis of aging (Zs.-Nagy *et al.* 1988a). This chapter summarizes the available evidence explaining the free radical induced membrane damage and the overall age-dependent decrease of the protein turnover of the cells (Zs.-Nagy 1987).

On the basis of the available experimental evidence, MHA can be described as a *circulus vitiosus*, the main points of which are summarized as follows.

Membrane Physicochemistry and Permeability

Starting during embryonic life, the membrane of all living cells is exposed to a continuous free radical induced cross-linking and the residual heat-induced damage. This damage manifests itself in the membrane physicochemistry. As a matter of fact, age-dependent changes of the membrane have been observed in lipid fluidity (Nagy *et al.* 1983a, 1983b), the asymmetry of the lipid layer (Schroeder 1984), the molecular weight distribution of the proteins (Nagy and Zs.-Nagy 1984), the lateral diffusion constant of the proteins (Zs.-Nagy *et al.* 1984, 1986a, 1986b, 1988b, 1989a; Kitani *et al.* 1988). Due to all these alterations, the cell membrane gradually loses its P_K (Zs.-Nagy *et al.* 1982a, 1985; Gyenes *et al.* 1984). An age-dependent loss of P_W is also expected, although has not been proven yet.

Intracellular Potassium Content

As a consequence of the loss of P_K of the membrane, the intracellular potassium concentration increases considerably (about 30–100%), if expressed on a mEq/kg water basis (Zs.-Nagy *et al.* 1977, 1979, 1985; Pieri *et al.* 1977; Lustyik and Zs.-Nagy 1985). Such an increase is beneficial from the point of view of the maintenance of the cell excitability; however, it exerts a strong condensing effect on the cytoplasmic and nuclear colloids (Zs.-Nagy 1978, 1979).

Intracellular Density

Under the influence of the increasing intracellular potassium concentration, the intracellular density of the cell colloids displays a parallel increase. This is reflected in a considerable loss of cell water content (Zs.-Nagy *et al.* 1982b, 1985; Lustyik and Zs.-Nagy 1985, 1988). An increase of the dry mass content from 20 to 27–30% by weight is quite a considerable change. It was shown that the colloidal mass is not only more condensed but also more cross-linked, since the colloid-osmotic pressure of the brain and liver cells considerably decreases with age (Zs.-Nagy *et al.* 1987). Moreover, the increase of the density causes an overall decrease of the enzyme activities in the sense of a theoretical enzyme kinetic model, the extent of which may reach even an order of magnitude from young to old age (Damjanovich *et al.* 1989).

Transcription and Translation

It is well known that the chromatin is especially sensitive toward the ionic strength of the medium; therefore, one can predict that the rate of transcription and translation is reduced simply because of the increased intracellular density and viscosity. Radioisotope experiments *in vivo* revealed that both the total and the mRNA synthesis rate decrease more than 50% between 2 and 26 months of age in the rat brain cortex (Semsei *et al.* 1982; Zs.-Nagy and Semsei 1984). Other available data (Zs.-Nagy 1987) strongly indicate that the rate of protein synthesis decreases with age in almost all experimental models studied so far.

Accumulation of Waste Products

It is evident from the retardation of both the RNA and protein synthesis that the protein turnover of elderly individuals cannot be maintained at the same speed as observed at younger ages. This explains why the so called age pigments (lipofuscin) are accumulated in the old tissues. Lipofuscin is accumulated apparently just because the protein synthesis is retarded and the necessary lysosomal enzymes are missing (Zs.-Nagy 1988).

Conclusions From the MHA

It is obvious that an age-dependent decrease of the protein turnover forces the cell membrane to perform its function for an ever increasing time in the presence of more and more damaged components. This involves that a self-destroying *circulus vitiosus* comes into being resulting in first a quantitative reduction and a complete functional breakdown of the given cell. If an organ consists of mainly postmitotic cells, like the brain, liver, etc., little or no chance exists for the replacement of the damaged cells, i.e., sooner or later the whole organ function becomes compromised, and the individual dies.

According to the MHA, the nature of the molecular damage is not qualitatively different in young and old systems. Even in quantitative terms, due to the higher metabolic rate of young systems, more harmful radicals are formed per cell unit time at younger ages. However, due to the lower physical density of young cells, the rate of protein synthesis can be maintained to such a high extent that even the growth of the system is possible. Maturation is achieved when a state of density in which the rates of damage and replacement are in equilibrium, i.e., growth is not possible any more. Lastly, in spite of a decreased metabolic rate observed in old age, primarily due to the increased intracellular density, the free radical induced damage becomes more and more deleterious in that fewer radicals produce relatively more macromolecular damage. Thus, the aging process will be accelerated. It may also be relevant that SOD has been reported to exhibit a salt dependence which would further render less efficient the defense mechanism against the superoxide radicals in old cells (Semsei and Zs.-Nagy 1984, 1985).

The MHA as outlined above has an advantageous feature. Namely, it can be tested from various points of view by using some pharmacological or dietary interventions *in vivo*. It is important to note that many drugs entering into the blood serum may also reach the cell membranes of most tissues (in case of the brain the blood brain barrier must be overcome). Basically, two types of experimental approaches are possible *in vivo* as detailed below.

ACCELERATION OF THE AGING RATE

The experimental possibility of accelerating the aging rate of the brain cells is of great theoretical interest, since it may clarify numerous questions raised by the MHA. On the other hand, such type of experiments can also be useful from the point of view of an anti-aging experimental strategy. Aging can be accelerated by either (1) weakening the defense mechanism against free radical attacks or (2) increasing the production of $OH^{\cdot}$ free radicals.

(1) Based on the well-known fact that vitamin E is one of the most efficient protective factors against lipid peroxidation (Donato and Sohal 1981), experiments were conducted in rats on a vitamin E deficient diet. It has been observed that this

diet, if established at the age of one month, causes an accelerated macroscopic aging of the rats which is accompanied by the same type of changes in passive permeability of the nerve cell membrane for K^+ and Rb^+ and in the intracellular ion and water content of the brain cortical cells as observed during the normal aging process (Bertoni-Freddari *et al.* 1981; Pieri *et al.* 1986).

(2) Experimental acceleration of aging was also achieved by increasing the OH˙ radical production through a Fenton reaction. As the blood brain barrier is extremely impermeable for iron, Fe^{2+} salts were injected in the cerebrospinal fluid of young rats. This intervention is extremely toxic. If sublethal doses of iron were injected repeatedly for three days, the synaptosomal fractions of the brain cortex displayed similar alterations as observed during the normal aging process (Nagy *et al.* 1985).

These results are consistent with the MHA. Since both the decrease of efficiency of the natural free radical defense mechanism (vitamin E deficiency) and the increase of the OH˙ radical production (overload with iron *in vivo*) accelerate the rate of brain cell aging, one could suggest that the active oxygen species may play the primary role in brain aging as predicted by the MHA.

DECELERATION OF THE AGING RATE

If the MHA is a basically correct hypothesis, one can expect that a properly designed, additional protection of the neuronal membrane components against OH˙ radical damage would retard aging. The term "properly designed" should be emphasized. Due to the extremely short lifetime of the OH˙ free radicals, one can envision protection against them only, if (1) the scavenger molecule has a considerably higher reaction rate with them than the target molecule to be protected and (2) the scavenger gets sufficiently close to the target and remains there as a component part for a sufficiently long time. Another important criterion is that the scavenger must not exert any deleterious side effect (toxicity) for the organism, in general, or in the immediate vicinity of the target molecule. Consideration of these criteria suggests that it is most probably a hopeless effort to start testing of various scavengers without having any particular knowledge about their molecular biology, binding sites, etc. Unfortunately, most of the studies on dietary antioxidants (Weber and Miquel 1986) have been performed without having such information.

The following lists the antiaging effects of two drugs. One is centrophenoxine (CPH) and a derivative CPH coded as BCE-001 (BIOGAL Pharmaceutical Works 1985). These experiments were performed not only considering the previously mentioned criteria, but the BCE-001 molecule itself was planned with the intention to increase the OH˙ radical scavenging ability of the CPH molecule. It should be stressed that the results obtained with these two drugs serve as examples to demonstrate the validity of the strategy suggested by the MHA, and obviously represent only the beginning in this type of research. In any event, the following results can be considered to be consistent with the hopes represented by the MHA.

Pharmacology of CPH and BCE-001

CPH is an ester of p-chlorophenoxyacetic acid (PCPA) and dimethylaminoethanol (DMAE) (Fig. 23.1). It was classified formerly in human therapy as a brain metabolic stimulant, and the ill-defined term ''neuroenergeticum'' was applied to it since it stimulated glucose uptake, oxygen consumption and carbon dioxide production of the brain *in vivo* and also *in vitro* in brain slices. Early publications on the effects of CPH described a number of beneficial effects of CPH in cases like cerebral atrophy, brain injury, postapoplectic disorders, chronic alcoholism, barbiturate intoxications, etc. It has also been observed that prolonged administration of CPH to healthy old animals significantly reduced the accumulation of lipofuscin in brain cells and myocardium. Furthermore, the median life span of the CPH-treated old animals increased significantly, and the learning ability of the old, treated mice improved as compared to their age-matched controls (Zs.-Nagy 1989b). On the basis of these results, CPH could be considered as a potential antiaging drug.

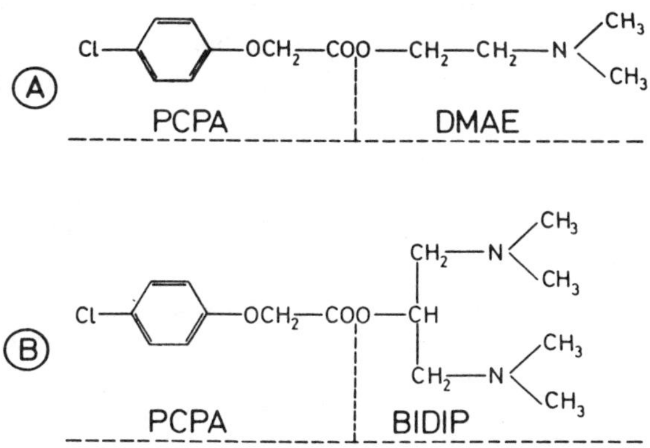

FIG. 23.1. THE CHEMICAL FORMS OF CENTROPHENOXINE (A) AND BCE-001 (B)
The PCPA moiety is identical in both drugs, however, in place of DMAE, BCE-001 contains BIDIP

The classification of this drug has recently changed, since the concept of ''nootropics'' has been introduced (Giurgea and Sara 1978). Today, CPH is one of the most frequently used representative of nootropics in various, mostly European, countries. Nevertheless, the mechanism of action of CPH on the age-dependent decline of the mental performance has never been clearly understood. It was supposed that the DMAE moiety of CPH enters the choline synthesis cycle (and thus improves the acetylcholine supply of the brain). However, an increase of choline availability by transforming a fraction of DMAE from CPH into choline (which has been shown to take place in the liver) (Bertoni-Freddari *et al.* 1982) cannot explain the effect of this drug, since a choline-rich diet alone does not result in the same effect (Zaniser *et al.* 1977; Jope and Jenden 1979).

Regarding the pharmacokinetics of CPH, after intravenous administration of equimolar doses of ^{14}C-labelled DMAE and CPH, much higher levels of DMAE were found in the brain after CPH treatment, as compared to DMAE alone since apparently the esterified form of DMAE with PCPA penetrates the blood-brain barrier more easily. CPH is hydrolyzed on both sides of the barrier *in vivo*; however, the DMAE moiety becomes phosphorylated in the brain and yields phosphoryl-DMAE which is in turn converted to phosphatidyl-DMAE, seemingly the end-metabolite of DMAE in the brain (Miyazaki *et al.* 1976). Phosphatidyl-DMAE is incorporated in the nerve cell membranes, and persists there for a relatively long time in the place of choline. The p-chlorophenoxy acetic acid moiety (PCPA) is excreted in the urine rather quickly. Although some fraction of DMAE administered alone or in the form of CPH was found in acid-soluble and lipid cholines in the brain, evidence is available that the trimethylation of DMAE does not take place in the brain but in the liver (Miyazaki *et al.* 1976). This fact suggested that its OH˙ radical scavenger ability shown *in vitro* may really be of significance also *in vivo*. Our laboratory has studied the effects of CPH since 1976 parallel with the development of the MHA. The conclusion was reached that the effects of CPH on the brain can be interpreted as an OH˙ free radical scavenging action of the DMAE moiety in the neuronal membranes (Zs.-Nagy 1989b).

Based on the results obtained with CPH (listed below), we designed the new drug coded BCE-001, with the intention to increase the OH˙ radical scavenging ability of CPH. BCE-001 is basically similar to CPH. The difference is that the PCPA moiety is esterified with 1,3-bis(dimethylamino)-2-propanol (BIDIP) instead of DMAE (Fig.23.1). BIDIP contains 2 dimethylamino groups suggesting that twice as many loosely bound electrons are present in this moiety, which can be useful in the neutralization of OH˙ radicals. As we demonstrate below, this property of the molecule proved to be biologically meaningful.

The OH˙ Radical-scavenger Properties of CPH and BCE-001

Protein Cross-linking Model. In this model OH˙ free radicals are generated by Fenton reaction, attacking and cross-linking the proteins (e.g., bovine serum albumine = BSA) added to the reaction mixture. As a consequence, the water solubility of the protein (originally 100%) gradually decreases. Therefore, it is sufficient to follow only the protein content in the supernatant in order to reveal the effect of the OH˙ radicals and the influence of radical scavengers like DMAE on this reaction. The molecular weight distribution of the still soluble fraction of BSA was also analyzed (Zs.-Nagy and Nagy 1980). These studies revealed that DMAE efficiently inhibits the polymerization of BSA induced by the OH˙ radicals, i.e., DMAE is a potent OH˙ radical scavenger under the given conditions. The polymerization of BSA could be detected not only as a precipitation of an insoluble, glue-like mass, but also in the still soluble rest of BSA in the form of di-, tri-, and tetramerized molecules (Zs.-Nagy and Nagy 1980). The covalent character of the newly formed intermolecular bonds has been demonstrated by chemical tests, such as treatment with concentrated (6 M) urea, etc.

BCE-001 behaved similarly to DMAE with the only difference that equimolar amounts of it displayed a roughly twofold protective effect against the polymerization of BSA (unpublished results).

ESR-spin Trapping Experiments. This technique applies to specially designed compounds (spin traps), the reactions of which with various types of free radicals are well known. They usually form some relatively long-lived radicals (spin adducts). The concentration of spin adducts can be quantitatively measured under controlled conditions by means of their paramagnetic properties by ESR spectroscopy (Floyd 1981, 1982; Floyd and Lewis 1983). Using this technique, one can obtain data regarding the competition for a given type of radical generated in the reaction mixture, and in some cases also the rate constants of the radical scavenging process can be estimated.

The spin trapping experiments demonstrated that the CPH molecule and both components of it display a strong affinity toward the $OH^{\cdot}$ radicals (Zs.-Nagy and Floyd 1984b). In the case of DMAE the reaction rate can be estimated at $0.8 \times 10^9\ M^{-1}\ sec^{-1}$. This value is quite comparable with that of the spin trap (DMPO) used (Floyd and Lewis 1983). Since most of the bio-organic compounds react with $OH^{\cdot}$ radicals at rates ranging from 10^7 to $10^{10}\ M^{-1}\ sec^{-1}$ (Walling 1975), DMAE really may exert a significant protection for numerous cell membrane components against $OH^{\cdot}$ free radicals. It is noteworthy that BIDIP displayed a reaction rate constant with $OH^{\cdot}$ free radicals about $1.7 \times 10^9\ M^{-1}\ sec^{-1}$ in identical test conditions (unpublished results) which is quite near to the theoretically expected two-fold increase, as compared to DMAE.

The $OH^{\cdot}$ scavenger ability of DMAE (Zs.-Nagy and Floyd 1984b) and BIDIP (unpublished results) have also been tested in some other spin trapping models using PBN and 4-POBN. In addition, proline or hydroxyproline were also tested as special spin traps (Floyd and Zs.-Nagy 1984). All these investigations supported the $OH^{\cdot}$ scavenger ability of DMAE and BIDIP. Therefore, these compounds, if incorporated into the plasma membrane of nerve cells can really be considered as site-specific $OH^{\cdot}$ free radical scavengers; i.e., their observed effects should be interpreted on this basis.

Although these experiments revealed also an $OH^{\cdot}$ radical scavenger capability of the PCPA moiety present in both the CPH and BCE-001 molecules, PCPA cannot be responsible for the nootropic effects of either of them, since no binding of this compound has been demonstrated in the brain. It cannot be excluded, however, that PCPA may have some physiologically meaningful effect in the blood or in some other tissues (e.g., kidney or liver) during its excretion.

Superoxide Radical Reactions of CPH

Known biochemical reaction systems (pyrogallol autoxidation, cytochrome c reduction and photoxidation of o-dianisidine) were used for detection of some typical superoxide radical-induced processes and the eventual superoxide radical scavenger properties of CPH and its components, DMAE and PCPA. It was found that the rate constant of the reaction of these compounds with superoxide radicals is only in the order of magnitude of $10^2\ M^{-1}\ sec^{-1}$; therefore, there is no reason to assume that either component or the CPH molecule itself would represent any efficient protection *in vivo* against superoxide radicals (Semsei and Zs.-Nagy 1985). BIDIP has not been tested by these methods.

The Main In Vivo Results With CPH and BCE-001 Treatments

Obviously, neither the presence of DMAE in neuronal membranes (Miyazaki *et al.* 1976) nor the *in vitro* $OH^{\cdot}$ radical-scavenging ability of this compound (Zs.-Nagy 1989b) prove directly that it acts as an $OH^{\cdot}$ radical scavenger *in vivo*. However, numerous experimental results, listed below, demonstrate indirectly that the presence of DMAE or BIDIP in the cell membrane is of physiological significance which can be attributed to their $OH^{\cdot}$ radical scavenger properties.

(1) If old rats had been treated with CPH for 60 days (Nagy *et al.* 1983b) or with BCE-001 for 20 days (unpublished results), the membrane lipid fluidity of synaptosomes of the brain cortex increased significantly (about the same extent) as revealed by fluorescence anisotropy measurements after DPH-labelling. Spin labelling techniques (Nagy *et al.* 1983a) confirmed the validity of the results obtained by DPH-labelling for both drugs (unpublished results).

(2) Synaptosomal membranes were protected considerably by CPH pretreatment against the toxic effect of *in vivo* acute Fe^{2+} overload in the cerebrospinal fluid of young rats (Nagy *et al.* 1985).

(3) The age-dependent shift of the molecular weight distribution of the proteins toward the higher values in the synaptosomes of the rat brain cortex was partially reversed in old rats by CPH-treatment (Nagy and Zs.-Nagy 1984).

(4) CPH and BCE-001 treatment reversed the age-dependent decrease of the lateral mobility of hepatocyte membrane proteins in old Wistar and Fischer 344 rats. BCE-001 produced a quantitatively larger increase of the protein diffusion constant under identical dosage and time of treatment than did CPH (Zs.-Nagy *et al.* 1989b).

(5) CPH treatment of old rats increases the passive potassium permeability of the neuronal cell membrane, i.e., it decreases the intracellular potassium content and rehydrates the cytoplasm of neurons considerably (Zs.-Nagy *et al.* 1979; Lustyik and Zs.-Nagy 1985). BCE-001 exhibited the same effect; however, lower dose and shorter time of treatment was sufficient to reach the same level of these alterations (unpublished observations).

(6) CPH treatment of old rats reversed the age-dependent deterioration of certain synaptic parameters as measured by electron microscopic morphometry in the cerebellar glomerulus (Bertoni-Freddari *et al.* 1982).

(7) An age-dependent decrease of the rates of total and mRNA synthesis was observed in the brain cortex of rats between 1 and 2 years of age (to 40–50% of the young-adult value) (Semsei *et al.* 1982). Both CPH and BCE-001

reversed this tendency. CPH treatment of 60 days reincreased these rates to 80–90% (Zs.-Nagy and Semsei 1984), whereas BCE-001 resulted in similar increases already during 40 days and values up to 113% were obtained when the drug was applied for 60 days (unpublished results.).

(8) CPH treatment reversed the age-dependent decrease of water solubility of proteins and the increase of the total protein content in the brain of old rats (Zs.-Nagy *et al.* 1981).

(9) CPH treatment can increase the median life span of laboratory animals, especially if the treatment starts at relatively young ages (6 months). It improves also the learning ability of several species (Zs.-Nagy *et al.* 1979; Zs.-Nagy and Semsei 1984). BCE-001 treatment administered from the age of 18 months increased the median life span of female CFY rats from 24 to 29 months (unpublished results.). CPH did not prove to be so effective on survival if started at such an advanced age.

(10) In a recent, double blind, randomized, human clinical trial, CPH treatment of 8 weeks improved the psychometric and behavioral performance in about 50% of patients with medium level dementia (DSM III, Category 1; ICD No. 299); the placebo group displayed improvement only 27% (Pék *et al.* 1989). A considerable rehydration of the intracellular mass was observed in the *verum* group at the expense of the extracellular liquid, meanwhile the body weight remained unchanged (Fülöp *et al.* 1990).

CONCLUSIONS

The main conclusions which may be of importance for future experimental gerontological and geriatric research are as follows:

(1) The experimental biological research is approaching a synthesis on the basis of which the understanding of the physicochemical reasons for the limited existence of living systems may become possible. The widest frame of this understanding actually is represented by the MHA suggesting that an interdisciplinary approach to cell aging is necessary, possible and hopeful at the same time. It describes a cellular mechanism explaining the effects of the oxygen free radicals with general validity and also offers good chances for experimental testing. The hopes for an eventual possibility of the prolongation of human life span are strengthened by the fact that according to the MHA, the rate-limiting process in cellular aging is the structural and functional deterioration of the cell membrane. This hypothesis can be tested with properly designed pharmacological interventions much more easily than in any other internal compartment of neurons.

(2) The experimental facts observed by applying special $OH^{\cdot}$ radical scavengers like CPH and BCE-001 are consistent with the assumptions and predictions of the MHA. It has been demonstrated by these drug effects that the alterations of the cell

parameters through a reversal of the age-dependent deterioration of the membrane structure and function is really meaningful in physiological terms, not only at cellular levels but also for the whole organism. The significance of these experimental results should not be overemphasized for immediate geriatric application since actually their most important message seems to be that a properly designed improvement of the defense against $OH^{\cdot}$ free radical attacks in the neuronal membrane is beneficial at least for lower animals.

(3) On the basis of the MHA, one can predict that even the future life-prolongation strategy can be based on the free radical theory of aging. However, the old, simple-minded approach according to which practically any kind of compounds displaying radical-scavenger ability *in vitro* were expected to exert a life prolonging effect, should be revised. Due to the known properties of the $OH^{\cdot}$ radical reactions, only a site-specific, nontoxic and physicochemically feasible radical protection offers the hope of success. It should also be stressed that in highly evolved living systems where the natural radical protection is *a priori* much more efficient than in rodents, for example, most probably only a multifactorial radical protection can be successful if one intends to improve the natural defense system.

REFERENCES

ADLIN, E. V. and KORENMAN, S. G. 1980. Endocrine aspects of aging. Ann. Intern. Med. *92*, 426–431.

BERTONI-FREDDARI, C., GIULI, C., LUSTYIK, GY. and ZS.-NAGY, I. 1981. *In vivo* effects of vitamin E deficiency on the intracellular monovalent electrolyte concentrations in brain and liver of rat. Mech. Ageing Dev. *16*, 169–180.

BERTONI-FREDDARI, C., GIULI, C. and PIERI, C. 1982. The effect of acute and chronic centrophenoxine treatment on the synaptic plasticity of old rats. Arch. Gerontol. Geriatr. *1*, 365–373.

BIOGAL Pharmaceutical Works. 1985. U.S. Pat. 4661618.

CHIO, K. S. and TAPPEL, A. L. 1969a. Synthesis and characterization of the fluorescent products derived from malonaldehyde and amino acids. Biochemistry *8*, 2821–2827.

CHIO, K. S. and TAPPEL, A. L. 1969b. Inactivation of ribonuclease and other enzymes by peroxidizing lipids and by malonaldehyde. Biochemistry *8*, 2827–2832.

CHIOU, S-H. *et al.* 1985. Specific cleavages of DNA by ascorbate in the presence of copper ion or copper chelates. J. Biochem. *98*, 1723–1726.

CUTLER, R. G. 1985. Peroxide producing potential of tissues: inverse correlation with longevity of mammalian species. Proc. Natl. Acad. Sci. USA *82*, 4798–4802.

CZAPSKI, G. 1984. On the use of $OH^{\cdot}$ scavengers on biological systems. Israel J. Chem. *24*, 29–32.

DAMJANOVICH, S., ZS.-NAGY, I. and SOMOGYI, B. 1989. Application of a molecular enzyme kinetic model for aging cells and tissues. Arch. Gerontol. Geriatr. *8*, 37–45.

DAVIES, K. J. A. 1987. Protein damage and degradation by oxygen radicals: I. General aspects. J. Biol. Chem. *262*, 9895–9901.

De LAAT, S. W. *et al.* 1984. Membrane fluidity in growth and differentiation. The neuroblastoma cell model. *In* Physiology of Membrane Fluidity, Vol. II, M. Shinitzky (ed.). CRC Press, Boca Raton.

DOBRETSOV, G. E., BORSCHEVSKAYA, T. A., PETROV, V. A. and VLADIMIROV, Y. A. 1977. The increase of phospholipid bilayer rigidity after lipid peroxidation. FEBS Lett. *84*, 125–129.

DONATO, H. AND SOHAL, R. S. 1981. Relationship of lipofuscin accumulation to aging. *In* CRC Handbook of Biochemistry in Aging, J. R. Florini, R. C. Adelman and G. S. Roth (eds.). CRC Press, Boca Raton.

DUNFORD, H. B. 1987. Free radicals in iron-containing systems. Free. Rad. Biol. Med. *3*, 405–421.

ELDRED, G. E. and KATZ, M. L. 1988. Possible mechanism for lipofuscinogenesis in the retinal pigment epithelium and other tissues. *In* Lipofuscin—1987: State of the Art, I. Zs.-Nagy (ed.). Akadémiai Kiadó, Budapest, and Elsevier Science Publishers, Amsterdam.

FENTON, H. J. H. 1894. Oxidation of tartaric acid in presence of iron. J. Chem. Soc. *65*, 899–910.

FLOYD, R. A. 1981. DNA-ferrous iron catalyzed free radical formation from hydrogen peroxide. Biochem. Biophys. Res. Commun. *99*, 1209–1215.

FLOYD, R. A. 1982. Observations on nitroxyl free radicals in arylamine carcinogenesis and on spin-trapping hydroxyl free radicals. Can. J. Chem. *60*, 1577–1586.

FLOYD, R. A. and LEWIS, C. A. 1983. Hydroxyl free radical formation from hydrogen peroxide by ferrous iron-nucleotide complexes. Biochemistry *22*, 2645–2649.

FLOYD, R. A. and ZS.-NAGY, I. 1984. Formation of long-lived hydroxyl free radical adducts of proline and hydroxyproline in a Fenton reaction. Biochim. Biophys. Acta *790*, 94–97.

FRIDOVICH, I. 1976. Oxygen radicals, hydrogen peroxide, and oxygen toxicity. *In* Free Radicals in Biology, Vol. I, W. A. Pryor (ed.). Academic Press, New York.

FÜLÖP, Jr., T. *et al.* 1990. Effects of centrophenoxine on body composition and some biochemical parameters of demented elderly people as revealed in a double blind clinical trial. Arch. Gerontol. Geriatr. (in press).

GIURGEA, C. and SARA, S. J. 1978. Nootropic drugs and memory. *In* Practical Aspects of Memory, M. M. Grüneberg, P. E. Morris and R. N. Sykes (eds.). Academic Press, London.

GOLDSTEIN, S. and CZAPSKI, G. 1986. The role and mechanism of metal ions and their complexes in enhancing damage in biological systems or protecting these systems from the toxicity of $O_2^{-\cdot}$. J. Free Rad. Biol. Med. *2*, 3–11.

GUTTERIDGE, J. M. C. 1988. Damage to biological molecules by iron and copper complexes. *In* Lipofuscin—1987: State of the Art, I. Zs.-Nagy (ed.). Akadémiai Kiadó, Budapest, and Elsevier Science Publishers, Amsterdam.

GUTTERIDGE, J. M. C. and XIAO-CHANG, F. 1981. Protection of iron-catalyzed free radical damage to DNA and lipids by copper(II)-bleomycin. Biochem. Biophys. Res. Commun. *99*, 1354–1360.

GYENES, M. *et al.* 1984. Age-dependent decrease of the passive Rb^+ and K^+ permeability of the nerve cell membranes in rat brain cortex as revealed by *in vivo* measurement of the Rb^+ discrimination ratio. Arch. Gerontol. Geriatr. *3*, 11–31.

HARMAN, D. 1956. Aging: a theory based on free radical and radiation chemistry. J. Gerontol. *11*, 298–300.

HARMAN, D. 1957. Prolongation of the normal life span by radiation protection chemicals. J. Gerontol. *12*, 257–263.

HARMAN, D. 1960. The free radical theory of aging: the effect of age on serum mercaptan levels. J. Gerontol. *15*, 38–40.

HARMAN, D. 1961a. Mutation, cancer and aging. Lancet *1*, 200–201.

HARMAN, D. 1961b. Prolongation of the normal life span and inhibition of spontaneous cancer by antioxidants. J. Gerontol. *16*, 147–154.

HARMAN, D. 1980. Free radical theory of aging: beneficial effect of antioxidants on the life span of male NZB mice; role of free radical reactions in the deterioration of the immune system with age and in the pathogenesis of systemic lupus erythematosus. Age *3*, 64–73.

IVY, G. O. and GURD, J. W. 1988. A proteinase inhibitor model of lipofuscin formation. *In* Lipofuscin—1987: State of the Art, I. Zs.-Nagy (ed.). Akadémiai Kiadó, Budapest, and Elsevier Science Publishers, Amsterdam.

IVY, G. O. *et al.* 1984. Inhibitors of lysosomal enzymes: accumulation of lipofuscin-like dense bodies in the brain. Science *226*, 985–987.

IYANAGI, T., YAMAZAKI, I. and ANAN, K. F. 1985. One-electron oxidation-reduction properties of ascorbic acid. Biochim. Biophys. Acta *806*, 255–261.

JOPE, R. S. and JENDEN, D. J. 1979. Dimethylaminoethanol (Deanol) metabolism in rat brain and its effect on acetylcholine synthesis. J. Pharmacol. Exp. Ther. *211*, 472–479.

KIKUGAWA, K. 1988. Involvement of lipid oxidation products in the formation of lipofuscin. *In* Lipofuscin—1987: State of the Art, I. Zs.-Nagy (ed.). Akadémiai Kiadó, Budapest, and Elsevier Science Publishers, Amsterdam.

KITANI, K. *et al.* 1988. Correlation between the biliary excretion of ouabain and the lateral mobility of hepatocyte plasma membrane proteins in the rat. The effects of age and spironolactone pretreatment. Hepatology *8*, 125–131.

LARRAMENDY, M., MELLO-FILHO, A. C., LEME MARTINS, E. A. and MENEGHINI, R. 1987. Iron-mediated induction of sister chromatid exchanges by hydrogen peroxide and superoxide anion. Mutat. Res. *178*, 57–63.

LUSTYIK, GY. and ZS.-NAGY, I. 1985. Alterations of the intracellular water and ion concentrations in brain and liver cells during aging as revealed by energy dispersive X-ray microanalysis of bulk specimens. Scanning Electron Microsc. *1985/I*, 323–337.

LUSTYIK, GY. and ZS.-NAGY, I. 1988. Age-dependent dehydration of postmitotic cells as measured by X-ray microanalysis of bulk specimens. Scanning Microsc. *2*, 289–299.

MCCORD, J. M. and FRIDOVICH, I. 1969a. Superoxide dismutase. An enzymic function for erythrocuprein (hemocuprein). J. Biol. Chem. *244*, 6049–6055.

MCCORD, J. M. and FRIDOVICH, I. 1969b. The utility of superoxide dismutase in studying free radical reactions. I. Radicals generated by the interaction of sulfite, dimethyl sulfoxide, and oxygen. J. Biol. Chem. *244*, 6056–6063.

MIQUEL, J., ORO, J., BENSCH, K. G. and JOHNSON, JR., J. E. 1977. Lipofuscin: Fine structural and biochemical studies. *In* Free Radicals in Biology, Vol. III, W. A. Pryor (ed.). Academic Press, New York.

MIYAZAKI, M. *et al.* 1976. Comparative studies on the metabolism of beta-dimethylaminoethanol in the mouse brain and liver following administration of beta-dimethylaminoethanol and its p-chlorophenoxyacetate, Meclofenoxate. Chem. Pharm. Bull. *24*, 763–769.

NAGY, K., FLOYD, R. A., SIMON, P. and ZS.-NAGY, I. 1985. Studies on the effect of iron overload on rat cortex synaptosomal membranes. Biochim. Biophys. Acta *820*, 216–222.

NAGY, K., SIMON, P. and Zs.-NAGY, I. 1983a. Spin label studies on synaptosomal membranes of rat brain cortex during aging. Biochem. Biophys. Res. Commun. *117*, 688–694.

NAGY, K. and Zs.-NAGY, I. 1984. Alterations in the molecular weight distribution of proteins in rat brain synaptosomes during aging and centrophenoxine treatment. Mech. Ageing Dev. *28*, 171–176.

NAGY, K., Zs.-NAGY, V., BERTONI-FREDDARI, C. and Zs.-NAGY, I. 1983b. Alterations of the synaptosomal membrane microviscosity in the brain cortex of rats during aging and centrophenoxine treatment. Arch. Gerontol. Geriatr. *2*, 23–39.

PFEFFER, S. R. and SWISLOCKI, N. I. 1976. Age related decline in the activities of erythrocyte membrane adenylate cyclase and protein kinase. Arch. Biochem. Biophys. *177*, 117–122.

PFEFFER, S. R. and SWISLOCKI, N. I. 1982. Role of peroxidation in erythrocyte aging. Mech. Ageing Dev. *18*, 355–376.

PÉK, GY. FÜLÖP, T. and Zs.-NAGY, I. 1989. Gerontopsychological studies using NAI (''Nürnberger Alters-Inventar'') on patients with organic psychosyndrome (DSM III, Category 1) treated with centrophenoxine in a double blind, comparative, randomized clinical trial. Arch. Gerontol. Geriatr. *9*, 17–30.

PIERI, C. *et al.* 1977. Energy dispersive X-ray microanalysis of the electrolytes in biological bulk specimen. II. Age-dependent alterations in the monovalent ion contents of cell nucleus and cytoplasm in rat liver and brain cells. J. Ultrastruct. Res. *59*, 320–331.

PIERI, C., GIULI, C., BERTONI-FREDDARI, C. and BERNARDINI, A. 1986. Vitamin E deficiency alters the *in vivo* Rb^+ discrimination of rat brain cortical cells. Arch. Gerontol. Geriatr. *5*, 21–31.

RICE-EVANS, C. and HOCHSTEIN, P. 1981. Alterations in erythrocyte membrane fluidity by phenylhydrazine-induced peroxidation of lipids. Biochem. Biophys. Res. Commun. *100*, 1537–1542.

ROTH, G. S. 1979a. Hormone receptor changes during adulthood and senescence: Significance for aging research. Fed. Proc. *38*, 1910–1914.

ROTH, G. S. 1979b. Hormone action during aging: Alterations and mechanisms. Mech. Ageing Dev. *9*, 497–514.

SAMUNI, A. *et al.* 1983. On the cytotoxicity of vitamin C and metal ions. A site-specific Fenton mechanism. Eur. J. Biochem. *137*, 119–124.

SCHROEDER, F. 1984. Role of membrane lipid asymmetry in aging. Neurobiol. Aging *5*, 323–333.

SCOTT, J. A. *et al.* 1987. Free radical-mediated membrane depolarization in renal and cardiac cells. Biochim. Biophys. Acta *899*, 76–82.

SEMSEI, I., SZESZÁK, F. and Zs.-NAGY, I. 1982. *In vivo* studies on the age-dependent decrease of the rates of total and mRNA synthesis in the brain cortex of rats. Arch. Gerontol. Geriatr. *1*, 29–42.

SEMSEI, I. and Zs.-NAGY, I. 1984. Effects of ionic strength on the activity of superoxide dismutase. Arch. Gerontol. Geriatr. *3*, 287–295.

SEMSEI, I. and Zs.-NAGY, I. 1985. Superoxide radical scavenging ability of centrophenoxine and its salt dependence *in vitro*. J. Free. Rad. Biol. Med. *1*, 403–408.

SHAW, J. M. *et al.* 1980. Phospholipid acyl chain oxidation in biological membranes and model bilayers. Fed. Proc. Fed. Am. Soc. Exp. Biol. *39*, 2098.

SHINITZKY, M. 1984. Membrane fluidity and cellular functions. *In* Physiology of Membrane Fluidity, Vol. I, M. Shinitzky, (ed.). CRC Press, Boca Raton.

SIMON, R. H., SCOGGIN, CH. H. and PATTERSON, D. 1981. Hydrogen peroxide causes the fatal injury to human fibroblasts exposed to oxygen radicals. J. Biol. Chem. *256*, 7181–7186.

STOEWE, R. and PRÜTZ, W. A. 1987. Copper-catalyzed DNA damage by ascorbate and hydrogen peroxide: Kinetics and yield. Free Rad. Biol. Med. *3*, 97–105.

TAPPEL, A. L. 1975. Lipid peroxidation and fluorescent molecular damage to membranes. *In* Pathobiology of Cell Membranes, Vol. I, B. F. Trump and A. U. Arstilla (eds.). Academic Press, New York.

TAUBER, R. and REUTTER, W. 1981. Turnover of plasma membrane proteins and glycoproteins in normal and regenerating liver and Morris hepatoma 7777. Eur. J. Cell Biol. *26*, 35–42.

YAMAGUCHI, T. *et al.* 1983. A study on the reaction of human erythrocytes with hydrogen peroxide. J. Biochem. *94*, 379–386.

WALLING, C. 1975. Fenton's reagent revisited. Acc. Chem. Res. *8*, 125–131.

WEBER, H. U. and MIQUEL, J. 1986. Antioxidant supplementation and longevity, *In* Nutritional Aspects of Aging, Vol. I, L. H. Chen (ed.). CRC Press, Boca Raton.

ZANISER, N. R., CHOU, D. and HANIN, I. 1977. Is 2-dimethylaminoethanol (Deanol) indeed a precursor of brain acetylcholine? A gas chromatographic evaluation. J. Pharmacol. Exp. Ther. *200*, 545–559.

ZSUPÁN, I. *et al.* 1987. The effect of OH˙ radicals generated by Fenton reaction on the growth and cartilage differentiation in limb bud cell culture. J. Submicrosc. Cytol. *19*, 445–455.

Zs.-NAGY, I. 1978. A membrane hypothesis of aging. J. Theor. Biol. *75*, 189–195.

Zs.-NAGY, I. 1979. The role of membrane structure and function in cellular aging: A review. Mech. Ageing Dev. *9*, 237–246.

Zs.-NAGY, I. 1986. Common mechanisms of cellular aging in brain and liver in the light of the membrane hypothesis of aging. *In* Liver and Aging—1986, Liver and Brain, K. Kitani (ed.). Elsevier Science Publishers, Amsterdam.

Zs.-NAGY, I. 1987. An attempt to answer the questions of theoretical gerontology on the basis of the membrane hypothesis of aging. *In* Advances in the Biosciences, Vol 64, E. Aloj-Totaro, P. Glees and F. A. Pisanti (eds.). Pergamon, London.

Zs.-NAGY, I. 1988. The theoretical background and cellular autoregulation of biological waste product formation. *In* Lipofuscin—1987: State of the Art, I. Zs.-Nagy (ed.). Akadémiai Kiadó, Budapest, and Elsevier Science Publishers, Amsterdam.

Zs.-NAGY, I. 1989a. Functional consequences of free radical damage to cell membrane. *In* CRC Handbook of Free Radicals and Antioxidants in Biomedicine, Vol. I, J. Miquel, A. T. Quintanilha and H. Weber (eds.). CRC Press, Boca Raton.

Zs.-NAGY, I. 1989b. Centrophenoxine as OH˙ free radical scavenger. *In* CRC Handbook of Free Radicals and Antioxidants in Biomedicine, Vol. II, J. Miquel, H. Weber and A. T. Quintanilha (eds.). CRC Press, Boca Raton.

Zs.-NAGY, I., CUTLER, R. G. and SEMSEI, I. 1988a. Dysdifferentiation hypothesis of aging and cancer: A comparison with the membrane hypothesis of aging. Ann. N. Y. Acad. Sci. *521*, 215–225.

Zs.-NAGY, I., DERECSKEI, B. and LUSTYIK, GY. 1987. Age-dependent changes in the osmometric behavior of rat brain and liver. Arch. Gerontol. Geriatr. *6*, 339–354.

Zs.-NAGY, I. and FLOYD, R. A. 1984a. Hydroxyl free radical reactions with amino acids and proteins studied by electron spin resonance spectroscopy and spin trapping. Biochim. Biophys. Acta *790*, 238–250.

Zs.-NAGY, I. and FLOYD, R. A. 1984b. Electron spin resonance spectroscopic demonstration of the hydroxyl free radical scavenger properties of dimethylaminoethanol in spin trapping experiments confirming the molecular basis for the biological effects of centrophenoxine. Arch. Gerontol. Geriatr. *3*, 297–310.

Zs.-NAGY, I. *et al.* 1982a. Age-dependent decrease of cell membrane permeability of rat hepatocytes as revealed by *in vivo* Rb^+-uptake and release. *In* Liver and Aging--1982, K. Kitani (ed.). Elsevier Biomedical Press, Amsterdam.

Zs. NAGY, I., KITANI, K. and OHTA, M. 1989a. Age dependence of the lateral mobility of proteins in the plasma membrane of hepatocytes in C57BL/6 mice: FRAP studies on liver smears. J. Gerontol. Biol. Sci. *44*, B83–B87.

Zs.-NAGY, I. *et al.* 1986a. Age-dependent decrease of the lateral diffusion constant of proteins in the plasma membrane of hepatocytes as revealed by fluorescence recovery after photobleaching in tissue smears. Arch. Gerontol. Geriatr. *5*, 131–146.

Zs.-NAGY, I. *et al.* 1986b. Age-estimations of rats based on the average lateral diffusion constant of hepatocyte membrane proteins as revealed by fluorescence recovery after photobleaching. Exp. Gerontol. *21*, 555–563.

Zs.-NAGY, I., LUSTYIK, GY. and BERTONI-FREDDARI, C. 1982b. Intracellular water and dry mass content as measured in bulk specimens by energy-dispersive X-ray microanalysis. Tissue Cell *14*, 47–60.

Zs.-NAGY, I. and NAGY, K. 1980. On the role of cross-linking of cellular proteins in aging. Mech. Ageing Dev. *14*, 245–251.

Zs.-NAGY, I. *et al.* 1981. Alterations in total content and solubility characteristics of proteins in rat brain and liver during aging and centrophenoxine treatment. Exp. Gerontol. *16*, 229–240.

Zs.-NAGY, I. *et al.* 1988b. Effect of perfringolysin O on the lateral diffusion constant of membrane proteins of hepatocytes as revealed by fluorescence recovery after photobleaching. Biochim. Biophys. Acta *939*, 551–560.

Zs.-NAGY, I., OHTA, M., KITANI, K. and IMAHORI, K. 1984. An automated method for measuring lateral mobility of proteins in the plasma membrane of cells in compact tissues by means of fluorescence recovery after photobleaching. Mikroskopie *41*, 12–25.

Zs.-NAGY, I., OHTA, M. and KITANI, K. 1989b. Effect of centrophenoxine and BCE-001 treatment on the lateral diffusion constant of proteins in the hepatocyte membrane as revealed by fluorescence recovery after photobleaching in rat liver smears. Exp. Gerontol. *24*, 317–330.

Zs.-NAGY, I. *et al.* 1977. Energy dispersive X-ray microanalysis of the electrolytes in biological bulk specimen. I. Specimen preparation, beam penetration and quantitative analysis. J. Ultrastruct. Res. *58*, 22–33.

Zs.-NAGY, I., PIERI, C., GIULI, C. and DEL MORO, M. 1979. Effects of centrophenoxine on the monovalent electrolyte contents of the large brain cortical cells of old rats. Gerontology *25*, 94–102.

Zs.-NAGY, I. and SEMSEI, I. 1984. Centrophenoxine increases the rates of total and mRNA synthesis in the brain cortex of old rats: An explanation of its action it terms of the membrane hypothesis of aging. Exp. Gerontol. *19*, 171–178.

Zs.-NAGY, I., TÓTH, S. and LUSTYIK, GY. 1985. Verification of the membrane hypothesis of aging on the identified giant neurons of the snail *Lymnaea stagnalis* L. (Gastropoda, Pulmonata) by a combined application of intracellular electrophysiology and X-ray microanalysis. Arch. Gerontol. Geriatr. *4*, 53–66.

SECTION VI

Nutrition and Aging: An Industry Perspective

CHAPTER 24

SUMMATION

IMPLICATIONS FOR THE FOOD INDUSTRY

G. E. LIVINGSTON, Ph.D.
Food Science Associates
Dobbs Ferry, New York

One of the goals which the organizers had in mind when they planned this conference was to inform the industries, both food and pharmaceutical, of the state-of-the-art of knowledge pertaining to dietary factors affecting aging processes in humans.

Some of the findings and techniques discussed at this conference might be of interest to members of industry. The role which diet plays in diseases such as cardiovascular disease, stroke, diabetes and cancer will not be discussed because the food and pharmaceutical industries have been adequately sensitized to these issues.

First and foremost, there is no question concerning the effect of caloric restriction on aging. The efficacy of this approach has been demonstrated in several species, in particular laboratory rodents. There are indications, but as yet no hard evidence, that caloric restriction may also be an effective means of increasing longevity in humans. Certainly underfeeding without malnutrition, particularly if accompanied by exercise, may improve the quality of life by retarding the onset of certain diseases associated with old age. Of all the findings discussed, caloric restriction has certainly received the greatest attention on the part of industry. I will let my colleagues from the food industry address the issue of how new food products might be developed which will provide full satiety and gustatory enjoyment to consumers while helping to reduce caloric intake.

As research intensifies in the whole area of nutrition and aging, industry will be looking for some agreement on the part of the scientific community as to biological markers of aging. Clearly, much research will be needed before such markers can be validated.

The food industry has been conscious for some years of the problem of osteoporosis, and many calcium-fortified new products have recently been introduced into the marketplace. The issue of whether aging bone loss can, in fact, be prevented by nutritional means has been raised here, as has the question of the influence of calcium and magnesium on bone aging. It appears that much more research is needed before we can answer these questions.

Zinc supplementation has been suggested as a possible means of preventing age-associated immune system deterioration. The food and pharmaceutical industries will certainly view this research with interest.

The Maillard reaction, which was the focus of many investigators during and after World War II, was revived at this conference in the form of a report that the reaction of glucose with proteins and nucleic acids may play a role in the aging process. One wonders if any of the research carried out in food systems to arrest or retard nonenzymatic browning may find some application in this area of interest.

Vitamin E was reported to slow down lipid peroxidation and development in neurons of the frontal cortex and of the hippocampus. Vitamin E has long been touted as a vitamin which could do many things from assisting one's sexual prowess to slowing down aging. It is good that we are now getting down to cases and that the issue of the role of free radical induced cross-linking in tissues aging and, therefore, the potential for oxygen scavengers in slowing down such processes is being scrutinized by responsible scientists.

The finding reported at this conference that circulating glucose levels can regulate memory storage processes will certainly spark industry interest in whether dietary management of glucose regulation may improve memory in the aged.

It is our objective to sort out the information resulting from the conference, set it into focus from the perspective of industry, and identify directions which might be pursued to ultimately be able to bring to the consuming public the benefits from knowledge of how nutrition may affect the process of aging.

RESEARCH AND DEVELOPMENT OF FOODS: CHALLENGES AND OPPORTUNITIES

R. J. CARBONELL, Ph.D.
Del Monte Foods
RJR Nabisco
Coral Gables, Florida

My personal concept of desirable longevity is not only survival for its own sake, but, more importantly, is an expectation of enjoying my golden years by being happy, active, useful to society, self-sufficient and able to maintain a good quality of life. Institutionalized longevity without a good quality of life is not worth striving for. I trust that in the pursuit of the purposes of your conference you have not overlooked the quality aspects of longevity.

An understanding of both the important contributions that have been made in the past and the important challenges and opportunities that lie ahead for the benefit of society is essential. First, I would like to review the area of nutrition and, more specifically, the relationship of diet to health and well-being. After all, health and well-being are what age and longevity are all about.

The fact that food and a proper diet are essential to health and well-being is not new. What is new is the current nature of this relationship. During the first half of this century, nutritionists, food scientists and food technologists focused primarily on diseases resulting from dietary insufficiencies. Indeed, they effectively helped eliminate the causes of malnutrition through fortification and enrichment programs, such as: iodine in salt; vitamin A and vitamin D in milk and margarine; niacin, riboflavin, thiamin and iron in flour; a wide variety of vitamins and minerals in breakfast cereals; vitamin C in numerous fruit juice type products; and, more recently, fluorides in water.

Unquestionably, these important changes in the nutritional value of the American diet made a significant impact in the control of diseases such as pellagra, rickets, goiter and tooth decay.

It is undeniable that the nutritionists and food scientists, who actually dealt with the nature of the foods we consume, had a fundamental impact on the healthfulness of the American food supply over the last half century or so. It is worth noting, however, that consumer choice played virtually no role in these dietary improvements. They resulted either from public-policy government mandates, or from self-imposed industry standards. In this country, in the United States, with the exception of some small pockets of extreme poverty, and some specific social problems—such as pregnant teenagers—we have succeeded in eliminating malnutrition, protein deficiency and most diseases related to vitamin and mineral deficiencies. We should also acknowledge American agriculture and its green revolution, and food technology's achievements in improving crop yields, reducing postharvest losses, establishing effective storage and distribution systems, extending shelf-life, and, most of all, assuring the safety and purity of our food supply. As a result of this, America has the world's most abundant, safest and cheapest food supply.

In parallel to this, medicine has made wonderful progress in eradicating or controlling most infectious and childhood diseases and their attendant high mortality rates. Thus, as we approach the new millenium, less than 12 years away from today, we find that we have significantly increased our life span, but we have not yet found the fountain of youth, nor a formula for immortality. As we enter the third millenium of the present era, we find that the main causes of mortality have changed. Instead of malnutrition, childhood and infectious diseases being forefront in our minds, we have found that, as we live longer than our ancestors did, inexorably, chronic degenerative diseases, such as cancer and cardiovascular disease, diabetes, osteoporosis, Alzheimer's disease, and the autoimmune deficiency syndrome known as "AIDS," now have taken the prominent place.

The main challenge facing us today is not to rest on the laurels of the past, but to go forward with further and novel dietary modifications, seeking to impact today's major mortality causes. In pursuing this challenge, we need to recognize that most chronic degenerative diseases are complex and multifactor problems. We must also reckon with the fact that perhaps an overriding issue is the host's genetic makeup, a factor we can yet do very little about given today's state of knowledge and society's policy standards. Yes, we need to deal with genetic predisposition to certain chronic diseases, and even with genetic immunity or resistance to some of them. However, beyond things we can do little or know enough about, there is much we can do to improve upon this situation.

Our knowledge of good nutrition and of the dietary vectors affecting chronic diseases is increasing tremendously. However, I must caution that our effectiveness now in impacting a favorable outcome is far different than it was when we were concerned in the past with malnutrition and other nutrition-related diseases. This situation stems from two circumstances that are peculiar to today's dietary problems. First, unlike the case of fortification, enrichment and fluoridation, we cannot correct today's nutritional problems through legislated or institutionalized solutions. Second, perhaps the most insidious problem we face today is overnutrition—overconsumption without moderation. Yes, we are the victims of our own success and, indeed, overconsumption is a much more difficult problem to control.

As a member of the food industry, I firmly believe it has an obligation to provide the consumer with alternative options to popular traditional foods that may impact today's chronic diseases.

In fact, we have been making some headway in the past 25 years. Two examples are: margarines that have no cholesterol and are low in saturated fat and cholesterol-free egg substitutes. Nevertheless, we must recognize that, while offering new and more healthful options to traditional foods is a necessary condition, it is *not* a sufficient condition to ensure an effective impact on chronic disease through improved dietary practices.

Today food science and technology alone cannot solve this problem without proper consumer education and effective marketing. We cannot dictate what people should or should not eat, or how much they should eat for that matter. Yes, we did force people to eat enriched bread, as all flour was enriched and there was no consumer choice. Bread was bread, before and after flour enrichment. But today, to make headway in the nutritional issues we face, consumer choice must not be ignored. Believe me, this can only be tackled effectively through intensive marketing and meaningful consumer education. The question is: Who is going to do it? Perhaps even a more appropriate question is: Would the regulators let the food industry do it? I must admit I don't know the answer to this question.

How do we stand when it comes to proper eating habits? Our knowledge of good nutrition and proper dietary habits has and is increasing tremendously. It is also true that many consumers have become a lot more cerebral about their eating, or pretend to be. On one hand, many American consumers understand that proper eating and exercise do have an impact on their health and well-being. But, on the other hand, this message does not seem to have penetrated effectively our society as a whole. A survey I saw recently indicated that about half the American public readily admits it has difficulty in following good dietary practices, even though it knows those practices have significant health implications. Most people who try dieting today seem to do so primarily for cosmetic or social reasons. I believe that the game being played of struggling to lose 20 pounds—just to gain them back—is more harmful than helpful. The most likely reason for this behavior seems to be that people eat to satisfy physiological needs, but overeat for psychological and social reasons.

Moreover, even when we deal with purely physiological needs, we may be dealing with desires that are not learned, but genetically inherited. We have seen how sweetness, for example, can trigger the sucking reflex in unborn children. The taste and craving for fat seems to have similarly deep roots. Another problem that probably has had a major impact on this issue is the extensive degree of confusion which has been planted in the consumer mind through the miriad of popularized diets which have gone on to become best sellers, often pursuing diametrically opposite approaches. It seems that our anxious public is eager to latch onto easy, quick-fix promises, failing to recognize that weight control is a difficult task often entailing dramatic behavioral modification.

Is there anything that food science and technology can do to impact on this picture? I believe there is. While we cannot dictate, or persuade Americans to eat what they ought to eat, and in the quantities they should, we have another alternative to pursue: make what they eat better for them by tailoring the components of food. Today, for many people, healthier foods simply mean foods with fewer calories and fat. I am sure you will agree that excess calories and fat represent today's most serious chronic dietary disease epidemic.

Your own conference amply recognizes this fact. Let me quote from some of the ideas presented here today.

Dr. Weindruch:	Dietary restriction of caloric intake increases life span in diverse species. In mice and rats dietary restriction extends maximum life span and opposes the development of most late-life diseases.
Dr. Harrison:	The only treatment known that retards aging in mammals is caloric or food restriction in short-lived rodents.
Dr. Richardson:	Dietary restriction, underfeeding not malnutrition, is the only experimental manipulation that has been shown to consistently increase the longevity of mammals.

Anything that makes weight control easier, particularly if it does not require a behavioral or traditional taste-standard modification to achieve it, is very likely to succeed in the market place and will help control this epidemic. While in the "good old days" we used to be penalized by words such as "imitation foods," nowadays we have the benefit of the magic words—"diet" or "lite foods." Therefore, we have already an ideal vehicle on which to launch and market tailor-made foods to help solve this dietary problem. I am not talking about reduced- or low-calorie foods that are really just aids to will power, such as thinner slices of bread or prepared entrees packaged in smaller portions. On the contrary, the real promise of tailor-made foods lies in the substitution of less desirable components and the increase of desirable components, while rendering a finished product that is *a reasonable facsimile of its traditional counterpart*. This is where the emphasis should be placed.

The closest technology can come to achieving this objective, the greater the likelihood of market success for a given tailor-made food. We really need to be able to produce tailor-made foods that the consumer believes are "the real thing," new foods that can be consumed pleasurably without requiring dramatic behavioral modification. Perhaps the best example of a successful tailor-made product fulfilling the requirements I have outlined is the one of diet sodas sweetened with aspartame. Aspartame-sweetened sodas have been an outstanding success. However, please recognize that the market potential of diet sodas was not fulfilled until there was a development in the ingredients area which allowed the production of a "reasonable facsimile" of a traditional product. Remember the bitter aftertaste of saccharine-sweetened diet sodas? Diet sodas are a good example of what I mean by a tailor-made product which is a reasonable facsimile of its traditional counterpart—not identical and undistinguishable, but equally pleasing, requiring no major behavioral modification. Their contribution in reducing caloric intake is undeniable.

Let us now turn our attention to another important component of the American diet, intrinsically, the highest caloric component of our food, namely fat. We have all known for at least two decades that high levels of fat intake, particularly of saturated fat, are undesirable in terms of blood serum lipid profiles and associated cardiovascular disease problems. Significant strides have been made in reducing animal fats from our diet. For example, through the substitution of margarines and cooking oils for butter and lard, increased consumption of poultry and fish, and the development of leaner beef and pork cuts through breeding and feeding programs. Yet, in spite of that, dietary fat intake remains much higher than prudent, at about 40% of total calories, instead of the more desirable 30% or less.

A recent report of the National Research Council (entitled *Designing Foods: Animal Options in the Market Place*) urged changes in federal regulations to encourage the production of reduced-fat meat and dairy products. According to this report, "animal products still contribute more than half the total fat, three-fourths of the saturated fatty acids and all the cholesterol" in the American diet. Here we have a real problem that needs to be tackled. Not only should we be concerned with the caloric contribution of fat to the diet, we also need to be even more concerned about intrinsic negatives, such as the association of total fat and saturated fat with serum lipids and cardiovascular disease, and recent negative associations with some forms of cancer. How can we tackle fat reduction? There have been a number of successful reduced-fat diet products in the market. These are primarily in the category of formulated foods and include, among others: milk, margarine spreads, salad dressings, toppings, puddings and ice cream. It is obvious, however, that these market actions are not enough to effectively attack our excessive fat consumption problem, as products of this type have been around for some time. The world is really waiting for two things: an effective fat substitute and further genetic improvement of red meats.

We need to be able to market a very wide range of tailor-made reduced- or low-fat foods. We need to be able to further replace the fats and oils used in cooking and food preparation. We must do this while being always mindful of the caveat we mentioned earlier—namely, the capability of yielding reasonable facsimiles of the traditional counterparts. I am pleased to note that now we see a dozen or so low- or non-caloric fat substitutes under development. However, as I see it, this is a very important challenge with yet no perfect answer. I am not only referring to the need to develop a universal fat substitute, which by itself would be of great significance, but to the need to further reduce the fat content of red meats and dairy products. To fully achieve the desirable consumption of not more than 30% of daily-intake calories as fat, we will be required to produce a consumer-acceptable, tailor-made "Big-Mac" hamburger, with half the fat calories of its traditional counterpart, obviously to retail for 99 cents. I am using this extreme example to emphasize my belief that biotechnology has a major role to play in tailor-made foods. No discussion such as this should be complete without mentioning biotechnology: it is today's true frontier of science and technology, and a potentially significant answer to the challenges and opportunities of the next millenium. The discovery of gene and DNA structure, and the development of gene mapping and recombinant DNA technology, potentially gives man the ability to make the natural raw materials he grows to have the exact composition he wants them to have.

Besides fat and calories, there are other important challenges and opportunities for food technology. For example, there are some elements of the diet we want to increase. Fiber is the primary example, since it has been linked to a variety of potential health benefits. Here again, the riddle is not entirely solved. Although it is generally recognized that a higher-fiber diet is preferable to a bland diet, there seems to have been both an overclaiming of benefits, particularly the conclusions of some early cancer studies, and the glossing over of some potential problems, such as possible reduction of the availability of some vitamins and minerals with some soluble fiber, and reduced availability of zinc and calcium with insoluble fiber. Moreover, while we have been quite successful in introducing fiber into breakfast cereals, now the problem is to address fiber in other foods. Insoluble fiber gives a gritty texture to liquids. It can also create problems of texture, flavor and oxidation in baked goods, and both soluble and insoluble fiber have a tendency to dry out the mouth.

Another potentially exciting area to consider is the effect of food on human physical and psychic performance. We already know that carbohydrate loading enhances the physical performance of marathon runners and certain other competitive athletes. We also know that a well-balanced breakfast improves the psychic performance of children in school. Food also appears to affect human performance in countless other ways. Take the "morning blahs" that affect our office workers. They just seem to run out of energy. Take the people who must have something to eat every two or three hours. Can we make foods such that the rate of release of energy is controlled, so that we get rid of the blahs? I believe we can. I am also sure that we will see increasing attention to the role of diet in the functioning of the body's immune system, a subject Professor Fernandes addresses in *Modulation of Immune Functions and Aging by Omega-3 Fatty Acids and/or Caloric Restriction*. This could put an entirely different dimension on how we have been looking at the diet, and I hope the attention this issue will receive will be both useful and timely.

I am convinced that my conclusion is valid: Nutrition and food science and technology can eventually bring us to the point where we can deal with all relevant factors in the relationship of diet to health, well-being and longevity. I am optimistic enough and confident in the talent represented in this conference to believe we will be able to do this in the future. This brings me to a pivotal question: If we develop this capability, how can we use it effectively? Unfortunately, there is still so much we don't know that we need to know before we can direct the tremendous force we are acquiring. For example, take an old subject, such as vitamins and minerals. We all know about the RDAs. Recently, they have been the subject of debate in the belief that they are too conservative. An interesting question in my mind is one of the time span over which the RDA's should be balanced: Over one meal? Over an entire day? Over a week? Do we need to be concerned about required *meal* allowances? On the other extreme, about required *weekly* (or longer) allowances? How do the RDAs vary from person to person (within a given sex and age bracket)? And, to get back to our favorite subject, take the case of overconsumption of fats and calories. If we succeed in marketing popular and acceptable foods that are reasonable facsimiles of their traditional counterparts and contain fewer calories and fat per serving, will people actually consume fewer calories? We do know that laboratory animals tend to consume a constant number of calories per day, even if we vary the caloric content of the food we give them. On the other hand, we also know that they will consume more calories if the fat content of their food increases, and vice-versa. I wish we knew the answer to this important question.

A very important aspect we need to consider is the potential beneficiary of our efforts—the American consumer. As always, he or she is very demanding. He or she expects us to produce foods that provide simultaneously a total package of nutrition, health benefits, sheer pleasure, indulgency without weight gain, with no risks, no problems, no incremental costs, and, preferably, they should be natural, vegetarian and organically grown. We know also that consumers are not completely consistent. They understand more than ever about good nutrition, but cannot always bring themselves to practice the lessons they have learned. Most of our consumers seem to be subliminally controlled by tradition and conservatism when it comes to changing their food preferences and dieting habits. They want improved foods, but remain very conservative about what they eat. They will avoid something that appears potentially risky for their diet, but will not necessarily add something that appears healthy. Nonetheless, we have a lot to tell our consumers about their diet. Although they are not easy to talk to and are more prone to listen to quacks and faddists, I sense they are more disposed to listen to us right now.

How are we doing so far in communicating with consumers? I believe that, at our best, we are beginning to do well. There's no doubt that the hypertension education program launched by the National Institutes of Health has made a lot of Americans very conscious of their blood pressure, and of the dietary and other influences that affect it. There is no doubt that nutrition and health education efforts, such as the American Health Foundation's "Know Your Body" program are being very impactful on the diet and health habits of future generations of Americans. On the other hand, as I mentioned before, there is a glut of popular books and articles about diet and health. Some are excellent, some are dreadful. How is the consumer to judge their value? I believe that the assertions about diet and health emanating from both government agencies and the food industry have generally been on a higher plane than most fad diet books. Although, occasionally, I see hints of health-hucksterism in some advertising, fortunately, these are mercifully rare. There is a residual credibility with the consumer that we must preserve at all costs. This would be true under any circumstance. But it is all the more important as we prepare to enter the era of tailor-made foods.

In conclusion, I believe we will soon possess unprecedented ability to alter the composition of popular foods to meet both our desirable dietary needs and the consumer's expectations. What is important at this juncture, however, is that we work together to make the era of proper nutrition into a healthier one for our nation, collectively, as well as individually, for ourselves. When I say "we," I mean all of us: the scientific community, the medical community, the food industry, the regulatory agencies and the consumers. There are still many difficult questions we have no answers for now, but we must begin the process. As a former food scientist and representative of the food industry, I am ready to join your ranks in the quest for a more healthful diet, for longevity, and, above all, for maintaining the quality of life.

NEW PRODUCTS FOR MODIFYING THE DIET

J. EDWARD HUNTER
Procter & Gamble Company
Winton Hill Technical Center
Cincinnati, Ohio

Dr. Carbonell has commented that the food industry needs to develop alternatives to traditional products that will assist consumers in making desirable dietary changes, such as altering the fatty acid composition or lowering the caloric density of their diets. Dr. Carbonell cited several examples of readily available foods that help consumers reduce their caloric intake. These include diet soft drinks sweetened with aspartame, low fat milk, reduced calorie salad dressings, and leaner beef. I would like to point out several additional examples of products developed recently by the food industry which were not discussed by Dr. Carbonell but which help to meet objectives he outlined.

First, let me note some examples of new products that enable consumers to modify the composition of specific nutrients their diets in ways that may benefit their health. For consumers who want to decrease their intake of saturated fatty acids, using a salad and cooking oil made with canola oil can help. Canola oil has the lowest level of saturated fatty acids among vegetable oils now available. Other compositional features of canola oil ultimately may prove to be beneficial from a cardiovascular health standpoint. These include its adequate but not excessive level of linoleic acid, its high content of the monounsaturated fatty acid, oleic acid, and its significant level of the Omega-3 fatty acid, α-linolenic acid. For individuals who want to increase their intake of fiber, there are many high fiber cereals available, including several containing oat bran which has been reported to be helpful in lowering blood cholesterol. For those who want to increase their intake of calcium, there are now calcium fortified fruit juices available as alternatives to dairy products.

There are also a few new products that can help consumers decrease their total caloric intake. The American Health Foundation recognized the Campbell Soup Co. this year for developing a line of dinners reduced in calories and fat. Fat substitutes such as polydextrose, Olestra, and Simplesse can significantly reduce the caloric content of certain foods. Polydextrose is a water-soluble amorphous solid prepared by high temperature polymerization of glucose under catalytic conditions. Polydextrose has a caloric value of one calorie per gram. It is used as a bulking agent and also has some utility as a partial substitute for fat in products like ice cream and cookies. Olestra is a fat substitute currently under review by the FDA. Olestra, also called sucrose polyester, consists of a mixture of hexa, hepta, and octaesters formed by the reaction of sucrose with long chain fatty acids. Olestra is not hydrolyzed by the lipolytic enzymes in the intestinal tract and thus is not absorbed. Therefore, Olestra contributes no calories to the food in which it is used. Olestra has the taste and consistency properties of conventional vegetable oils. Simplesse is another recently introduced fat substitute under review by the FDA. Simplesse is made from milk or egg protein and contains approximately four calories per gram. This is about one half the caloric density of conventional fats.

In summary, the food industry has been and continues to be responsive to consumer needs by developing food products that can help modify the diet in potentially helpful ways.

DIETARY MANIPULATION FOR THE AGING

RIDA ALI, Ph.D.
Bristol Meyers International
New York, New York

Nutritional modulation of aging and longevity is a lifelong process which is closely related to lifestyle and economic status of the individual. It represents both a challenge and opportunity to the food industry. With the aging of the population in the industrialized nations, the need to develop food products that address some of the nutritional concerns aiming at improving the quality of life for the aged, and with the advancing of our knowledge to affect longevity. Based on available evidence regarding the effect of caloric restriction on aging and longevity, an area of immediate concern, which requires collective effort (academia, governmental agencies and industry), is to re-examine physiological relevance of the recommended dietary allowances for the population over 50 years of age. Appropriate adjustment may be required to reduce recommended caloric intake with advancing in age at the rate of 10% of adult intake for every additional decade of life span in order to achieve 20-30% reduction in recommended caloric intake for the population 80 years and older.

The challenge to the food industry in this regard is to develop appropriate food products with reduced caloric density, yet capable of achieving satiety through bulk filling. The obvious tool available is in the application of dietary fiber in a variety of forms and textures to reduce caloric density of food, yet maintain consumer appeal and acceptability.

Another area of relevance to nutritional modulation for the aged is to pay greater attention to nutritional supplementation particularly with calcium, iron and zinc which have been shown to be negatively affected by the process of aging. Finally, basic *in vitro* and *in vivo* research to study the aging phenomenon at the cellular and subcellular level in appropriate models should continue to provide better understanding of the cause-effect relation between nutrition and aging. This research may lend us a more direct approach to improve quality-of-life and longevity through dietary manipulation and intervention over the life span of man.

CALORIC RESTRICTION AND HUMANS

AMY SAMUELSON, Ph.D.
Nabisco Brands
East Hanover, New Jersey

The data presented at this provocative meeting strongly suggest that caloric restriction can ''safely'' decrease many biomarkers of aging and, concomitantly, increase longevity in laboratory models. Two questions arise which I have to grapple with as a nutritionist and researcher involved in new food product development. First, can these results be extrapolated to humans of all ages and both genders? Second, if so, what can and should be done by Food Companies to try to insure compliance to low-calorie, nutrient-dense diets.

My answer to the first question is that the jump from laboratory animals to humans cannot be made, and that an appropriate human model should be developed and tested. In this regard, I found Dr. McCarter's proposal of a setpoint theory interesting, since the idea of body weight and metabolic setpoint is currently being examined in the obesity field to explain how obese individuals defend their increased body weight when diet-challenged, that is, how these individuals defend their genetic potential. In the caloric deprivation field, it may explain how diet-*reduced* individuals defend life, another form of genetic potential.

Although I do not think the results presented at this conference are immediately transferable to Nutrition Public Policy, I do believe that they should be followed closely, and further research should be done to define more specifically the physiologic mechanisms involved in increased longevity resulting from caloric deprivation. Once the mechanisms are established, it may be possible to bring about the same effects by methods such as exercise which do not require general and radical deprivation by the public in an area where even modest deprivation is hard to effect; that is, limiting food intake. In virtually all societies, food and eating have great psychosocial associations and benefits which are not readily relinquished.

Another possibility, is the creation of novel low-calorie food ingredients and nutrient-dense formulations. But these developments are also radical, the technologies here are far from perfected, and the beneficial effects on longevity are as yet completely untested. It may be that consumption of these novel ingredients will itself cause disease and thereby shorten life span, or may not affect biomarkers or mechanisms of aging in an advantageous way.

In summary, I see the caloric deprivation model of aging as a useful probe to define the physiologic controls of the aging process. Once these are known, I would hope that lifestyle changes which are less invasive, and both more conservative and easy-to-implement than severe calorie restriction, will prove effective.

INDEX